Award-winning writer, television broadcaster and author of numerous bestsellers, **Leslie Kenton** is described by the press as 'the guru of health and fitness' and 'the most original voice in health'. A shining example of energy and commitment, she is highly respected for her thorough reporting. Leslie was born in California, and is the daughter of jazz musician Stan Kenton. After leaving Stanford University she journeyed to Europe in her early twenties, settling first in Paris then in Britain where she has since remained. She has raised four children on her own by working as a television broadcaster, novelist, writer and teacher on health and for fourteen years she was an editor at *Harpers & Queen*.

Leslie's writing on mainstream health is internationally known and has appeared in *Vogue*, the *Sunday Times*, *Cosmopolitan* and the *Daily Mail*. She is the author of many other health books including: *The New Raw Energy* and *Raw Energy Recipes* – co-authored with her daughter Susannah – *The New Ultrahealth*, *The New Joy of Beauty*, *The New Biogenic Diet*, *Cellulite Revolution*, *10 Day Clean-Up Plan*, *Endless Energy*, *Nature's Child*, *Lean Revolution* and the *10 Day De-Stress Plan*. She turned to fiction with *Ludwig* – her first novel. Former consultant to a medical corporation in the USA and to the Open University's Centre of Continuing Education, Leslie's writing has won several awards including the PPA 'Technical Writer of the Year'. Her work was honoured by her being asked to deliver the McCarrison Lecture at the Royal Society of Medicine. In recent years she has become increasingly concerned not only with the process of enhancing individual health but also with re-establishing bonds with the earth as a part of helping to heal the planet.

THE NEW
AGELESS
AGEING

The natural way to stay young

LESLIE KENTON

VERMILION
LONDON

1 3 5 7 9 10 8 6 4 2

First published in the United Kingdom in 1995 by
Vermilion
an imprint of Ebury Press
Random House
20 Vauxhall Bridge Road
London SW1V 2SA

Random House Australia (Pty) Limited
20 Alfred Street, Milsons Point, Sydney,
New South Wales 2061, Australia

Random House New Zealand Limited
18 Poland Road, Glenfield,
Auckland 10, New Zealand

Random House South Africa (Pty) Limited
PO Box 337, Bergvlei, South Africa

Random House Canada
1265 Aerowood Drive, Mississauga,
Ontario L4W 1B9, Canada

Random House UK Limited Reg. No. 954009

A CIP catalogue record for this book is available from the
British Library

ISBN: 0 09 178520 0

Photoset by Deltatype Ltd, Ellesmere Port
Printed and bound in Great Britain by Cox & Wyman Ltd,
Reading, Berkshire

Papers used by Ebury Press are natural recyclable products
made from wood grown in sustainable forests.

For Gloria Hunniford
who ages agelessly,
with admiration and affection

Acknowledgements

Many friends and colleagues have contributed to make this book possible. So have a number of brilliant and humanitarian doctors, age-researchers and other scientists. It would be impossible to thank them all properly. There are a few to whom I am particularly indebted: Johan Bjorksten, Herman Le Compte, Linus Pauling, Ralph Bircher, Dagmar Leichte von Brasch, Phillip Kilsby, Stephen Levine, Bob Erdmann, Gordon and Barbara Latto, I.I. Brekhman, Robert O. Becker, Julian Kenyon, Alan Cott and Lilla Bek. I am especially grateful to Monica Fine who offered to help me research the book in her own spare time, to Yvette Brown who laboured long over the updating process, to my daughter Susannah who set aside several days of her holiday to correct my apauling (appalling) spelling and to edit the text, and to my son Dr Jesse Kenton-Smith, known in the family as 'the scientist', for meticulously vetting my own inadequate language of science.

Leslie Kenton
Pembrokeshire 1995

Contents

Part One
HIEROGLYPHS OF AGEING

Part Two
ELIXIRS OF LIFE

Part Three
THE AGELESS BODY

Introduction

Pick up any book on ageing and you are likely to be dazzled by the scientific confusion into which you've been plunged: a score of complex and contradictory theories expounded in hundreds of polysyllabic words, none of which has much meaning to the man or woman who simply wants to know what he or she can do right now to protect him or herself from premature ageing and degeneration, to maintain youthful good looks and to live a long and productive life. The talk is of free radicals, cellular clocks, hormones, enzymes, heredity and immunity. And the disagreements are rampant. On the one hand you have highly respected conservative scientists claiming there is no way we can lengthen life appreciably. On the other you find Nobel prize winners who insist not only that it can be done but that it can be done with relative ease now. Then there are the real eccentrics – I call them the 'immortalists' – who believe that death itself is little more than a mistake, an event which we have been programmed to expect and which therefore becomes a self-fulfilling prophecy. Alter your expectations, they say, and you can alter reality. There is no reason why you cannot live forever, they insist – yes, you – right now. So get on with it.

Amidst so much confusion where do you find sense? Is there strong evidence that we can alter the individual rate at which we age? Can we live longer? And not just longer but *better* – a healthier, happier, more productive and creative life? Can we look younger in five years than we do right now? Are the knowledge and the tools available now to give us control over the rate at which our body ages? And what about rejuvenation? Is it just another of those old-fashioned notions which went out with romantic Forties films – a notion which hard science has banished to the scrap pile of fantasy?

Or can you use natural means to transform an ageing body into a younger one? And, if so, where do you begin?

These are a few of the questions which were plaguing me twenty years ago as I began to research the scientific literature into ageing and rejuvenation. What set them off? What led me to spend hours in dusty medical libraries ploughing through esoteric papers on longevity, the immune system and anti-oxidant nutrients? Why did I set out to interview scientists all over the world who had spent their lives studying the process of ageing?

The notion of writing a book about ageing had never entered my head. Yet I found myself passionately committed to the research. I *needed* to know; and it was a need which sprang from no abstract sense of scientific curiosity: each spring as I looked into the mirror I would notice that a few more tiny lines had appeared. Sometimes when I went out for a run I'd sense a certain stiffness in my muscles which wasn't there last year. Or was it? In short, ageing for me, as it is for most people, was a highly personal experience. I knew that I was doing it, and I figured there was nothing I could do about that. But by heaven I was going to do it *slowly!* I was going to find a way to live which kept me looking good and supported the needs of my body and mind at a high level of vitality and awareness well into my forties . . . sixties . . . nineties.

Now, after two decades of digging and mulling over contradictory facts and figures, trying out endless techniques and rejecting many which seemed worthless before trying more, I believe my search has been well rewarded. Oh, don't get me wrong. I have found no fountain of youth – no magic pill which you can take one morning and make biological time stand still. But I have come upon a great many techniques which I believe really work to keep you young and even to make you look and feel younger. Much to my surprise, I have also discovered that, amidst all those contradictory theories about why and how the body ages, and what can be done to slow down the process, there are unifying principles which we can put into practical use right now. There is necessarily a good deal of complex information to be digested in Part One of *Ageless Ageing.* Bear with me though, for it is background knowledge which will give you real understanding of the practical applications discussed in the later chapters of the book.

One of the things that worried me most in the beginning was the fact that so many of the anti-ageing techniques – from the use of high doses of anti-oxidant nutrients to the ancient practice of fasting – seemed quite contradictory. How, I asked myself, could massive doses of ascorbic acid have a similar effect to a high-raw spring-clean diet when it came to revitalizing the body, softening lines on the face and restoring high levels of energy? What possible relationship was there between the diet and lifestyle of the much studied long-lived peoples of the world – the Hunzas, the Vilcabamba Indians in South America, the Georgians in former Soviet Russia – and the pill-popping anti-ageing culture that has grown up in the United States? These were some of the issues which troubled me. Wrestling with them gradually forced me to look at the ageing process in an entirely different way.

I realized that ageing is far more than simply biological degeneration. That to begin to understand it, even to begin to answer some of my questions about why degeneration takes place and what can be done to slow it down, I would have to explore the nature of a living organism as an energetic system: a system with the remarkable property, unique to life itself, of sustaining a very high degree of order within a universe which the second law of thermodynamics tells us very clearly is *entropic* – that is, a universe in which everything tends to degenerate towards chaos. There *was* magic in it all. Gradually the sense of this magic took hold of me and wouldn't let me go.

When I began my research I had no idea just where it would take me. I certainly never suspected that a desire as narcissistic as wanting to prevent wrinkles on my own face would lead me to a view of age-retardation which has so deepened my respect for the living body and so expanded my sense of awe at the splendour of life processes that my original goal has often been almost forgotten. Oh yes, I've found ways of slowing down the wrinkle-formation on the skin, of restoring firmness and youthful contours to the body, of increasing vitality and encouraging the body to function in a more youthful way on a cellular level. And, make no mistake, I have used them well; but in the midst of it all I have come to be aware of something which to me seems infinitely more valuable. I have come to stand in awe of the order and the perfection that is life. I have come to believe that for too long we have been fascinated by the elegance of scientific laws which govern inert matter yet we have remained blind to the natural laws which govern our own bodies and our consciousness. They are more obscure laws to be sure, but they are every bit as inexorable as the laws of the cosmos. And they are laws which many farsighted people – from the physicians of ancient China to those who belong to the long tradition of natural healing in Europe – have examined, delineated and made use of to heal and to rejuvenate their patients.

Slowing down the ageing process depends greatly on exploring and then making use of these laws. For when in ignorance or disregard we transgress them, accelerated biological degeneration and a tragic waste of human potential is our reward.

It is ten years ago that *Ageless Ageing* was first published. At that time much of what it contained not only in the realm of high-tech free radical biochemistry but also in relation to natural therapies seemed strange and surprising. Now, however, talk of free radicals and oxidation damage has become commonplace – even the good skin care creams are now full of free radical scavengers. Meanwhile the natural therapies, once considered by many to be eccentric, have also entered mainstream health care.

In *The New Ageless Ageing* I have sought to simplify, clarify and bring up to date information and techniques for slowing premature ageing and improving the quality of life in the hope that this will make these techniques easier to use and more widely available.

Get to know the natural laws and couple them with the latest biochemical techniques for protecting the cells of the body from age-related damage, and I believe you create a force for ageless ageing which has not yet been known in the recorded history of man.

But that's the end of my story. Let's begin at the beginning.

PART ONE

HIEROGLYPHS OF AGEING

1
Why Ageless Ageing?

HOW LONG YOU live rests largely in your own hands. So does how *well* you live, how much vitality you have and how good you will look in twenty years' time. They are not, as most people still believe, accidents of fate. Neither are they heavily dependent on the kind of medical care you get, nor on your genetic inheritance – although both certainly have a part to play. Instead they depend mostly on two things: first, your lifestyle; second, how much use you make of some of the recently discovered tools for protecting your body against degeneration. Together these two form an integrated approach to ageless ageing which has two branches. The first branch I call *natural law*. It is based on what appear to be the biological laws of life. It centres around becoming aware of the quite specific needs of your *mind-body-spirit* for optimum health and vitality and then on supplying them. These include psychosocial, physical, nutritional, environmental and spiritual needs which, when fulfilled, keep you in a state of maximum wellness year after year. The second branch of an integrated approach to ageless ageing, which I call *high-tech*, depends on making intelligent and effective use of the tools for age-retardation which have recently come to light thanks to research done in scientific disciplines such as free radical bio-chemistry, submolecular biology, biophysics and electrobiology.

Making ageless ageing work for you is simply a matter of exploring these two aspects of age-retardation in all their depths and then putting them into practice both to extend your life and to enhance its quality.

In the process it should soften lines on your face and prevent many new ones from forming, firm your muscles and help restore youthful contours to a body which is losing them, increase your vitality, and in many ways quite literally rejuvenate you by restoring your immune system to better functioning, lowering blood pressure which has become elevated, strengthening your heart and lungs and improving your body's use of oxygen at a molecular level – a major measure of biological age.

The First Branch – Natural Law

This two-pronged approach to retarding ageing is something which so far very few people, either within the scientific community or outside of it, have yet put into practice. Yet good solid information about how each branch can retard ageing, prolong youthful good looks and extend life is now available to anyone who is willing to take the trouble to dig for it and daring enough to make a few changes in the way he or she eats, thinks and lives to put it to work. The natural law branch – that of supplying an organism with all of its needs and living with an awareness of the biological laws by which we appear to be controlled – forms the foundation of every major tradition of natural health and healing throughout history, from ancient Taoist medicine in China and the Ayurvedic tradition of India to nineteenth-century European nature-cures and the jazzy 'holistic' approach to health becoming popular in this last quarter of the twentieth. It largely determines how susceptible you are to 'premature' ageing – a widespread phenomenon which makes faces wrinkle and arteries harden and which can be halted by such things as correcting any subclinical nutritional deficiencies which you may have, by altering your diet and by changing your lifestyle.

What modern scientific exploration has done for the first branch is to validate what natural traditions of health and healing have always taught – for instance it has shown how and why eating a low-calorie diet of natural foods, getting enough of the right kind of exercise, and enhancing your psychosocial well-being can strengthen immunity, slow ageing and preserve mental clarity and emotional balance. Laboratory and clinical studies have also been able to define better than ever before what the specific factors are that make up a natural lifestyle for ageless ageing, to show why they are important, and to present us with statistics that indicate that abiding by the natural laws of health we can live longer. We know for instance that non-smokers are less likely to end up with lung cancer, that exercise improves cardiovascular strength and makes you less likely to fall prey to a heart attack, that a low-salt diet should help protect you from high blood pressure. At one time these things would have to have been taken on faith; now many of them have been scientifically proven. Having said that, for every hard statistic we have about what helps prevent disease, degeneration and early death, there are still a hundred well-tried and -tested but as yet 'unproven' techniques – tools and morsels of anti-ageing wisdom buried in the natural health and healing traditions – which can be put to use.

Learn about them, put natural law anti-ageing to work for you, and you should be able to live a longer, more creative, more energetic and more satisfying life, starting right now. Only when you do will you be able to live up to your psychobiological potential – something that as yet very few of us ever reach. This is the first step towards ageless ageing. Unless you choose to take it, no amount of fancy biochemical manipulations are going to do the trick for you. For some people this step alone may be enough. It has enabled such well-studied long-lived cultures as the Hunzas in Kashmir, the Georgians and the Vilcabamba Indians in South America to live active lives while most of our grandparents lay ailing in hospital beds. For it has great power.

High-Tech Secrets

The second anti-ageing branch – the *high-tech* scientific approach – is different. It is entirely dependent on scientific discoveries which have taken place, mostly within the last fifty years. These discoveries include a growing understanding of the role that the immune system plays in the rate at which we age, a knowledge of how certain natural and artificial chemicals known as the anti-oxidants can be used to prevent age-related damage on a cellular level and to strengthen immune functions, and how specific nutrients such as the free amino acids can be used to alter the chemistry of the ageing brain or firm sagging muscles, as well as an awareness of how specific pathways between mind and body enable your feelings, attitudes and expectations to play a major role in determining the rate at which you age. The use of anti-oxidant nutrients in animal experiments (one branch of the high-tech approach) as dietary supplements has been shown substantially to retard the basic biological process of ageing and to improve general well-being throughout the animals' lives. Human beings too can make use of them. We can also put into practice some of the recent findings about how dietary restriction boosts immune functions, rejuvenates the immune system and retards degeneration. Discoveries such as these have led even the most conservative scientific researchers to estimate that in the early years of the next millennium we should be able to prolong life far beyond the proverbial three score and ten. For, unlike natural law anti-ageing, which can banish the 'premature' factors in the ageing process, the high-tech approach aims at longevity by attempting to extend 'maximum' lifespan as well. (More about the implications of this later.) In effect it is involved in exploring the processes of ageing and degeneration in very specific terms – from the wrinkling of skin to the disruption of a cell's genetic material which is implicated both in ageing and in the development of cancer. Even more important, science is discovering specific and effective remedies for counteracting these processes of ageing and degeneration.

So when it comes to combating ageing, we live in exciting times. But we also live in fragmented times. It is always tempting to believe that thanks to the latest discoveries in free radical biochemistry we should be able to load up on anti-oxidants from the local health food store while we continue to smoke sixty cigarettes a day, to sunbathe relentlessly, to eat rich desserts, to burn the candle at both ends, and still live for ever. Alas, it just ain't so – no matter how much a few sensational books and articles on the subject would have us believe otherwise. To get maximum benefits from what is currently known about age-retardation we need to fuse natural law and high-tech into a single power for de-ageing. Used together they can not only have you looking good and feeling good twenty-five years hence, they can go a long way towards alleviating human suffering. For there are bonuses to ageless ageing: the very same tools, techniques and lifestyle changes which will keep you young-looking and full of energy will also go a long way towards preventing the degenerative diseases of civilization which have reached epidemic proportions in Britain and in the United States. That in a nutshell is what ageless ageing is all about.

Lay the Ghost

Most of us hold a lot of false notions about ageing and life expectancy – ghosts which need to be laid before we can make ageless ageing a workable part of our lives. Two are particularly common. The first is the idea that degeneration – including a loss of good looks and the onset of long-term illnesses such as arthritis, coronary heart disease and cancer – is a 'normal' experience of growing older. The second is the belief that the 'miracles' of modern medical science have already significantly lengthened our lifespan. Both commonly held views are untrue. They are supported neither by vital statistics nor by biological evidence.

Degenerative diseases and the untold suffering they bring are by no means an inevitable part of getting older. Wild animals do not experience the slow and painful degeneration which takes so many forms in our society. They have been called 'diseases of civilization' – illnesses which orthodox medicine is unable to prevent and which lie behind the current crisis that medicine is experiencing. Neither, according to epidemiological and anthropological studies, do primitive cultures living on a sparse diet of natural foods suffer from this kind of degeneration. Throughout history most medical traditions – from China and India to ancient Sumeria – have taught that degeneration is not a normal part of ageing: that, provided we recognize the biological laws by which we are constituted and live with respect for them, we can live to a great age free of arthritis, heart attacks, cancer, lung diseases and the rest. These traditions have also taught that great age can be matched by great vitality so that we should be able – as an editorial in the *Journal of the American Medical Association* suggested not long ago – 'to die *young* late in life'.

There are people who already do this. Not only the well-studied long-lived cultures, but aware individuals living in the urban environments of the high-tech west. I know a number personally – men and women of seventy or eighty or ninety who not only have the vitality of people fifty years younger than they, but who look wonderful and whose energy and creativity are an inspiration to everyone they come in contact with. Given an understanding of the basic laws of nature and the needs of our body as well as the means to care for it, there is no reason why, barring some untoward accident, we should all not also be able to 'die young late in life'.

Stretching Statistics

The second big 'fiction' about ageing – the belief that medicine has already been able significantly to extend life – is as unfounded as the notion that degenerative diseases are inevitable. It is true that the average life expectancy of a baby born in Britain today is around seventy-three whereas in 1900 it was only fifty. (In North America the statistics are respectively seventy-three and forty-seven.) But that is almost entirely due to a decrease in infant mortality thanks to improved child-bearing methods and better sanitation. Every baby who dies at birth drastically reduces *average* lifespan. Because we have fewer babies and children dying now than we had at the turn of the century, statistics show that *average* life expectancy has increased. But this figure gives little idea of real *life* expectancy. For statistics also show that once beyond childhood we have little chance of living much longer than our grandfathers did.

It is important to understand the distinction between *median* lifespan, which is often used to indicate life expectancy, and *maximum* lifespan, which is a major goal of ageless ageing. *Median* lifespan measurements give you an indication of the age by which half of a population of people or animals have died. In ancient Rome this measurement was twenty-two years, by 1850 it had risen to forty. At the turn of the century it hovered around fifty. It was sixty-seven by 1946 and now, thanks mostly to this drop in infant mortality, it is around seventy-three. But neither mass immunization nor high-technology hospital procedures have had much impact on the *real* life expectancy of somebody who has already reached adulthood. For they have had little impact on *maximum* lifespan, which is an important measure of ageing. Despite miracle drugs, kidney transplants, and the other dramatic medical techniques for saving life, medical science has found no way of holding back the basic biological process of ageing.

How Long Can We Live?

Rather like the proverbial fisherman's tale, stories about how long man is capable of living tend to get more and more exaggerated. Moses, we are told, lived to be 120, Noah to 950 and Methuselah to 969. But scientific investigation has been little able to confirm such figures. What then is the maximum lifespan of man?

This is not an easy question to answer. In laboratory animals it is relatively simple. You take, say, a hundred rats, feed them the best quality of diet you can find and provide them with optimal environments and then you wait for the last one to die. That last death gives you your figure. For non-laboratory animals, such as bulls and elephants, turtles and thoroughbred horses, the procedure is to collect verifiable records of the oldest of a species. In the case of man these records are hard to verify. For while history abounds with stories about people who have lived to 200 years or more, we have no proof that this is so. Systematic birth and death records have only been kept in the past century and in many societies in the world these personal statistics are still not recorded. Scientists – such as Harvard Medical School's Alexander Leaf – who have travelled the world have often come back with stories of isolated communities which are well stocked with centenarians. The Andean village of Vilcabamba in Ecuador was found to boast nine individuals over 100 and one of 123 in a community of only 819, while in the Republic of Georgia in the Caucasus mountains, 8890 centenarians were reported, 150 of whom were said to be between 120 and 170. But recently some scientists have become very suspicious of these reported ages and insisted that they have been highly exaggerated by the peoples themselves for whom vigorous old age is a status symbol. Dissenters insist that maximum human lifespan as of right now is probably between 110 and 120.

Two truths emerge from research into maximum human lifespan. The first is that whether it turns out to be 200 or only 110, practically none of us comes anywhere near to approaching it. The second is that these long-lived peoples whose diet and lifestyles have by now been so well studied, by any standard, are able to live remarkably long, healthy and vigorous lives. At age 90 or 100 men are still siring children, riding horseback and taking daily dips into icy water – things that few of us westerners would dream of doing past middle age. We can learn a lot from them.

Go For The Best
To most people in the west old age brings ghastly images of decrepitude – not pictures of vigorous and sexually active old men and women intensively involved in work and looking forward to what comes next. The potential for creativity and enjoyment which is wasted in age-degeneration in the developed countries of the world is shocking. So is the cost to the state in providing medical treatment, hospitalization, food and care for people for whom ageing has become a nightmare of physical pain and emotional isolation. Few of us even come close to fulfilling our psycho-biological potentials. Instead we look forward to a steady and inexorable increase in morbidity and mortality from one disease to another. The exciting thing about the principles of ageless ageing is that if we begin now to apply them we will not only be able to extend our lives but to improve their quality beyond all recognition. For all of the major causes of death and disability appear to be secondary to the progressive degeneration of ageing. And the same principles which help keep your skin smooth, your muscles firm and your vitality high can also reduce the incidence of chronic disease and postpone degenerative illnesses so that if they occur at all, they come only very late in life.

To arrest the diseases of civilization with which medical science has been fruitlessly wrestling we are going to have to take preventative action – action which draws on the optimum health practices implicit in natural law anti-ageing as well as on recently discovered high-tech scientific techniques for protecting the body from degeneration. One American medical expert, Ernest M. Gruenberg, put it rather well when he said:

> Now we recognize that our life-saving technology of the past four decades has outstripped our health-preserving technology and that the net effect has been to worsen the people's health, we must begin the search for preventable causes of the chronic illnesses which we have been extending . . . We will not move forward in enhancing health until we make the prevention of nonfatal chronic illness our top research priority.

What has become increasingly apparent is that to do this one needs to confront the ageing process itself. As famous age researcher Johan Bjorksten says, we must aim to 'give as many people as possible as many more healthy vigorous years of life as possible'. He continues, ' . . . every one of the major diseases tabulated is age-dependent. To attack the problems of these diseases separately, as is now the preponderant course of action, is akin to trying to stop a haemorrhage by closing all of the capillary vessels separately rather than ligating the main artery.'

Longer *And* Better

The ways and means of ageless ageing are as diverse as are the disease conditions which it makes it possible for us to avoid. Some belong within the realm of natural law. These include low-calorie-high-potency ways of eating, exercise techniques, mental tools to alter expectations, as well as sun, air and water treatments. Others are pure high-tech science based on the latest free radical biochemistry. Together they can work wonders for the way you look and feel. For the pursuit of ageless ageing – with all that it implies – goes far beyond a narcissistic desire of the over-privileged middle classes for eternal youth. It reaches deep into the well of human possibilities for health, joy and lifelong creativity. It can lead us to a time when, instead of our elderly being a burden to their families and to the state, like the long-lived Hunzas, Georgians or

Vilcabamban Indians they will be able to contribute their experience, energy and wisdom to society. These are treasures which we can't afford to waste.

2
Story Without End

THE HISTORICAL SEARCH for ageless ageing as a means of prolonging active life is a tale full of haunting legends, elegant alchemical theories, exciting successes and grandiose failures. It begins when, racked with grief over the death of his friend Enkidu and fearful of his own impending death, the Sumerian hero Gilgamesh sets himself to search for the herb of eternal life. No sooner does he find it than this magical plant is devoured by a serpent as he swims in a beautiful lake and the secret is lost for ever. Another chapter was written in ancient Greece: on returning from the voyage in search of the Golden Fleece, Jason entreated his bride Medea to use her magic powers to rejuvenate his aged father Aeson. The process took her nine days. She purified the old man with sulphur, fire and water. Then she prepared her formula of 'pebbles from the farthest Orient, hoarfrost gathered under the moon, wings and flesh of the infamous horned owl, entrails of a werewolf, the skin of the Cynyphian water snake, the liver of a long-lived stag, the head of a crow nine centuries old and a thousand other things.' So successful was Medea's brew that Aeson's beard changed from grey to black, his body lost its lean and withered look and he took on the state of a man forty years his junior. And so powerful was Medea's rejuvenation mixture that its very smell transformed her dragons, causing them to slough off their old skins and to become young again.

Man has continually pined for the fountain of youth and been fascinated by the idea of ageless ageing. Down through the Middle Ages and beyond we have numerous records of special practices and potions designed to rejuvenate the body or to extend life. It was this longing which spurred the ageing conquistador Ponce de Leon to make his sixteenth-century voyage to the New World. It was the exceptional longevity of the famous seventeenth-century British peasant Thomas Parr which has not only made him a paragon of healthy old age but which turned him into an object of fascination for the British court.

Parr's life and death are no legend. They have been well documented historically. A man who had lived his whole life on a spartan diet of cheese, fresh fruit and a little bread, Parr was summoned at the amazing age of 152 to the court of King Charles I where he was lavishly feasted in the hopes of learning the secret of his longevity. But overindulgence proved too much for the frugal peasant. He sickened and quickly died. No less a scientist than William Harvey, discoverer of the circulatory system, performed the autopsy on Parr's body and wrote up the case. Harvey relates in his report that he was astonished at the peasant's superbly youthful brain and organs.

Brains, Brawn and Sex Organs

Modern ageing research goes back to the end of the nineteenth century by which time the discovery of the endocrine system had led some scientists to ask themselves if glandular secretions were not substances which could be used to regenerate fading youth, to restore flagging vitality and to prolong life. In the spring of 1889, an eccentric seventy-two-year-old physiologist named Charles Edouard Brown Séquard carried out some revolutionary experiments in which he injected himself with extracts taken from the testicles of dogs. Delighted with the results, Brown-Séquard reported that the tone of his muscles had improved and that he felt thirty years younger. Unfortunately his experiments were taken seriously neither by his family nor by the scientific community who insisted his 'results' were based on nothing more than an overactive imagination. They made him a laughing stock. He died a few years later in scientific disgrace. Yet a number of colleagues were intrigued by his work. Many experimenters began to look into glandular extracts as a workable means of rejuvenating the body and to experiment with other hormone-related techniques which might be useful against age.

One long-standing myth about ageing is the notion that much vitality is lost in men through ejaculation. Soon after Brown-Séquard's downfall, a Viennese endocrinologist named Eugen Steinach decided to restrict this 'vitality loss' by tying off the sperm ducts, in effect performing a vasectomy, on animals, following the theory that in doing so male sex hormones would be redirected back into the bloodstream and would rejuvenate the organism. An impeccable technician, Steinach carried out elaborate experiments with rats. All his tests appeared to confirm the theory although no scientist either then or now has yet been able to explain why. Unfortunately for humans, so far there have been few reports of increased vitality in men who have undergone vasectomies.

From Apes into Man

As interest in Steinach's work declined, a new star appeared on the rejuvenation horizon. He was a Russian (or at least so he said) named Serge Voronoff. An effervescent gentleman with a fascination for youth, Voronoff believed that you should be able to rejuvenate the body by giving testicular transplants. Working with farm animals, particularly rams and bulls, he succeeded in bringing back their potency and restoring their ability to sire offspring in old age. Voronoff quickly became a favourite amongst the agricultural community. Then in the spring of 1928, using anthropoid apes as donors of testicular tissue, he carried out his first ape-to-man transplant. This was followed by another 162 such operations in the next two years. Voronoff rapidly became the talk of Paris – famed for his 'monkey-gland' rejuvenation. And although medical colleagues at the time ridiculed his techniques, by the late Twenties even Europe's orthodox medical profession had moved to a position of acknowledging that the eccentric surgeon's technique did have some therapeutic effect. A conference of a thousand leading surgeons in Austria agreed that while 'rejuvenation' as such was a misnomer (it is still a word which makes most scientists squirm), 'the gland transplantation operation devised by Dr Serge Voronoff afforded transient regeneration'.

Modern Cell Therapy

The work of Steinach and that of Voronoff with his curious glandular transplants served as inspiration for another famous and highly controversial 'youth doctor' – Swiss surgeon Paul Niehans. Aware of the problems of foreign-tissue rejection, Niehans turned to foetal glands taken from unborn sheep and developed a technique of fresh-cell therapy. Selecting specific organs, glands and tissues which had been determined by examination of the patient and tailored to his specific needs, Niehans injected these fresh cells into people to heal and to rejuvenate them. The technique has attracted wide interest from the rich and famous who claim it makes them look and feel younger. It has even been used to treat mental retardation in the young, often with considerable success. But since so far no one has ever done controlled studies to show that it works, the British and American orthodox medical profession insist vehemently that it doesn't. Niehans died, after an active, and very lucrative, professional life, at the age of eighty-nine. His clinic, La Prairie in Vevey, Switzerland, continued with some variations on the original theme, to offer cell therapy at very high fees.

Errors in Cell Immortality

Meanwhile another line of investigation was being followed in the United States by the brilliant French physiologist and Nobel laureate Alexis Carrel. In 1912 at the Rockefeller Institute in New York, Carrel initiated a study using fibroblast cells – connective tissue cells widely distributed throughout the organism – from a chicken embryo. This experiment was instrumental in forming scientific opinion about the ageing process for almost fifty years. Carrel grew the cell structure in a glass vessel, nourishing it with a crude embryo extract. To the amazement of the scientific community, it far outlived even Carrel himself. The cells went on multiplying for more than thirty years at which point technicians terminated the experiment. Thanks to Carrel's long-lived chicken cells, the scientific community came to believe that ordinary cells in a living organism were immortal. Many scientists assumed therefore that there must be some substance in embryonic tissues with an ability to maintain youth and life. This belief, which was sustained for almost half a century, triggered a vast number of research projects in search of this natural youth serum – the elixir of youth.

The belief persisted until another famous age-researcher, Leonard Hayflick, carried out experiments which showed that cultured human fibroblasts *in vitro* are only able to divide about fifty times before they die out. This process takes but a few months in the laboratory. Hayflick discovered that when fibroblasts get to the limit of their dividing they do not suddenly just stop but the time needed for them to reach maturity gets longer as they approach their limit of fifty doublings. This eventually leads to the development of a group of cells which never reach confluence no matter how long they are incubated or how often the nutrient medium in which these cells are grown is renewed. In the end the cells undergo a variety of degenerative changes and then die. Looking more closely at Carrel's accomplishment it became apparent that his results were the outcome of a basic error. The embryo extract on which his cell culture was nourished was 'impure'. Inadvertently it had become contaminated with live chicken cells. One of Carrel's laboratory technicians even admitted later to Hayflick that she knew of the contamination, but so strong was the scientific community's commitment to the notion of cell immortality and to its search for the elixir of life which the belief implied, that she dared not voice criticism.

A Maximum Lifespan?

It was while doing cancer research at the Wistar Institute in Philadelphia that Hayflick happened upon the chance discovery that fibroblast cells appear programmed to die. Since then this finite lifetime of cultured human cells has been confirmed by researchers looking at fibroblasts as well as at other normal cell types including liver, smooth muscle, skin and brain. But, in keeping with the paradoxical nature of age research throughout history, it is now being contradicted by other scientists who claim that adding specific nutrients to such a culture can prolong its life – perhaps indefinitely.

The Nasty Immortals

One of the interesting offshoots of this cell research has been the discovery that, unlike normal cells which divide only until their limit is reached, some cells are actually immortal – they seem able to divide forever. These are cancer cells. By now a number of malignant strains have been cultured, mostly from animals. But the most famous of all is a human cell line which was derived in 1952 from cultured tissue taken from the cervix of a woman called Henrietta Lacks. It is known as the HeLa culture. Parts of this famous cell proliferation are still being studied in laboratories all over the world. Meanwhile the limit of about fifty divisions possible for normal cells on which many age-researchers agree has come to be known as the 'Hayflick limit'. And this fifty-division figure is important because, provided of course that Hayflick's findings turn out to be valid for cells *in vivo* – living cells within the body – they could be used to calculate mathematically the potential average maximum lifespan of any species. Employing Hayflick's mathematics, the average human lifespan should be somewhere between

100 and 120 years – although many age-researchers insist this figure is far too low. But low or not, few of us ever get anywhere near this. Why? With this question, elaborate contemporary research into the mechanics of ageing began. And, in an attempt to answer it, gerontologists have developed complex, often contradictory and sometimes confusing hypotheses.

The Language of Ageing

Theorists tend to fall into two camps. Some believe that the causes of ageing are fundamentally cellular: these scientists spend their time searching within the cells for the location of the trigger for Hayflick's limit. Is it in the cytoplasm – the cell's gel-like interior? In the mitochondria, the minute organelles – the cell's powerhouses for energy? In the lysosomes – the cell's rubbish dumps which, when they happen to split open, pollute the cytoplasmic ocean with their toxic wastes? Or perhaps in the cell's nucleus itself? The fault could well be in the DNA molecule – life's coded blueprint. After all, they point out (as Hayflick himself showed), when you separate the nuclei from the cytoplasm of young cells and then recombine them with older cytoplasm, it is always the age of the nuclei, not the cytoplasm, which determines when their limit of doubling has been reached.

Other age-researchers – equally esteemed – disagree with the 'cell-focusers'. They believe that the primary causes of ageing are general, not cellular. Some scientists insist that a mechanism in one of your body's centres of control – such as the endocrine glands, the brain, the nervous system – triggers the production of some as yet unknown substance which signals your cells to die. Others believe that ageing is the result of wear and tear to the organism as a whole. The former speak of 'death hormones' and genetic clocks while their colleagues talk instead of stress, loss of *adaptive* energy and overload.

Thirty years ago the 'cell-focusers' and the 'generalists' seemed poles apart. Now, thanks to the vast amount of intellectual cross-fertilization in the discipline of gerontology and to rapid developments in the field of free radical biochemistry and immunology, most age-researchers have come to believe that there is no single factor which can be pinpointed as the cause of ageing. What has become obvious is that ageing is a multi-dimensional process involving many repairing and destructive mechanisms both at a cellular level and systemically – in the body as a whole. Even more important, there now appears to be a strong relationship between age-degeneration being studied at a cellular level and the ageing of the body as a whole so that in a sense both the cell-focusers and the generalists are right. They are only looking at the phenomenon of ageing through different sets of binoculars. And, just as the practices involved in *natural law* anti-ageing and the newly discovered tools of *high-tech* anti-ageing appear to work best when they are applied together, the whole process of ageing – with all that it implies – makes better sense when you try to look at it from a number of different angles at once. On a cell-focusing level these include investigating recent discoveries in the areas of free radical biochemistry, electrobiology and submolecular physics. On a whole-body level they take in an awareness of the role that stress plays in age-degeneration, how ageing is related to a decline in immune functions, and new advances in the realm of psychoneuro-immunology – the study of how the mind affects the body's immune system. Each of these areas of scientific study has something to offer to an understanding of why your body ages. They also have much to contribute in developing a personal lifestyle for ageless ageing. Some of them can even offer ways of reversing age-related changes you may have experienced already. Let's look at the cell and at free radical biochemistry first.

3
Mysteries of the Cell

THE SMALLEST STRUCTURAL unit in your body is the cell. It is truly a remarkable entity simply because it is *alive*. It moves, grows, reacts, protects itself and even reproduces. And so far, despite the most elaborate and learned research attempting to understand the nature of that aliveness, it remains a mystery. No matter from what perspective you view ageing, you are ultimately looking at changes in life energy which take place over a period of time. A major goal of ageless ageing on a cellular level is making sure that everything functions properly to ensure good energy production and to keep the life machinery of cells ticking over as the years pass, much as it does in a healthy person of say twenty-five. To understand just how complex a task this is and just what is involved in fulfilling it you need to understand something about the structure and function of these miracles of nature – the cells from which your body is built.

The Cell as an Energy Factory
Each cell – and there are trillions of them in the human body – is like a factory complex. The famous American biochemist Roger Williams describes this very well when he says:

> Every cell has its own power plant from which it derives its energy. The burning process from which energy is derived is a highly ordered, many-step process in which many different catalysts are involved. Each catalyst (enzyme) is protein in nature and is made up of hundreds of amino acids (and often vitamins) put together in exactly the right way. The power plant makes it possible for every cell to be highly dynamic. Something is happening every microsecond. Complex chemical transformations – filtering, ultrafiltering, emulsify-

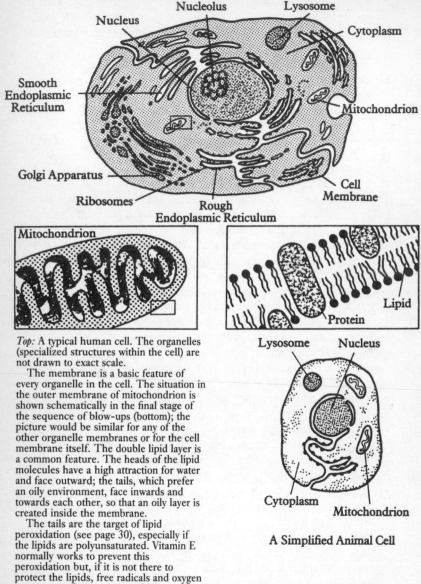

Nucleolus

Nucleus

Lysosome

Cytoplasm

Smooth Endoplasmic Reticulum

Mitochondrion

Golgi Apparatus

Ribosomes

Cell Membrane

Rough Endoplasmic Reticulum

Mitochondrion

Lipid

Protein

Lysosome

Nucleus

Cytoplasm

Mitochondrion

A Simplified Animal Cell

Top: A typical human cell. The organelles (specialized structures within the cell) are not drawn to exact scale.

The membrane is a basic feature of every organelle in the cell. The situation in the outer membrane of mitochondrion is shown schematically in the final stage of the sequence of blow-ups (bottom); the picture would be similar for any of the other organelle membranes or for the cell membrane itself. The double lipid layer is a common feature. The heads of the lipid molecules have a high attraction for water and face outward; the tails, which prefer an oily environment, face inwards and towards each other, so that an oily layer is created inside the membrane.

The tails are the target of lipid peroxidation (see page 30), especially if the lipids are polyunsaturated. Vitamin E normally works to prevent this peroxidation but, if it is not there to protect the lipids, free radicals and oxygen can cause a chain reaction which ties them together and disrupts the membrane. This impairs the function of the organelle and possibly damages the cell as a whole.

ing, dispersion, aggregating, absorption – are continually in progress. Tearing down, building up, and repairing are constantly going on.

He continues:

> Cells have their own ways of designing and making blueprints; 'printing' and duplicating are very much in evidence. Cells also have their own versions of assembly lines. They have transportation systems; sorting, pumping, and streaming; and molecules riding piggy-back on others are common processes. Intricate mechanisms, including feedbacks, are used by cells to regulate their numerous activities. Cells have communication systems – messages and messengers. They have the equivalent of both an intercom system and devices for sending and receiving messages to and from the outside. Cells are equipped with sewage and disposal systems. They even have in effect pollution-control mechanisms whereby toxic molecules are converted into others which are relatively harmless.

This marvellous creation of nature – the tiny cell – is superbly *ordered* in its functions and structure. On this order depends your body's youthfulness and longevity. But because it is so complex each part of the cellular mechanism is also highly subject to disorder. And when a cell becomes deranged, its entire function can be seriously impaired. Multiply one deranged cell times the thousand million million cells in your body and you experience what is known in modern medicine as degenerative disease and ageing.

Cellular Order – Foundation of Ageless Ageing

At its outer edge each cell is surrounded by a protective membrane built mostly from lipids or fats. Through this membrane all nutrients and oxygen must pass to keep the cell alive and all wastes must be eliminated. Inside the cell lies a gel-like ocean of cytoplasm which contains a variety of subcellular bodies – fat protein complexes – called *organelles* which take part in cell functions. The organelles include microsomes which make new proteins, lysosomes which are like automatic waste collectors whose job it is to keep the cytoplasmic ocean unpolluted, and mitochondria – minute energy factories. Each cell also has a nucleus in its centre.

Here all the genetic details of its structure and functions are carefully locked away in molecules of DNA, so that when a cell gets ready to divide, another nucleic acid called RNA carries the DNA's coded instruction to get the correct amino acids for the synthesis of new proteins.

Just like the cell itself, every organelle it contains is encased within a protective membrane. These membranes are very important to the integrity of a living cell and to protecting the body as a whole from ageing and illness. If they are disrupted, chaos can ensue: wastes can leak into the cytoplasm and cause the cell to poison itself, enzymes contained in the mitochondria can cause serious biological disruption, and damage to the DNA within the nucleus in turn can lead to a missynthesis of protein and the production of a mutant or damaged daughter cell. In fact all of these detrimental changes appear to take place as your body ages. Preventing them and protecting the integrity of each individual cell within any biological system is the central issue in preventing age-degeneration. And one of life's great paradoxes is that amongst the worst threats to cellular order and integrity on many different levels is the one element without which we cannot live even for a few minutes: oxygen.

The Two Faces of Oxygen

Two billion years ago – give or take a few million years – a profound change took place on earth which dramatically affected evolution: plant life came into being. These first primitive plants started to release oxygen into the atmosphere by breaking down water in the presence of sunlight through a process called photosynthesis. In the beginning this 'new' element oxygen was lethal to almost every living organism. The few creatures who managed to survive could do so only by continually adapting to its presence in their system. Slowly these early simple animals evolved ways of doing this. They created protective mechanisms against oxygen toxicity. And they found ways of using oxygen to create energy – so successfully in fact that by now oxygen has become the potent impetus behind most metabolic processes that fuel complex forms of animal life.

Yet oxygen's toxicity is still with us. Expose yourself to levels of oxygen beyond what you are used to and you can become ill. For instance breathe in pure oxygen at 1 atmosphere for a few hours and you will develop inflammation in the trachea. Stay in such an

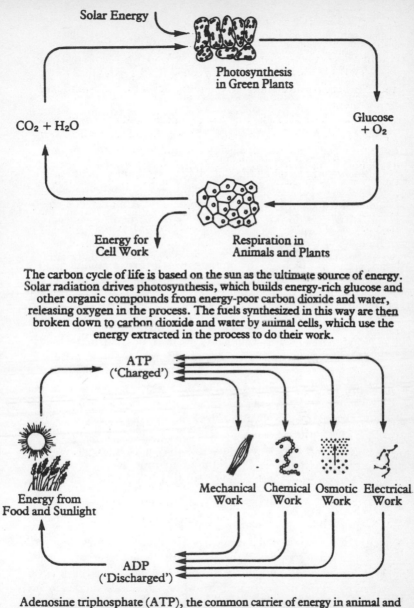

Solar Energy

Photosynthesis
in Green Plants

$CO_2 + H_2O$

Glucose
+ O_2

Energy for
Cell Work

Respiration in
Animals and Plants

The carbon cycle of life is based on the sun as the ultimate source of energy.
Solar radiation drives photosynthesis, which builds energy-rich glucose and
other organic compounds from energy-poor carbon dioxide and water,
releasing oxygen in the process. The fuels synthesized in this way are then
broken down to carbon dioxide and water by animal cells, which use the
energy extracted in the process to do their work.

ATP
('Charged')

Energy from
Food and Sunlight

Mechanical
Work

Chemical
Work

Osmotic
Work

Electrical
Work

ADP
('Discharged')

Adenosine triphosphate (ATP), the common carrier of energy in animal and
plant cells, is formed in the mitochondria (animals) and chloroplasts (plants).
It supplies energy for muscle contraction, protein synthesis, transfer of nerve
impulses, etc. The 'discharged' adenosine diphosphate (ADP) thus formed is
'recharged' by solar or food energy.

atmosphere for days on end and, ironically, soon you will die from a condition called *anoxia* which means lack of oxygen. Even the oxygen we take in through the air we normally breathe is still highly toxic to many essential life processes on a cellular level, because oxygen tends to combine with other substances and to wreak havoc with delicate cell structures causing *disorder.* It is a disorder which is central to the whole process of ageing.

Atoms, Molecules, and Energy Exchange

In biochemical terms all the stuff of life – from the genetic material in your cells to the air that you breathe – is built out of atoms and molecules arranged in infinite combinations. Although contemporary physicists do not rely completely on particulate concepts of atoms, generally speaking a molecule is only a combination of atoms, and atoms are made up of a number of particles, the most important of which are the protons (which carry a minute positive electrical charge) and neutrons, both of which are found in the centre of the atom, and the electrons (each of which carries a small negative charge) which spin around in orbitals on the outside. Oxygen is the most important molecule we ever deal with.

What makes energy-yielding metabolism possible in the human body is the ability we have evolved through evolution to convert nutrients taken in through foods we eat into chemical energy to fuel life processes by burning it. This is a process known as *aerobic metabolism.* And it is a highly efficient means of energy production and release. Specifically it involves the transfer of electrons from one molecule to another. In scientific terms this occurrence is generally known as an *oxidation-reduction* or a *redox* reaction. So important are redox reactions both to life processes in general and to helping to slow age-degeneration that it is important to take a closer look at them.

Whenever an electron is transferred from one atom or molecule to another this complementary oxidation and reduction takes place between the two interacting species of molecules. In fact the word *oxidation* is a description of the process in which a molecule or atom loses an electron and the term *reduction* refers to the process whereby an electron is gained. So when molecules interact in any redox reaction one substance is *oxidized* (the molecule loses an electron) while the other is *reduced* (it gains an electron). For some time physicists have tended to view electrons not only as subatomic particles but also as basic units of energy. And the energy-producing metabolism which our bodies carry out can be described in biochemical terms as the oxidation or removal of electrons from reduced carbon compounds and the reduction of or transfer of these electrons by suitable carriers to their ultimate acceptor oxygen. It is a process which creates water as its by-product.

So long as we live these redox reactions are ceaselessly taking place. They are the basis of the oxygen-based metabolism which keeps us alive. And we need vast amounts of energy to stay alive. This we get by oxidizing biological substances – burning food as fuel. It is a burning which takes place not in some haphazard way as it would in a furnace. Instead it is ordered with superb precision: enzymes act as catalysts and oxidations occur in a carefully modulated series of small steps which are able to liberate the maximum amount of energy present for effective use while causing the minimum amount of disturbance to the cell. Energy which is liberated by such a process needs to go through many intermediate compounds which serve as electron-carriers in order to provide the control necessary. For if electrons were to reduce oxygen directly and not go through these intermediate steps then we would be unable to harness the energy released for useful purposes.

The trouble is that a number of highly reactive, potentially toxic and destructive species of molecules are generated in the process. They are known as *free radicals* and they put us as human beings in the curious position of being dependent upon oxygen for our life energy and yet also susceptible to its toxic effects – what in biochemistry is known as *oxidizing stress* or *oxy-stress*. It poses a continual challenge to the integrity of our cells and tissues and it appears to be a central cause of ageing.

Friendly and Unfriendly Free Radicals

Free radicals are species of atoms or molecules which are highly reactive simply because they are electrochemically unbalanced. In stable molecules and atoms you'll find the positively charged protons and the negatively charged electrons in perfect balance so that the electrical charge the atom or molecule carries can be said to be nil. The molecule is neutral. Free radicals are different. Instead of having the usual orbitals occupied by pairs of electrons which spin in opposite directions these renegades have an odd number. Therefore they carry a small electrical charge. Most retain a single unpaired electron in an outer orbital. This not only creates the electrical charge; it also gives the molecule astounding instability and makes it react with other atoms and molecules with which it comes into contact. It is a relatively simple matter to turn a stable non-radical molecule or compound into a free radical species simply by bringing it in contact with another free radical from which it gains or to which it loses an electron. The whole exchange takes place in microseconds. Once a free radical is present it tends to propagate by generating other free radicals from chain reactions with the stable non-radical species which happen to be present.

Free radicals, which are common in all biological systems, are essential for the maintenance of life. Indeed free radicals are formed naturally during a wide variety of biological processes from respiration to the carrying out of enzyme activities which are a normal part of cell metabolism. However free radical reactions are also responsible for many of the things that go wrong with the body on a cellular level. For when these free radical reactions get out of hand they can precipitate a relentless process of destruction and degeneration in the body as a whole.

Molecular Rapists

Gerontologist Alex Comfort once compared a free radical to a convention delegate away from his wife: 'a highly reactive chemical agent that will combine with anything that's around'. Other researchers believe free radicals can be better likened to rapists whose union with other molecules, willing or unwilling, is nothing less than a clear attack. Free radicals can cut other molecules down the middle, chop pieces off them, distort cellular information and generally wreak havoc with living systems. They can cause injury, inflammation and destruction to parts of cells, cell walls and to collagen fibres, the body's most important structural protein.

An important source of free radical harm in relation to ageing occurs through a process called *lipid peroxidation*. Lipid is simply the scientific word for fats and oils. Lipids are found all over our bodies: in the blood; stored as potential energy in the cells; joined to certain proteins called lipoproteins and as a part of steroid hormones. Lipids are particularly important to individual cells because they largely make up the membrane which separates a cell from its surrounding medium. The lipids in our bodies come from the foods we eat – saturated and unsaturated fatty acids. In fact it is absolutely necessary that we take in an adequate supply of unsaturated fatty acids for life and health. The trouble is that unsaturated fatty acids have a strong tendency to react with oxygen in the body to form chemical compounds known as peroxides. Peroxidation also occurs in the presence of oxygen in the atmosphere. This is what makes cooking oils or peanut butter turn rancid. Like free radicals, once formed in the body peroxides then tend to join with yet more lipids and to propagate yet more peroxides and free radicals. These, it appears, cause serious damage to organelles in the cells and to cell membranes, allowing cellular pollution and reducing the electrical potentials – thus lowering body vitality in yet another way. Protect your body from oxy-stress – free radical and peroxidation damage – and you will dramatically slow down the rate at which you age.

Free Radical Revolution
Recent findings in the field of free radical pathology – the study of free radicals 'gone wrong' – are nothing short of revolutionary. They make it possible for the first time in scientific terms to formulate a *unified* theory of disease. Thanks to free radical biochemistry, doctors well versed in the subject are beginning to make sense of a lot of what until now appeared to be contradictory clinical and epidemiological observations, and to create a scientific rationale both for the treatment and for the prevention of a number of the major causes of degeneration and death: arteriosclerosis, cancer, arthritis, dementia and other age-related diseases. Free radical damage now appears to underlie the pathology of all of these conditions despite the difference in their manifestations in the body.

This discovery is perhaps the most important medical finding in the past fifty years. The discovery that oxy-stress – free radical damage and peroxidation – can bring about disease and degeneration in the body and the development of ways and means of counteracting it are providing scientists with coherent and workable methods both for preventing illness – from allergy to many serious mental disorders – as well as for restoring much of the degenerative damage which is associated with ageing. The free radical concept can also explain how many of the natural law therapies (which we will be exploring in later chapters) work to slow down ageing and reverse pathological changes in the body – from chelation therapy and anti-oxidant supplementation to diet and lifestyle changes which are traditionally used to restore health to a chronically ill person. And, although it will take another decade before free radical biochemistry becomes fully integrated into the work of the average doctor, it is already being used successfully by health practitioners, anti-agers and cosmetic scientists to bring about life-enhancing change.

Elmer M. Cranton and James P. Frackelton – two physicians who are experts in the field of free radical biochemistry and its clinical applications – put it beautifully in the *Journal of Holistic Medicine*, when they wrote: 'The field of free radical biochemistry is as revolutionary and profound in its implications for medicine as was the germ theory and science of microbiology which made possible development of effective treatments for infectious diseases.' Methods for detecting and measuring the presence of free radicals in living systems have only just been developed. What they show is that the reason why many of the natural treatments for ageing and illness work is the fact that, in the words of these two scientists, ' . . . physical exercise, applied clinical nutrition and moderation of health-destroying habits, all have common therapeutic mechanisms which reduce free radical damage.' Free radical damage, for the moment at least, appears to be at the very foundation of what is known about ageing. If you want to counteract it you need to understand how and what to do about it.

4
Shoe-Leather and Cross-Linking

PROTEINS ARE MADE up of *amino acids* – the most important of all known substances in the organic world. For amino acids are the basis of life. They are used to build cells and to repair tissue. Your immune system – from its white blood cells to interferon – depends upon amino acids. Your bones and teeth are made with chains of amino acids in which minerals have been laid down. In your body over 50,000 different proteins are made from amino acids. Every enzyme is a protein. So, largely, are the hormones which direct organic functions, the muscle tissue which gives your body form and strength, and the vascular tissue which carries nutrients to the cells. Your cells' genetic materials – DNA and its messenger nucleic acid RNA – while not themselves proteins, are deeply involved in the process of protein synthesis. On the integrity of all these proteins you are entirely dependent for life and health.

When free radicals react with molecules of protein in the cell or in the tissue, these long-chain proteins can become *cross-linked*, which means they become molecularly bound together and tangled. As a result tissues lose their suppleness, skin wrinkles, veins and arteries become hardened and more inclined to build up deposits of cholesterol, your chances of developing cancerous growths increase and the genetic material in your cells, which is necessary for cell division and tissue repair, becomes garbled. Cross-linking is a phenomenon which is fundamental to age-degeneration – both at a deep internal level where it can cause arteriosclerosis and brain degeneration and superficially since it appears to be the major reason why skin wrinkles and sags. Prevention of excessive cross-linkage in your body is essential to any effective programme of ageless ageing.

During the Second World War, Finnish chemist Johan

Bjorksten was working for an American photographic company. In the midst of carrying out a routine task one day, he realized that the changes which take place in the gelatins of film and plates are akin to those which take place in our cells when we age. These changes are the result of chemical bonds being formed – cross-linking – between thin protein molecules which make up the gelatin. They are also, he remarked, similar to the changes deliberately brought about in order to turn animal hides into strong leather. This cross-linking is responsible for the enormous difference in the way a finished piece of leather feels as compared with the skin of the animal from which it was taken. It was Bjorksten who coined the word cross-linking. He then went on to explore it as a central cause of ageing and to develop what is perhaps the most comprehensive theoretical approach to age-retardation of any scientist in the world today.

Factory Slow-Down

To understand how cross-linking interferes with cellular metabolism and leads to degeneration, Bjorksten explains that protein molecules – the most important chemical parts of the living body – are like long spirals. In all of them, along the chain there are points which can tie in very easily with other molecules or atoms. In fact it is thanks to these many 'sensitive' parts on the protein molecules that proteins are able to carry out so many useful tasks in the body and why they are so necessary to life processes. But when 'cross-linkers' such as free radicals or highly reactive oxygen molecules come along, rather like small rods with hooks at each end, they can hook into these sensitive points on the protein molecules. And when they do this – with each end on a protein molecule – they bind proteins together. When two or more protein molecules are joined together in this way they can no longer move as freely. When they become linked up to many protein molecules in many places they finally get so jumbled up that they can no longer do their job efficiently. Going back to our analogy of the cell as an energy factory it is easy to see what happens. Bjorksten once explained it this way to his child:

> Imagine you are in a big room, where thousands of people are working. Each day some evil person comes in and slips a pair of handcuffs on a pair of people so that it ties them together. That makes it difficult for them to work, doesn't it? . . . Now if

this goes on so that at the end of every day a couple more handcuffs are put on so that one handcuff is put on one person and the other end of it on another person, then you can see that things get more and more messed up . . . Finally everything becomes so confused that nothing can get done, and the whole work or whatever they are doing in that hall has to stop. Think of the handcuffs as cross-linkers, and the people as those important protein molecules. When a person is young and in his prime, he hasn't many protein molecules that are handcuffed together to slow down the work of his body. But as he gets older more and more of the cross-linker 'handcuffs' slide into place and the work of his body slows down and he gets old and weak.

Wrinkles and Radiation

The damage that free radicals and cross-linking can do to the collagen, elastin and reticulin in connective tissue is particularly worrying from a cosmetic point of view. It makes your skin sag and your muscles lose their firmness. Collagen, which is often considered the mortar of the cells, makes up more than 40 per cent of your body's protein. When collagen and other connective proteins are young they have almost a gel-like quality to them. They lend structural support to all the living cells. For these cells to be nourished, oxygen, moisture and nutrients have to pass through the collagen network. Through this network too are eliminated the cells' waste products. Collagen which has become cross-linked as a result of free radical attack impedes proper cell nutrition and waste elimination, thereby lowering cell vitality and eventually the vitality of the whole organism.

Apart from natural body agents which cause a small amount of cross-linking to take place – even in the collagen of a baby – in order to give structure to muscles, the vascular system and skin, a wide variety of external factors also cause cross-linking to occur. They include industrial pollutants, polyvalent metals such as lead, cadmium, mercury and so forth, sodium nitrite (which is used to preserve luncheon meats), radiation (including the sun's ultraviolet light and x-rays), cosmic radiation and nuclear radiation in our food and atmosphere. When you are young your body produces enzymes which break down excess cross-linkages when they take place. Then, there is an excellent 'balance of power' which keeps our skin and muscles and veins and capillaries strong but flexible and supple. But as the years go by cross-linkage tends to occur faster than these enzymes can undo it – probably both because enzymes tend to be reduced with age and also because we tend to accumulate more and more cross-linking substances in our system as we get older.

Cross-linking appears to be largely responsible for the loss of elasticity in our body's tissues – the wrinkling and sagging skin that comes with age, as well as the increased brittleness of rigid tissues which is also a characteristic of age. It's also implicated in the decline in the percentage of bound water in the tissues which, because of the important role water appears to play in energy transfer in the body, can decrease vitality in tissues and organs, another characteristic of advancing age. Animals kept on very low-calorie diets show dramatically increased lifespans. This, according to Bjorksten and others, is probably because a low-calorie diet creates a minimum of metabolic by-products which can act as free radicals and cross-linkers. The more you can avoid cross-linkage the smoother will stay your skin. If we can find a way of dissolving cross-linkage after it occurs then we would have a rejuvenation treatment *par excellence.* This has been (and still is) a major goal of ageless ageing.

Damaged DNA

Free radicals and the by-products of lipid peroxidation can also react with DNA, the cell's genetic material, and RNA, which carries the genetic messages, to disrupt genetic information so that abnormal proteins are synthesized. As yet no one has been able clearly to understand how this takes place. What is known is that when genetic material is altered in this way cells no longer reproduce themselves accurately. This appears to be a major factor in age-degeneration as well as in the development of cancer. Bjorksten believes also that cross-linkages are formed between parts of DNA's spiral helices – although other researchers disagree with him. In any case there is strong evidence that disruptions in genetic information do take place as we age, resulting in mis-synthesized proteins. The level of RNA decreases in middle age and it appears that RNA's susceptibility to misprogramming also increases. This may be the result of a reduction in protein and enzyme manufacture.

Missynthesized proteins cause problems in many ways. When the right protein is not made then the purpose for which it is

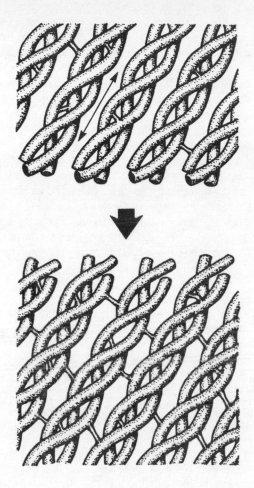

Collagen and the cross-linkage of collagen. In this model of one type of connective tissue, each of the tube structures represents a chain of amino acids; three such chains twisted together in a spiral (a triple helix) are considered as a unit of collagen. Many of these units are joined end to end to form long, continuous threads; in turn, these continuous threads are stacked side by side to form larger strands. A small section of one of these strands is shown here.

During youth, only a moderate amount of cross-linking ties the collagen threads to each other (top). As a result, the collagen threads slide past each other, and the connective tissue is quite elastic. With increasing age, however, progressively more cross-linkages are formed, so that the sliding of threads past each other is greatly restricted (above), with the result that the connective tissue is less elastic.

intended does not get fulfilled and either the function or a structure of an enzyme is changed or impaired. Missynthesized proteins tend to be bigger than normal proteins and to crowd them out, competing with them for available nutrients. They can also create wastes which pollute cells and, since the body needs to produce new proteins to replace them, can greatly lower a cell's vitality and drain its resources. Nucleic acids in the cell nucleus have a quite remarkable ability to repair themselves. But in order for this to happen there must be an adequate supply of ascorbic acid, amino acids, the B vitamins – especially folic acid, B2, B6, B5 and choline – as well as zinc, manganese and chromium. A number of studies show that the sulphur amino acids, selenium, ascorbic acid and vitamin E working together promote DNA and RNA repair. This is one of the reasons why these nutrients are included in the list of natural substances taken as nutritional supplements for ageless ageing. To preserve genetic information intact it is necessary to protect DNA and RNA from lipid peroxidation and free radical attack.

Anti-oxidant Defences
This is a challenge for which our exquisitely organized life processes have a double-barrelled answer, in the form of complex anti-oxidant defence systems. The body in its wisdom has devised a number of mechanisms to protect itself from oxy-stress. Our first line of defence comes in the form of special enzymes called free radical scavengers – with names you will find commonly mentioned in any treatise on age-retardation. They include: superoxide dismutase (SOD), glutathione peroxidase and catalase. Each enzyme has a specific and very important task to perform; all of them are involved in the processes of protecting living material from damage. The second line of defence is made up of the anti-oxidant nutrients we take in through our foods and which serve as free radical 'quenchers', mopping up reactive molecular species including *singlet oxygen* – an oxygen molecule containing only one atom instead of the usual two – and neutralizing their ability to cause damage. They include ascorbic acid, beta-carotene, vitamin A, certain amino acids, vitamin E and selenium. One of the most profound findings in biomedical research in the last few decades is that anti-oxidants are also anti-cancer agents.

About anti-oxidant nutrients we will be talking a great deal – not only because they help protect your body from accelerated ageing and degeneration but because, as free radical biochemistry has now demonstrated, they have an important role to play in the treatment of many serious illnesses including environmental and food allergies. Also, the same anti-oxidant nutrients which protect from oxy-stress have an ability to improve immune functions – another important factor in slowing down the ageing process. They can also be used for their anti-inflammatory properties. So important can these substances be for improving health that many doctors who use them in high doses for healing serious illness in their patients have now begun to incorporate similar high doses into their own lives for preventative purposes.

External Threats

Were the body's own metabolic processes the only trigger for free radical production and cross-linking we would probably have little worry about age-related degeneration nor about supplying extra anti-oxidants for prophylactic purposes. Our own protective mechanisms might be enough to protect our cells, proteins and lipids from damage. But a myriad of external factors can also initiate and accelerate free radical reactions. Our environment is full of external triggers. These include radiation of all sorts – from the sun's ultraviolet rays to emanations from nuclear power stations and even the electromagnetic fields set up by high-tension electrical installations. They also include air pollutants such as ozone, nitrogen dioxide, and sulphur dioxide; cigarette smoke, solvents, pesticides and drugs; heavy metals such as lead, cadmium and aluminium; as well as certain foods, particularly those which are lacking in freshness. The eating of too much food, and the toxic residues from illness or prolonged emotional stress, also tend to increase free radical reactions and cross-linkage. Even oxygen in the air we breathe brings about free radical damage, not only because the majority of free radical reactions involve oxygen but because oxygen in certain forms actually behaves like a free radical itself. Two forms of activated oxygen – singlet oxygen and hydrogen peroxide – although technically not free radicals themselves, nonetheless share with them a similar capacity to damage biological tissue and therefore to age the body.

The Fire, the Heat and the Screen

One useful way to look at the nature of free radical reactions and the cross-linking they cause, and understand how the body is able to protect itself from free radical damage, is through an analogy devised by an American scientist whose major focus has been on oxy-stress as an underlying cause of environmental allergies. An expert on clinical ecology, Steve Levine likens it to sitting in front of a fireplace watching logs burn. The burning of the wood gives off the energy needed to heat the room – akin to redox reactions which burn fuel for cell energy. And, thanks to the fact that in front of the fireplace is placed a good protective screen, the sparks which are emitted as part of the wood-burning process do no damage to our carpets or clothes. Think of the screen as the body's anti-oxidant defence systems. Think of the sparks as free radicals and other activated species of molecules. They are of course a normal outcome of cellular metabolism just as sparks are a normal occurrence when burning. Both are the inevitable result of inefficiencies in the burning process. If the burning process were total – completely efficient – then there wouldn't be any sparks.

Free radicals are destructive and ageing to an organism only if the 'protective screen' – our anti-oxidant defence system – is damaged or worn, or if the number of sparks formed by the fire overwhelms the screen and sends it crashing to the floor, which is what happens in serious chronic illness and degeneration. The numerous parts of your body's anti-oxidant defence system must absorb the potentially damaging sparks – the free radicals and other activated molecular species. But when we are overwhelmed by environmental chemical exposure, or emotional stress, or the trauma of infection, then there is an increase in sparks. And our metabolic machinery, which is basically burning fuel and deriving energy, ultimately has to deal with the sparks of metabolism. An inability to do this can result in illness, fatigue, degeneration and ageing.

Cellular Age Control

Age control on a cellular level entails preventing peroxidation of the foods we eat and inhibiting lipid peroxidation in the body, avoiding as much as possible the triggers for oxy-stress in our environment, and preventing free radical damage and cross-linking by strengthening the body's anti-oxidant defence system. Many researchers believe, as Bjorksten does, that we may also be able to use certain chemical or nutritional agents to *dissolve* cross-linked proteins and repair free radical damage which has already occurred as well. Bjorksten has actually discovered a means of doing this – a special strain of *Bacillus cerus* which is proteolytic (protein-digesting). It can reverse the cross-links formed, for instance, in the tanning process, so that hide returns to its original soft shape even after having been turned into leather. But the enormous amount of research time and money necessary to develop such a find into a safe form of treatment which can be brought on to the market has so far made this impossible.

Meanwhile biochemists continue to probe the secrets of the body's anti-oxidant system. They have discovered that it is an overtaxing of this system – an excess of oxy-stress – which leads to the widespread incidence of both food and environmental allergies. Meanwhile, although the average doctor is still unaware of it, strong evidence is emerging that free radical damage is the underlying cause of the so-called diseases of civilization which plague our society, from coronary heart disease to cancer. This is an exciting area of research which holds out many promises for healthier lives and slowing down the rate at which we age. The two-branched approach to ageless ageing relies heavily on new discoveries in free radical biochemistry, and in later chapters I deal with making use of anti-oxidants, amino acids, diet and exercise to lower oxy-stress and slow the rate at which you age. But it is by no means the whole story. For there is always the danger that, lost in his world of electron microscopes, the free radical biochemist may lose his ability to see the wood for the trees. Even when I am most entranced by the elegance of the theories and the exciting implications of what can be achieved using natural anti-oxidant nutrients to protect the body from age-degeneration (and as you will see in subsequent chapters it is a great deal) I am still brought back to an awareness of the fact that, after all, we are dealing not just with a collection of cells, atoms and molecules but with a complex self-adjusting organism with as yet largely undefined control systems. And when attempting to penetrate the mysteries of ageing and the magic of age-retardation, we have also to view the organism as a whole. When you step back from a microscope two important, closely related areas of focus loom large on the horizon – stress and the immune system.

5
Immune Power

THE IMMUNE SYSTEM is a complex network of specialized cells and processes which form your body's natural defence against invasion, poison and disease. There are two aspects to it: *humoral* immunity, and *cell-mediated* immunity. How well it is working determines to a large degree how rapidly you age. The immune system is like an enormously complex and highly organized secret police in a totalitarian country which – together with its special branch of armed militia – has the job of ensuring that absolutely everything foreign, everything which does not carry the marker of 'self', is kept out. It guards against foreign proteins, viruses, bacteria and aberrant cells.

It is humoral immunity which creates antibodies as a response to invading viruses, chemicals, bacteria and foreign substances. These invaders are known as antigens and your humoral system manufactures a specific antibody to handle each antigen. Each antibody is only capable of recognizing and getting rid of a specific antigen. Over the years your body collects a vast log of thousands of antibodies which create your lifelong *immunologic memory*, all of which is encoded in proteins.

Cell-mediated immunity, on the other hand, is centred around the actions of specialized cells, the most important of which are T-cell and B-cell lymphocytes – more about these in a moment. Just as a cell membrane must remain intact to protect the integrity of the cell, so your immune system must maintain its high-protection surveillance to ensure the integrity of your body as a whole. Build a strong immune system and you create a powerful resistance to ageing and illness.

As you get older two very dangerous things can happen to the immune system. First, its function can decline so that it is no longer an effective military force against invasion and aberrant cells. Second, rather like a secret police without proper control from the top, it may go haywire and fail to distinguish between self and non-self so that it not only is no longer able to protect you, it can begin to attack and destroy the body's own protein. This not only leaves you vulnerable to invasion by disease-provoking microbes, it can also make you prone to a number of specific diseases known as the auto-immune disorders. They include multiple sclerosis, rheumatoid arthritis, rheumatic heart disease, and systemic lupus.

Immunity – Free Radical Damage and Age Decline

The complicated system by which 'self' and 'non-self' are recognized appears to be regulated by a collection of genes found very close to one another on a single chromosome. It is a collection called the *major histocompatibility complex* (MHC). Interestingly enough, some of the enzymes such as SOD and probably catalase – which, you may remember, are the body's natural free radical scavengers – are also found in the same chromosome. Even mechanisms such as the repair of damaged DNA appear to be influenced by the MHC. Two well-respected age-researchers, Roy Walford at the UCLA (University of California at Los Angeles) Medical School and Ed Yunnis at Harvard, have shown that the MHC is an important regulator of the rate at which we age. How well it works is closely determined both by the actions of free radicals and by how much decline has taken place in the immune system as a whole. The functions of the body's anti-oxidant defence systems and those of the MHC and immunity appear to be inextricably intertwined. Take action to improve one and you improve the other as well. If science can find a way of preventing immune functions from declining and of preventing the immune system from acting against the 'self' of which it is a part, it will also go a long way towards slowing down or even reversing the ageing process. Immune dysfunction is a major pacemaker of ageing.

At the National Institutes of Health in the United States, researchers have been able to measure just how dramatic is the decline in immunologic efficiency as an animal ages. They discovered that when mice were subjected to measured doses of disease organisms designed to stimulate the immune system, the old mice demonstrated a response that was only 10 per cent of that of young mice. In other words, their immune systems had

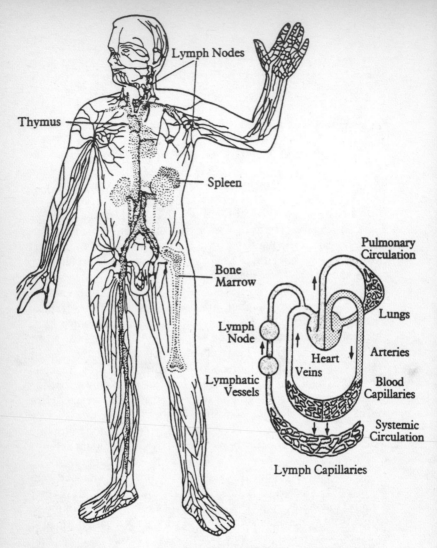

Lymph Nodes

Thymus

Spleen

Bone
Marrow

Lymph
Node

Lymphatic
Vessels

Pulmonary
Circulation

Lungs

Arteries

Heart
Veins

Blood
Capillaries

Systemic
Circulation

Lymph Capillaries

The immune system consists of the lymphocyte cells and the antibody molecules which they secrete. The cells and antibodies pervade most of the body's tissues, being delivered there by the bloodstream, but they are concentrated in the tree of lymphatic vessels and the lymph nodes stationed along them, the bone marrow (which is in the long bones, only one of which is illustrated), the thymus and the spleen. The lymphatic vessels collect the cells and antibodies from the body's tissues and return them to the bloodstream at the subclavian veins in the neck. Lymphocytes are manufactured in the bone marrow and multiply by cell division in the thymus, the spleen and the lymph nodes. *Right:* A highly schematic representation of the relation of the blood vessels and the lymphatic vessels.

experienced a 90 per cent decline. Translated into human terms one could say that at age seventy you are ten times more susceptible to disease and age-degeneration than you were at twelve years old.

The Master, the Police and the Militia

Just above your heart in the chest cavity is the master gland of immunity – the thymus. It is a gland which, until recently, was largely ignored because scientists believed that the thymus was only involved in the growth process and after that was simply redundant to the body. This theory they justified by the fact that the thymus tends to shrink dramatically after about the age of fourteen.

We now know however that not only is the 'thymus-redundancy theory' wrong, the thymus is probably the single most important part of the body in protecting you from both illness and ageing. This small pinkish-grey body under your breastbone oversees your state of health from birth to death. The levels of hormones which this gland produces – called thymusin – appear to be related both to the state of your endocrine system, with all its hormones, and to many brain chemicals as well as to how rapidly you are ageing. It is from the thymus that instructions come to the lymph nodes and the spleen to fight off bacterial invasions and to reject foreign cells. These tasks it relegates to the two major protective forces of the immune system – the secret police and the militia.

The thymus and its T-cells are the secret police. They make up about half of the resources for defence in your body. Another group of white blood cells called B-cells, whose main purpose is to protect your body against most bacterial threats and a few viral infections, make up the other half. They are the armed militia. These two branches work together but differently to provide constant vigilance against external threats – from bacterial invasions to chemicals which cause free radical damage, peroxidation and cross-linking. Where the T-cells produce their single *lymphokines*, B-cells make *antibodies*.

T-Cells, B-Cells and Integrity

The thymus sends instructions to the lymph nodes and the spleen to fight off bacterial invasions and to reject foreign cells. It issues these instructions via a group of hormones which act as messengers to your body's defence system. They mobilize T-cell *lymphocytes* – your body's 'warrior cells' – and set them to work battling the thousands of potentially lethal micro-organisms, cancer-inducing ultraviolet radiations from the sun or toxic chemicals from our highly industrialized environment. These warrior cells then produce another group of hormone-like substances called lymphokines which are considered the immune system's natural drugs. One of these lymphokines is interferon – now famous because of its demonstrated ability to fight cancer – but there are a number of others with strange titles like SIRS and IL-2.

When B-lymphocytes or B-cells locate a foreign organism they start producing antibodies against it. When T-cells spot an invader they produce their lymphokines to kill the organism or destroy a cancer cell directly. These T-cells can call upon another kind of cells too, called *macrophages*. The word means 'big eaters', since they are able to engulf and destroy bacteria or malignancies, or they can help B-cells to produce more powerful antibodies. By acting as 'suppressors', they also protect your body against the possibility that your B-cells and other T-cells attack its own tissue, which is what happens in the case of the auto-immune diseases such as arthritis. So important to health is the thymus-mediated T-cell system that it is considered the brain of the immune response. If there is any imbalance between the different types of T-cells, or if there are too few of them, your immune system falters and you become susceptible to the auto-immune diseases, early ageing and sickness.

Lymph Magic

At any moment there are about a trillion lymphocytes in your body ready for action. They weigh a total of 2lb and they are constantly dying and being renewed at a rate of almost 10 million a minute. The B-lymphocytes, whose major task it is to produce antibodies – important weapons in the militia's armoury – are highly efficient. Every second they release trillions of antibody molecules into the bloodstream. Lymphocytes can monitor your body's internal environment and maintain its stable functions thanks to their ability to flow around the body in the bloodstream and to pass through capillary walls into the interstitial fluid, maintaining close contact with the tissue cells, and to their ability to pass along the lymph vessels which carry fluids throughout the body. Flowing within the lymph system, they pass through lymph nodes – lymph vessels with filters – which work together with the cells to wipe out many disease carriers. The lymph system and all of the hardworking lymphocytes it carries are vital to the health of the body and to resisting age-degeneration. It helps keep you clean and safe internally by detoxifying the body of all the chemicals, bacteria and other toxic products which can cause free radical damage, peroxidation and cross-linking. That is why a major focus of natural law age-retardation has always been to use diet, exercise and various natural treatments such as hydrotherapy to encourage lymphatic drainage and stimulate circulation.

Ageing and T-Cell Decline

To prevent ageing the body must not only ensure good lymphatic and B-cell functions. It must also keep T-cells in top condition so they can protect against bacteria, fungi, viruses, foreign cells and allergens and so they can help the body resist cancer and the auto-immune diseases. But as we get older the thymus gland tends to produce less and less thymosin – the hormone required for T-cells to function normally – and a decline in T-cells takes place. Defective T-cell function also occurs in most of the degenerative diseases such as rheumatoid arthritis, cancer, multiple sclerosis, diabetes mellitus and ulcerative colitis. Any loss of T- or B-cells indicates a decline in our immunological defence system and makes us increasingly vulnerable to degeneration and less capable of coping both with cancer and with destructive changes that occur in the vascular system.

A standard medical laboratory test – the T- & B-Cell Test – is used when organs are transplanted because physicians must artificially decrease T- & B-cell count just enough to keep the patient's body from rejecting the transplant but not so much that it would result in his death. The same test has now begun to be used as a means of determining how rapidly a normal person is ageing and as a means of indicating what kind of nutritional or hormonal treatment may be needed to slow any decline which has taken place.

There are a number of possibilities which science has so far investigated as means of slowing ageing and prolonging life by improving immune functions. Some researchers have discovered that (at least with cold-blooded animals) if animals are kept at a lower temperature than normal their immune functions are protected from decline and they live significantly longer than normal. Others have begun to use injections of the thymosin hormones to boost immunity in cancer patients, to increase people's resistance to stress, to improve brain functions, and to slow ageing. Animal experiments also show that putting mammals on a diet which is low in calories and protein yet provides a high degree of nutritional support from vitamins, minerals and other nutrients, can actually rejuvenate a flagging immune system and prolong life. (More about that in Chapter 10.) But perhaps the most relevant approach to improving immune status and cutting down on auto-immune responses so far developed centres around the use of relatively high doses of specific immune-supporting nutrients. And it is no accident that most of these nutrients, vitamins and minerals happen also to be anti-oxidants which offer protection against oxy-stress – free radical damage, peroxidation and cross-linking. For a close relationship between immunity and cross-linkage reactions has now been well established.

Nutrients Can Protect Immunity

T-cells contain a high concentration of ascorbic acid – vitamin C. In fact the concentration of this vitamin in the cells known as neutrophils and macrophages is 150 times greater than in your blood plasma. No wonder neutrophil activity is suppressed when vitamin C is deficient in the body. When these protector cells go to work killing infection – another oxidative reaction in the body – they mop up all the vitamin C available like miniature sponges. The vitamin therefore reduces damage from the neutrophil *oxidative burst*.

As we age our level of ascorbic acid drops progressively; so does our resistance to illness. And when illness strikes – say in the form of a virus or a bacterial infection – ascorbic-acid levels in T-cells quickly drop. The more severe the sickness the lower the drop. Smoking also causes T-cell ascorbic-acid levels to fall. But experiments with both animals and human beings indicate that large supplements of vitamin C will actually improve the ability of T-cells to protect the body both from the intensity and from the length of an illness. Even more important is what occurs when these supplements are given *before* illness strikes. Research shows that vitamin C helps protect the immune system from degeneration. Many of the B complex vitamins such as vitamin B1, B2, B3, B6, pantothenic acid, B12, and folic acid are also particularly important in maintaining a sturdy immune system and preventing age-degeneration. So is the element chromium. In animals, a folic acid deficiency decreases T-cell count by up to 80 per cent. In humans folic acid deficiencies are commonplace – particularly among women.

The vitamin E content of lymphocytes and neutrophils is 10 to 20 times that of red blood cells so it is little wonder that vitamin E has also been shown to enhance immune functions and improve resistance to disease and ageing. These benefits have now been demonstrated in over a hundred studies. And people with high levels of vitamin E get significantly fewer infections than those with average levels. Its main joy is to prevent lipid peroxidation – to protect the fat-based membranes and parts of the body from free radical damage. Vitamin E is the most important anti-oxidant within each of the body's 30 trillion cells. When animals are deficient in this vitamin the membranes of lymphocytes become damaged and immunity becomes depressed.

Research shows that adding vitamin E supplements to the diets of animals deficient in it will enhance immunity – and it also does this when given to animals who are not deficient in vitamin E. Vitamin E also helps protect against damage caused by the oxidative burst which takes place when macrophages and neutrophils attack invaders and cope with injuries. Much evidence now suggests that supplements of 800–1,600mg of vitamin E daily (800–1,600 IU (international units) of d-alpha tocopherol) during stress can greatly help protect the body from damage and degeneration. And vitamin E appears to be non-toxic in these amounts.

Beta-carotene also boosts immunity. Ever since the National Cancer Institute in the United States carried out large-scale trials demonstrating that beta-carotene prevents cancer, this nutrient has been making headlines. A precursor to vitamin A (that is, a substance which is turned into vitamin A in the body) beta-carotene has shown itself to be much more. Beta-carotene triggers the release of a chemical from the macrophages called *tumor necrosis factor*. As two powerful studies show, 30, 45 or 60mg of beta-carotene increase lymphocyte response and natural killer-cell responses to immune challenges in the diets of normal, healthy human beings.

The minerals zinc and selenium have also been shown to enhance immunity. Selenium works together with vitamin E as an anti-oxidant. It also contributes to an important anti-oxidant enzyme in the body called *phospholipid hydroperoxide glutathione peroxidase*. In animal studies selenium supplements added to the diet have been shown to increase immune strength by 400 per cent. Zinc deficiency has been shown to bring about a rapid decline in T-lymphocyte function. In a Belgian human study researchers discovered that using zinc to supplement the diet of people with normal zinc status and normal immunity significantly enhanced lymphocyte responses too.

Another very special nutrient, *coenzyme Q10* has also been shown in hundreds of studies to improve cell-mediated as well as humoral immunity.

The Role of Slow Viruses

In an effort to discover why, as we age, the immune system has increasing difficulty in distinguishing between self and non-self and tends to begin attacking the body's own protein, scientists have recently been investigating the possible role that a certain kind of virus – known as a slow virus – may play in ageing. Viruses are known to produce three kinds of clinical disease. Some, such as those involved in colds, for instance, appear to leave no permanent damage behind them. Others, such as the virus involved in poliomyelitis, are different. Although they cause rapid initial damage to the organism they also leave behind the damage when they are gone. A third group which appears to play an important role in degenerative diseases and ageing are the *slow viruses*. With incubation periods which can be measured in years, perhaps in decades, these virus infections appear to bring about slow, destructive changes over a long period of time. They are able to enter the body at one time but may not cause damage until years later. Slow viruses may be able to alter the genes in an organism although they don't inhibit the synthesis of RNA – the genetic messenger. They can live within cells for many years without destroying the cell although they can do damage to the cell's outer membrane and its organelles. Such damage can make the cell appear to the immune system to be 'non-self' so that cells are attacked by the immune system. Some viruses also appear to depress the immune system's ability to produce antibodies that will destroy other viruses. Many researchers now believe that the auto-immune diseases associated with age-degeneration are really the effect of slow viruses. It is an area which is currently being closely investigated.

The Psychology of Immunity

Another area of investigation which appears to be particularly important in finding ways of preventing immune-system decline and ageing centres around the influence that brain and behaviour have on immunity. The ability of the immune system to respond to foreign material or to attack depends upon thymus functioning, which in turn relies on impulses from a centre of the brain called the hypothalamus which triggers immune-system activity. The functioning of the hypothalamus is highly responsive to emotions and mental imagery and is highly stress-responsive. Grief, shock, fear and anger can all strongly suppress immune functions and encourage rapid age-decline. Positive emotions have been shown to have the exact opposite effect by enhancing immunity and making the body highly resistant to degeneration. We will look at this phenomenon more closely in Chapter 28 and also at some of the ways it can be used for ageless ageing. Meanwhile, let's investigate the area of age-research which appears to tie together both free radical biochemistry and immunity. Let's look at ageing in relation to stress.

Overleaf
The principal participants in the functioning of the immune system (see pages 42–51). At lower right are shown the results of the body responding or failing to respond to damage. At lower left the immune response is shown in more detail.

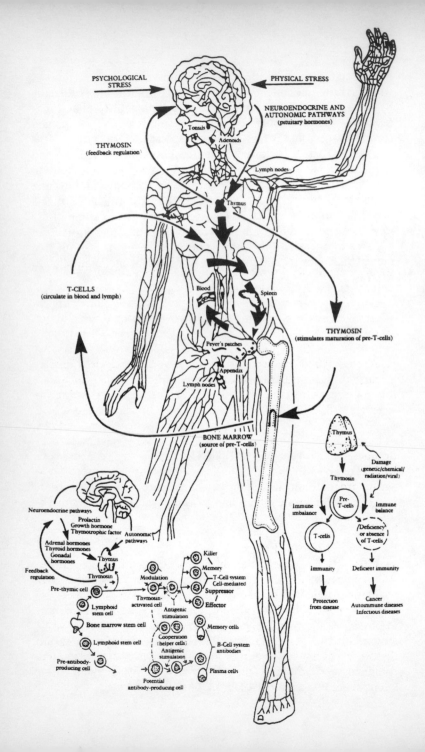

6
The Stress of Ageing

EVERYBODY KNOWS ABOUT stress. It is a word which is bandied about in the media – something we are all familiar with from long experience. Stress, the journalists tell us, is the kind of harassed feeling you get when you have too much to do in too little time or when some taxi-driver is rude to you or when you are grieved about the death of a close friend or the fate of your career. Or is it?

In truth, few concepts are as misunderstood as stress. Before we can even begin to create a lifestyle which works for ageless ageing, we need to clear up a few of the misunderstandings which surround the popular use of the word and to investigate what 'stress' in scientific terms really is and how it relates to ageing. For a real understanding of stress can not only draw together recent findings in free radical pathology and immune functions in relation to age-degeneration and how to prevent it, it is also the unifying principle which explains why, when the longstanding natural law approach to age-retardation and its high-tech counterpart are used together, you are able to create a lifestyle for ageless ageing which is as yet unequalled.

Einstein, Selye and Energy
In 1905, while exploring the characteristics of inanimate nature, Albert Einstein gave the world access to a vast reservoir of energy which until then had been unavailable for use. He developed the *theory of relativity*. In the beginning this theory was only of concern to physicists and mathematicians. Eventually it led to the use of atomic energy. But the practical significance of Einstein's scientific discovery was not realized until forty years later. Since then it has completely revolutionized the way we view reality. Einstein had a strong sense that without a belief in the inner harmony of the world

there could be no science. He also knew that the energy to which his theories gave man access could either be used for ill or good. And he struggled long and fiercely for peaceful applications of atomic energy.

What Einstein did for inanimate nature, another scientist of Austro-Hungarian origins, Hans Selye, has done for animate nature. In the late 1930s Selye developed his *theory of stress*. In it he revealed a central law of animate nature. He showed that living organisms have access to an enormous reservoir of vital energy – what he called *adaptive energy*. On learning to draw on it and using it wisely the biological future of each individual life depends. Like Einstein's theories, which at first were only of interest to the scientific community, Selye's stress concept was first only applied in highly technical ways by specific branches of science and medicine. In fact, only recently has it begun to be used in a practical way. Probably the most practical application of all is in the area of ageless ageing and longevity.

Another thing which Einstein and Selye had in common was an awareness of the unity implicit in both the animate and inanimate worlds and a belief that all energy must be used wisely and well if man is to live in a life-enhancing rather than a life-destroying way.

The two scientists never met. But when early articles about Selye's work began to appear in the scientific press, Einstein was one of the first to recognize their importance. He wrote a letter to Selye in which he suggested that a *unified theory of medicine* might be able to be created. That was Selye's dream too – a dream on which he worked eighteen hours a day for fifty years until his death in October of 1982. Now, thanks to scientists who are building upon Selye's original research, and a growing number of doctors who are searching for ways of putting it into practice, such a unified theory is becoming a reality. It is a theory in which new findings in free radical biochemistry, electrobiology, immunology and psycho-biology all come together – a theory which is of central importance to anyone interested in ageless ageing.

First Beginnings

Born in Vienna in 1907, Selye began his medical studies at the University of Prague in 1924. The following year he and his fellow students were shown a number of patients, all in the early stages of various infectious diseases. His professor then pointed out the specific characteristics of each disease. But what intrigued Selye was not so much the differences which were obvious between the various diseases but rather their similarities. Regardless of the specific illness from which a patient suffered, they all felt and looked sick: they had diffuse joint pains, intestinal disturbances, coated tongues and they showed a loss of appetite and weight. In Selye's words:

> The patients had a common syndrome, but the professor attached very little significance to the signs that were common to all these diseases because they were 'non-specific' and hence 'of no use' to the physician in making a correct diagnosis or prescribing the appropriate treatment.
>
> I began to wonder why patients suffering from the most diverse diseases have so many signs and symptoms in common. Whether a man suffers from severe loss of blood, an infectious disease or advanced cancer, he loses his appetite, his muscular strength and his ambition to accomplish anything; usually the patient also loses weight, and even his facial expression betrays that he is ill. What is the scientific basis of what I thought of at the time as the '*syndrome of just being sick*'? Could the mechanism of this syndrome be analysed by modern scientific techniques?

It was a question which plagued the young scientist for more than ten years. During that time he continued his medical education at the Universities of Paris and Rome, returned to Prague to take both a medical degree and a degree in chemistry there, and became a research fellow at Johns Hopkins University in the United States and then at McGill University in Montreal.

It was in his laboratory in the biochemistry department at McGill that all of his ideas began to come together. Trying to isolate a new hormone from the ovaries of cattle, Selye was testing ovarian extracts by injecting them into rats and then looking for evidence that the rats' organs showed unexpected changes which could not be attributable to any hormone already known. Much to his delight, he found that three important changes were taking place: (1) the rats' adrenal cortex became enlarged; (2) their thymus glands, spleens, lymph nodes and other lymphatic structures all shrank; (3) bleeding ulcers developed in their guts. At first Selye assumed that these changes were the reaction to a new hormone in the extract. But soon, working with other substances as well, he discovered that every toxic substance – whether from living tissue or not – which was injected into the rats would bring about the same three changes. His mind shot back to medical school and his notion of a *syndrome of just being sick* and he realized that with these toxic drugs and extracts he had just created an experimental replica of the sickness syndrome. This he described in a classic paper which appeared in *Nature* in 1936. It was called, 'A Syndrome Produced by Various Nocuous Agents'. Later it was renamed the *General Adaptation Syndrome* (GAS) or the universal biological stress syndrome. He began to investigate it in depth.

Three Stages of GAS

He found that an organism, including the human body, experiences the same non-specific reactions whenever it is *stressed* – that is, whenever it is faced with a challenge to its integrity. The challenge which Selye calls the *stressor* – can be a biological or chemical agent, such as bacteria or an environmental poison, excessive heat or cold, overwork or intense emotion, or physical injury or shock, to name just a few possibilities. Selye defined stress as *the non-specific response of the body to any demand made upon it*. All of these stressors trigger the GAS, the purpose of which is to maintain the structure and function of an organism in a steady state of *homeostasis* – the tendency of the body to maintain normal internal chemical and functional equilibrium – and by doing so, to preserve its life.

Working at first with animals, Selye discovered that the GAS occurs in three well-defined stages: *alarm*; *resistance* or *adaptation*; and *exhaustion*. The first stage – alarm – is the body's calling of its defensive forces to arms. During this stage the body's immune system is challenged, overall resistance is lowered, the sympathetic nervous system fires, brainwaves change, muscles prepare for action, circulation to the muscles increases and the adrenal glands secrete hormones. All of this is a kind of biological preparation to 'fight or flee'. The second stage – that of adaptation or resistance – follows close behind it, unless of course the noxious agent or stressor is so virulent that it destroys life. During the stage of adaptation many of the body's systems are stimulated into increased activity in order to meet the challenge presented and to protect the body from harm. In effect resistance is raised and symptoms which first appeared in the alarm stage often disappear. This second stage of the GAS can last for a long or a short time depending on individual make-up and on the intensity of the reaction to the stressor. But it cannot go on for ever. If the stressor or noxious element remains, sooner or later the third stage is reached – exhaustion. By the time the third stage of the GAS is reached, the body's adaptive qualities have become exhausted and its weakest systems start to break down. Chronic fatigue and illness are the hallmarks of the exhaustion stage. If they continue then eventually the body dies.

'The three stages', wrote Selye, 'are reminiscent of childhood (with its characteristic low resistance and excessive responses to any kind of stimulus), adulthood (during which the body has adapted to most commonly encountered agents and resistance is increased) and old age (characterized by loss of adaptability and eventual exhaustion).'

Is Adaptation Energy Finite?

This triphasic nature of the GAS gave Selye the notion that the body's adaptability or adaptation energy is finite. Experiments showed that when animals are exposed to cold, or intense physical effort, or haemorrhage and other stressors, they can withstand them only so long. After the first alarm reaction the organism starts to resist. How long it can continue before exhaustion sets in depends upon its innate adaptability and on the intensity of the stressor.

Neither Selye nor any of his colleagues could define exactly what this adaptation energy is which is lost, but they knew it was not merely caloric energy – for food intake is normal during the period of resistance. One would expect, so long as an organism is fed, that it would go on for ever. But it does not. Adaptation energy appears to be finite. As Selye says:

Our reserves of adaptation energy could be compared to an inherited fortune from which we can make withdrawals; but there is no proof that we can also make additional deposits. We can squander our adaptability recklessly, 'burning the candle at both ends', or we can learn to make this valuable resource last longer, by using it wisely and sparingly, only for things that are worthwhile and cause least distress.

So far nobody has yet discovered a way of synthesizing a 'fuel' for adaptation processes, although there are strong indications that nutrients such as amino acids, minerals and vitamins can be employed to restore flagging resources. But then when Einstein developed his theory there was no fuel for atomic stations either. The fuel was discovered only when a real demand appeared for making practical use of the great physicist's discoveries. There are already ways known of lending support to the body's adaptation energy. In Chapter 27 we will look at some of them which Russian scientists have been researching in recent years. There are certainly many ways of slowing down its energy expenditure – from eating a low-calorie-high-potency diet, learning to let go of unnecessary worries and tensions and strengthening the body through regular, vigorous exercise, to using anti-oxidant nutrients and free amino acids which can even alter your physical and mental response to many stressors. For – and this is one of the most important truths to come out of Selye's half century of work with stress – it is not the stressors which are dangerous to life, it is the way in which you respond to them. More about this later.

Selye believed that stores of adaptation energy cannot be replaced and, while we know now that there are certain substances that appear to strengthen adaptive energy (see Chapter 27), in principle he appears to have been right:

> . . . we have no objective proof that additional deposits of adaptation energy can be made beyond that inherited from our parents. Yet, everyone knows from personal experience that, after complete exhaustion by excessively stressful work during the day, a good night's sleep – and, after even more severe exhaustion a few weeks of restful holidays – can restore our resistance and adaptability very close to what it was before. I said 'very close to', because complete restoration is probably impossible, since every biological activity leaves some irreversible 'chemical scars' . . . I look upon the irreversible process of ageing as something very similar. The stage of exhaustion, after a temporary demand upon the body, is reversible, but the complete exhaustion of all the stores of deep adaptation energy is not; as these reserves are depleted senility, and finally, death ensue.

Work, Stress and Ageing
Selye recognized that a close relationship between work, stress and ageing exists. Ageing, he said, is *the result of the sum of all the stresses to which a person has been exposed during a lifetime.* It corresponds to the

stage of *exhaustion* of the GAS which is an accelerated version of normal ageing. Again in Selye's words; 'Each period of stress, especially if it results from frustrating, unsuccessful struggles, leaves some irreversible chemical scars which accumulate to constitute the signs of tissue ageing.' The biological wear and tear on the body is the result of stress and *the accumulation of the irreparable part of this attrition is ageing.*

This wear and tear manifests itself in biochemical terms as the accumulation of undesirable by-products of metabolism such as cross-linked proteins, the kind of ageing pigments which create brown spots on the surface of the skin and which clog the brain, heavy mineral deposits around arteries, joints, and in the crystalline lens of the eye. It shows itself in declining elasticity of connective tissue as a result of oxy-stress and free radical damage and in a loss of cells throughout the body. To prevent the wear and tear of ageing and to preserve precious adaptive energy therefore becomes the goal. It is a goal which in part is achieved by how well we adapt to the stressors to which we are subjected and in part by eliminating or rendering impotent as many unnecessary stressors as possible. Let's look at the first challenge first.

The Adaptive Response

Stress, Selye believed, is neither good nor bad. It is simply a fact of life. And, although stress has been linked not only to rapid ageing but also to many diseases such as ulcers, kidney disease, heart disease and arthritis, it is not stress which is the cause but our reaction to it, especially when the reaction is negative – that is, one of *dis-stress*. Selye always insisted that ' . . . stress is the spice of life. Being associated with all types of activity we could avoid it only by never doing anything. Who would enjoy a life of "no runs, no hits, no errors"? It is still not completely understood that *stress depends not upon what happens to an individual but upon the way he reacts.*' Illnesses such as emotional disturbances, stomach upsets, allergic reactions, rheumatoid arthritis, sinus problems and sleeplessness as well as circulatory disorders and heart and kidney diseases can all be triggered by what Selye calls 'faulty adaptation reactions.' The so-called stress-related illnesses are in fact not the direct result of any particular stressor but rather of these faulty reactions. And the reason why a particular stressor – say the death of a close relative – can cause quite different illnesses to develop in different people is due to each individual's inherited systemic weaknesses.

The Choice: Active or Passive?

The stereotype stress reaction of the organism to whatever demand is made on it can occur either in an active or a passive way. When you respond actively to a stressor, *catatoxic* hormones such as adrenaline are secreted into your blood. They trigger immune reactions and raise blood pressure. They cause blood sugar and fatty acid concentrations to rise, all of which mobilizes your organism 'to fight or to flee'. When on the other hand you respond passively, syntoxic hormones are secreted which are exactly the opposite in their biological effects. They tell your organism 'no struggle, no mortal enemy is facing you' and they reduce immune reactions.

The choice of responding to a specific stressor is made by one's consciousness. Selye says:

> Suppose you meet a helpless drunk who showers you with abuse but is quite unable to do you harm, nothing will happen if you ignore him, in other words if you choose the syntoxic reaction. But if you don't estimate the situation correctly, then your organism will make a catatoxic reaction and throw itself into a state of preparedness. Stress hormones will go to work at full capacity. The result may be a fatal brain haemorrhage or heart attack, even if the drunk didn't touch you. This would be nothing less than *biological suicide.* Death is caused by choosing the wrong reaction. On the other hand if the man who attacks you is a homicidal maniac with a gun in his hand and you respond passively you are likely to end up with a hole through your head. It is clear that, contrary to common opinion, *Nature does not always know what is best, both on a cellular and an interpersonal level, we do not always recognize what is and what is not worth fighting.*

One of Selye's favourite personal maxims used to be 'Fight for your highest attainable aim but never put up resistance in vain.'

When I first met Selye, at an international conference on stress in Monte Carlo, I was astounded by his vitality and his enthusiasm. I knew that six years before he had contracted a type of cancer called reticulosarcoma which is fatal in 99.5 per cent of cases. Yet he'd survived it. I was told also that only a few months before he had been given two artificial hips as well. Yet I have never seen a human being more alive. His eyes sparkled. When he spoke his voice was rich with emotional depth. His intellect was as sharp as any I have ever encountered and when he walked with his two canes he moved more rapidly than most people do on two good legs. In medical school Selye developed the habit of rising at 4 a.m. and working all day until 6 p.m. virtually without a break. It was a habit which continued throughout his life. He travelled the world lecturing, wrote, researched, and indefatigably pursued his interests. Yet he showed no signs of 'being under stress'. When I asked him why, his reply was simple. 'I love it. It isn't how much stress you are subjected to but how you respond to it. This determines whether it causes you to break down or brings you joy.'

The Individual Stress Response

Each person differs in his reaction to stressors. And what is a stressor to one may not be to another, although certain stressors such as burning or physical trauma affect everyone. We also differ in how much stress we can take before reaching the exhaustion stage. This depends both on how we have been conditioned to respond to difficulties and on the amount of adaptation energy we have been born with. One person will have a great deal – he may be on the move continually and is able to withstand a great deal of stress – while another, when faced with the same stressors, quickly reaches the GAS exhaustion stage. Selye himself had high tolerance to stress and adaptation reserves which were quite phenomenal – in no small part due to his passion for life and work. He used to say, 'If you are a racehorse you have to be a racehorse but if you are a turtle and you try to behave like a racehorse you are asking for trouble.' The point is that once adaptive energy is used up as a result of the wear and tear of stress it appears to be very difficult to restore it. This is exactly what happens as the body ages. To make use of Selye's findings for ageless ageing, each of us needs to become aware of our own stress patterns and optimum stress levels, remembering that it is as bad for a racehorse to be made to function as a turtle as it is for a turtle to be pushed into behaving like a racehorse. We also need to examine carefully how our adaptation energy is being used and if it is being used up unnecessarily, either by the way we are responding to emotional situations or by exposure to powerful stressors in our environment or our lifestyle which result in high levels of oxy-stress and damage to the body on a molecular level.

Free Radicals and the GAS

Recently, biochemists have begun to relate Selye's GAS specifically to oxy-stress. Research is beginning to show that this is probably the mechanism behind the development of both ecological illnesses such as food and chemical sensitivities as well as overall degeneration. So on a molecular level as well it appears that the 'rain barrel' concept of stress applies: each organism can only cope with so much free radical and peroxidation damage and cross-linking (from whatever cause or causes they may come) before its limit of adaptive energy is reached. At that point the rain barrel of stress spills over, causing biological destruction and rapid ageing.

In a very real sense, on the use of adaptation energy depends the ecology of the human body in the same way that on the use of natural resources and the protection of life depends the ecology of the earth. And the decision about how it is going to be used rests with each of us. As the highly respected Russian age-researcher I.S. Khorol has said:

... according to stress-conception 'adaptation energy' is the main source of creation. The only holder of this source is a man... no machine will be able to surpass man if he doesn't himself exhaust or destroy this source by careless treatment of his own nature. Einstein dreamed of creation of a unified theory of *inanimate* nature. Selye's investigations are aimed at the general laws of *animate* nature. But modern science has proved that there is no insuperable barrier between the two. We believe that some day these theories will be created. We believe that they will come together in a unified metatheory of the Universe, that will allow people to build our future quite reasonably and harmoniously.

7
Information Lost

DESPITE THE POWER of free radical theory and the new immunology, despite the fact that they have now been shown to provide a scientific basis for the treatment and prevention of the many causes of disability and death, they still have a couple of major drawbacks. First, they tend to be self-limiting. The understanding of the ageing process which they provide and the practical applications which they make possible are strictly contained within biochemical parameters. Yet, no matter how much some longevists would have us believe otherwise, life processes can by no means be fully explained according to biochemistry. Second, despite the new unified theory of ageing, many scientists working with a biochemical approach to ageing and to age retardation still have a strong tendency to be mechanistic and reductionist. They take an analytical and fragmented point of view – what I call the 'robot approach' to man. It treats the body as an obedient machine which adheres to all the laws of chemistry and physics, and they often neglect to consider the living system as a whole which is far greater than the sum of its parts.

Ignoring this reality can limit practical applications for ageless ageing to lists of anti-oxidant nutrients – both natural and artificial – which you swallow to cut down free radical and oxidative damage and special sunscreens which you smooth on your face to protect from ultraviolet rays, to the exclusion of wider issues. For when age researchers break living things down into their constituent parts, somewhere along the line life itself slips through their fingers – that which they are most concerned about preserving and enhancing. Too many approaches to ageing still don't show enough awareness of the fundamental role which lifestyle – how you eat, think, exercise, breathe and how you are oriented spiritually – plays in either slowing down or speeding up the processes of degeneration. And often because the high-tech approach to age-retardation has as yet found no explanation for many clinically tried and tested tools for increasing vitality, it tends to ignore them altogether. These include such practices as periodic spring-cleaning of the body, the use of *adaptogens* – substances which increase the body's ability as a whole to withstand stress and ward off exhaustion – and the vitality-enhancing properties of a low-calorie-high-potency diet based largely on fresh foods.

To get full benefit from what is now known about life processes and age-retardation we must make good use of the biochemical model of ageing but we also need to go beyond it. How? First, by asking a few provocative (and largely unanswerable) questions such as 'What is the nature of life energy anyway?' and 'How can we preserve it?' Second, we need to take a look at theoretical models now at the leading edge of science which can be applied to the ageing process. They include models built on information theory as applied to biology and on the new physics. These new scientific paradigms can be useful, not only in gaining a broader understanding of the ageing process, but also in devising a more comprehensive and effective approach to ageless ageing.

Laws to be Broken

The biochemical view of ageing which we have been looking at is based on the assumption that life can be explained through an understanding of the laws of chemistry and physics. It looks at the way in which inorganic chemicals are used in a biological system to perpetuate the living state. Indeed this is the whole point and purpose of biochemistry and molecular biology – the major scientific models involved in most theories of ageing. The only problem is that the living body breaks all the rules.

In physics, the laws of thermodynamics focus on energy changes. These laws are really an attempt to understand events in the universe by studying the kind of energy changes which accompany them. The second law of thermodynamics is particularly important for our purposes. It is called the *law of entropy* and states very simply that, left to their own devices, things become disordered: iron rusts, buildings crumble, dead flowers decay and so forth. This is stated scientifically by saying that everything tends towards *maximum* entropy – a state of maximum disorder in which all useful energy is decreased. But what is so remarkable about living organisms (and what has been a great puzzle to some of the world's finest scientific minds) is the fact that, despite the second law of thermodynamics, living organisms are able to remain highly ordered. Our bodies are maintained in a state of fantastic improbability despite the innumerable destructive processes continually going on in and around us. Indeed there is every indication that in many ways we are continually involved in creating even more order. This we do both individually in the repair functions of our cells and enzymic systems and from an evolutionary point of view since living creatures differentiate into ever more complex and highly structured organisms.

Order to the Highest Degree

In a way which no one has ever been able to explain fully, unlike things in the inorganic world, living organisms are superbly ordered to maintain their systems. This is something which makes virtually no sense within the paradigms of physics and chemistry. Where by rights there should be little difference in the chemical and physical processes taking place in a living body and those of a corpse – since both follow the same scientific laws – in reality there is every difference in the world. In life, events are able to maintain the system in quite exceptional harmony (in scientific terms a high degree of negative entropy) despite the fact that events leading to maximum entropy in the universe as a whole are running wild to destroy it. In the words of Nobel laureate Albert Szent-Györgyi who has spent most of his life trying to penetrate this mystery of life energy:

Life is a paradox . . . the most basic rule of inanimate nature is that it tends towards equilibrium which is at the maximum of entropy and the minimum of free energy. The main characteristic of life is that it tends to decrease its entropy. It also tends to increase its free energy. Maximum entropy means complete randomness, disorder. Life is made possible by order, structure, a pattern which is the opposite of entropy. This pattern is our chief possession, it was developed over billions of years. The main aim of our existence is its conservation and transmission. Life is a revolt against the statistical rules of physics. Death means that the revolt subsided and statistical laws resumed their sway.

Age = Maximum Entropy

Since ageing appears to be the process which transports our body from a highly ordered internal state towards maximum entropy, to protect our body from ageing we need quite simply (or perhaps not so simply) to give it all the help we can to maintain that order. This can't be done only by manipulating chemicals in the system, for that won't go far enough. To be effective and complete, any anti-ageing programme needs also to be holistic. It needs to take into account as many of the factors acting on an organism for good and ill as possible and to treat the living organism not as a machine but as a highly evolved and elaborate self-maintaining organic unity.

One of the first scientists to do this was physicist and Nobel laureate Erwin Schrödinger. He took a close look at the scientific contradictions implicit in the living state and concluded that so long as the human body is alive it avoids decaying into an inert state of equilibrium (death) through metabolism – by eating, drinking and assimilating information from the environment. As far back as 1944 Schrödinger wrote:

> Every process, event, happening – call it what you will; in a word, everything that is going on in Nature means an increase of the entropy of the part of the world where it is going on. Thus a living organism continually increases its entropy – or as you may say, produces positive entropy – and thus tends to approach the dangerous state of maximum entropy, which is death. It can only keep aloof from it, i.e. alive, by continually drawing from its environment negative entropy . . . What an organism feeds upon is negative entropy . . . which is in itself a measure of order. Thus the device by which an organism maintains itself stationary at a fairly high level of orderliness really consists in continually sucking orderliness from its environment.

The body is often described as an *open living system*. As such we are constantly processing *information* which comes to us not only through the kinds and combinations of foods we eat and the way we prepare and process them but also from the air we breathe, the ideas on which we allow our minds to play, the electromagnetic environment in which we live and so forth. In other words, we need a constant supply of the right quantity as well as the right kind of information from the outside world to keep our bodies functioning optimally. Schrödinger believed, as a long tradition of natural medicine both in Europe and the Orient has taught, that to maintain a high degree of vitality and to protect the body from degeneration, we need to 'suck order' from our environment.

Although a number of scientists have noted the importance of Schrödinger's concept of living organisms feeding on negative entropy, and it is mentioned in standard textbooks on biophysics and biochemistry such as Bray and White's *Kinetics and Thermodynamics in Biochemistry* and *Metabolic Pathways* by Pardee and Ingraham, it is still largely ignored by most nutritionists, biochemists and other researchers concerned with slowing down the rate at which we age. A few eminent scientists such as Ludwig von Bertalanffy, author of *Robots, Men and Minds*, British scientist and philosopher Michael Polanyi, and the Russian biochemist I.I. Brekhman at the Far East Scientific Centre of the Academy of Sciences of the CIS, Vladivostok, have, however, taken it very seriously indeed.

Information Loss and Degeneration

Brekhman refers to information in relation to his main interests, food and the adaptogens – natural medicines with a long history of use which scientific research has shown have non-specific abilities to strengthen an organism's vitality and even to prolong life. Until recently man's interaction with nature has been seen only in terms of the constant change of *materials* and *energy* – the one a measurement of chemistry and the other a measurement of physics. Now, thanks in part to the development of cybernetic concepts, some farsighted scientists such as von Bertalanffy and Brekhman are beginning to add *information* to these categories. 'But this is not', as Brekhman points out, 'the kind of information about the external world which is received by the sensory organs and the nervous system and termed *relative*, *free*, or *semantic information*. It is information reflecting the degree of diversity and complexity of internal structure inherent in physical bodies. It is called *absolute*, *connected* or more frequently, *structural information*. From this we can see that there is a constant exchange of substance, energy and information between man and the natural environment.' To retard the process of ageing and degeneration, then, both the quantity and quality of this information must be as close to the ideal needs of our organism as possible.

Such paradigms have a number of important implications when it comes to the nutritional control of ageing. They make it clear that slowing down the ageing process demands more than simply supplying megadoses of those vitamins, minerals and other natural substances which lend support to your body's anti-oxidant and immune systems. They imply that it is necessary to approach the whole question of food not only from the point of view of energy (calories) and materials (specific proteins, vitamins, minerals, fatty acids, etc). (If that were the case we would have nothing to worry about except the number of calories, how much carbohydrate, fat, etc we were consuming. But such an approach can never support a high level of well-being.) And they are stimulating some researchers to explore how nutrition for age-retardation is also dependent on the complexity of the way all of this energy and material is woven together by nature. For, as the eminent American biochemist Roger Williams has said, the body also extracts *trophic factors* from the molecular balances of the entire food. Now, not only do specific nutrients which can be measured chemically – vitamins, minerals, protein, etc – appear important for age-retardation, so does the complexity of the way they and other (as yet unidentified) factors are combined in a particular food. This contributes to the *quality* of energy in terms of the information which the food carries. Brekhman and others have shown that the heating and processing of foods which we carry out can decrease the quality of structural information which they bring to an organism and thus their health supporting and age-retarding properties. Fresh foods appear to contain a higher degree of the structural information which the body can beneficially use than do cooked or processed foods. So do a number of natural medicines such as ginseng and eleutherococcus which can be enormously helpful in any serious programme for ageless ageing (see Chapter 27).

In experiments Brekhman has shown that foods high in structural information enable animals to carry out physical tasks for significantly longer periods than processed foods low in structural information, even when the foods compared are equal in calories and therefore, by orthodox biochemical standards, supplying an organism with the same amount of energy. Brekhman and other Russian scientists are particularly interested in those natural pharmacological substances which appear to supply a high degree of structural information to an organism and therefore to help support a high level of health and energy. They are now attempting to quantify the action of a plant substance or food on the body in terms of what he has called *significant units of action* (SUA) which is a way of measuring how long an animal can continue to carry out a piece of work when fed a particular food. One of the implications of his work in human terms is that how well your nutritional habits support your system for ageless ageing depends not only on how many of the anti-oxidant nutrients and immune-enhancing nutrients you take in, but also on the ability which nature has to provide the right kind of structural information for high-level wellness in foods which are grown on healthy soils and have been little processed. This can never be gained artificially by measuring chemicals and swallowing pills alone.

Information Sources for Order

Of course food is not by any means the only kind of information which we take in and which is necessary to support the needs of the body for ageless ageing. We also need stimulation to the nervous system from changing environmental conditions, information taken in through the water we drink and the air we breathe, and even from the effects of body movement. All of these things act as stimuli to an organism. In terms of ageing their effects can be either good or bad. We need to make use of everything possible to ensure they are good. This is something which advocates of natural law anti-ageing have been doing for generations in two main ways. First, by applying stimuli to enhance bodily responses and increase vitality. It is on this principle that most of the natural methods of healing from Kneipp water therapy to aerobic exercise are based. Second, by examining the quality of information which is coming to a person in terms of the environment in which he lives. If it is the right kind of information, if the air you breathe is rich in the elements such as negative ion particles known to produce a sense of harmonious well-being in most people, then it is something which belongs in any holistic programme for ageless ageing. If it is not – if, instead, it is full of industrial pollutants, and depleted in negative ions – then the opposite is true and you need to take action either to change it or to protect yourself from the negative effects of the kind of information your body is being forced to process. As a medium for information-transfer to living systems, nothing at the moment is more interesting as a possibility (nor less explored by most age-researchers) than *electromagnetism*.

8
The Body Electric

LIFE, WE HAVE been taught, is simply a collection of biochemical processes. The human body is nothing more than a machine which runs on fuel from the foods you eat and the air you breathe. It is as simple as that. But is it? New developments in information theory and high-level physics as applied to biology are leading many scientists to question this assumption. Some quite fascinating research into the electric and electromagnetic properties of living tissue are beginning to create new paradigms for life processes – paradigms which, like the unified theory of ageing now developing from Selye's work, are so revolutionary they threaten to shake classic biochemistry at its foundations. The new scientific models indicate that life and health are not just a matter of chemistry. The chemical changes in a living system which have been so carefully charted, from the way in which your body burns glucose to make energy to how it repairs damaged tissue when you are cut or burnt, now appear to be not primary but *secondary* events – events which may be controlled by an electronic dimension of reality that until now science has almost completely ignored.

Where classic chemistry and high-technology medicine have tended to be mechanistic in their approach to health and healing and to ignore the enigmas of life, the new electronic view of reality (a view which is now well supported by burgeoning experimental evidence) embraces many of them. Not only will it have profound implications for healing, growth, ageing and consciousness in the next twenty years; it also brings in its wake a new vision of the nature of life itself and a new awareness of the potential dangers of twentieth-century electromagnetic technology to health and life.

The Body as Chemistry

Your body is a living organism which needs a vast amount of energy to carry out the chemical and physical work necessary to keep you alive. It gets this energy by oxidizing biological substances – burning food as fuel. This burning occurs not in some haphazard way as it would in a furnace. Instead it is ordered with superb precision: enzymes act as catalysts, and *oxidations* take place in a superbly modulated series of small steps which are able to liberate the maximum amount of energy present for effective use while causing the minimum amount of disturbance to the biological order of cells and tissues. In scientific terms oxidation is defined as the loss of electrons from the outer orbits of an atom or molecule. This electron loss can either occur singly – that is one electron at a time – or in pairs, and paired electron loss can either take place in one step where both electrons are transferred at the same time, or two steps, where one electron is transferred at a time and a free radical species (see page 29) is momentarily formed as a *transient intermediate*.

One of the major problems for science has always been to unravel the precise mechanisms by which living tissues control this release of energy and orchestrate the myriad complex adjustments necessary to keep an organism functioning with only very small changes in temperature and minimal disruption to the life processes which are going on in an organism at the time. It is really quite a feat when you consider that in all the cells of your body there is a continuous process of repair and maintenance in which the chemical components are disassembled and resynthesized, day in, day out, throughout your whole life. And thanks to the remarkable organization implicit in the living state, the entire architecture of your body's cells can be replaced without disturbing the normal activity, an example of superb order – negative entropy carried to the nth degree. How? These are questions for which the biochemist has no answer. They can describe the living machinery itself in terms of proteins, nucleic acids and nucleoproteins. And they can describe at length how electrons and nuclei form atoms, atoms molecules, amino acids peptides, peptides proteins and so on, but ask them to describe the nature of life's organization – the basic principle by which two things are put together to produce something new, a thing quite different from the qualities of its constituent parts – and they are at a loss for words. They can chart the enzyme functions and alterations which control the energetic transformations on a cellular level but there still remains a very important, and until now almost completely unanswerable, question: what controls the controllers? This too is a question biochemists have been unable to answer.

Life processes which cannot be explained within a particular scientific discipline have a long history either of being ignored or misinterpreted. Yet these unanswered questions are central to an understanding of the ageing process. For when control processes go awry, disorder invades the organism and degeneration ensues. They are also biology's most intriguing problems. And therefore problems which make many biochemists very uncomfortable indeed simply because they are unanswerable in biochemical terms. Where can one find the answers? Or at the very least, where should we be looking?

Electricity, Semiconduction and Living Cells

The eminent scientist, Albert Szent-Györgyi, who won a Nobel prize for his work on oxidation and for isolating vitamin C, asked himself this question more than fifty years ago. He has spent almost every working moment of his life since in an attempt to answer it. He is often quoted as having posed the question at a dinner party: 'What is the difference between a living rat and a dead one?' By rights, according to the laws of classic chemistry and physics, there should be no fundamental difference. Szent-Györgyi's own reply is simple yet revolutionary – 'Some kind of electricity.'

Szent-Györgyi observed more than a quarter of a century ago that the molecular structure of many parts of a living cell, rather like crystals, might be able to support semiconduction of electricity. It is a notion which, outside Russia where it has been vigorously researched ever since, has been largely ignored by orthodox scientists.

Semiconduction takes place only in materials which have a highly ordered molecular structure, such as in crystals, where atoms are arranged in neat geometrical lattices, enabling electrons to move with ease from the orbit of one atom or molecule to another. Szent-Györgyi postulated that molecules of protein in cells and tissues can boast this kind of molecular order, each offering a temporary 'hole' for mobile electrons, and that they may be linked together in long chains in the body in order that electrons can flow in a semiconducting current over great distances without any loss of energy taking place. This kind of protein semiconduction would enable energy to be passed along as *information* rather than being absorbed and stored in foods as chemical bonds – which is what takes place in the process of photosynthesis by which plants translate the sun's energy into the foods which we then eat and get energy from. In effect Szent-Györgyi is looking at a living organism not from a biochemical point of view (which is the point of view most age-researchers have exclusively taken) but from an electronic one.

In the past thirty years, thanks to the miracles of electron microscopes, researchers looking at living cells and tissues have discovered that structures of crystal-like organization and complexity do indeed exist in living organisms. Meanwhile the exponential leap in knowledge which has taken place within the realm of solid-state physics has brought about advances in electronics, such as the development of transistors used in computers (something that was believed before to be totally impossible), which make the notion of electronic processes based on solid-state properties of highly organized structures in living organisms very feasible indeed.

The *Élan Vital*

Of course Szent-Györgyi was not the first one to consider that living things might have electrical or electromagnetic properties. Mystics and healers have long insisted that the transmission of thought, and laying-on-of-hands healing, are possible thanks to some kind of ill-defined electronic or electromagnetic phenomenon. And in the eighteenth and nineteenth centuries electricity looked to many scientists like the miracle find which would revolutionize philosophy and healing.

Luigi Galvani, the famous Italian anatomy professor after whom the word 'galvanism' was coined, discovered as far back as 1794 that there is a 'current of injury' – an electrical charge generated at the site of damage in living organisms which is proportional to the severity of the wound. He tried to link electricity with the mysterious *élan vital* as the healing force – that enigmatic vital impulse of life which Bergson believed was the creative principle immanent in all organisms and responsible for evolution. Thirty years later in Pisa another Italian scientist, Carlo Matteucci, proved conclusively that this current of injury was real. He was able to measure it using the newly invented 'galvanometer'. But their findings and the findings of others experimenting with the relationship between electricity and living processes became enmeshed in a passionate philosophical debate between *mechanists* and *vitalists*, and were largely ignored.

The Mechanists vs. the Vitalists

It was a debate the outcome of which formed the basis of classic chemistry and physics as well as the drug-based approach to medicine which has become the hallmark of treatment in the twentieth century. It went something like this. The vitalists (many of whose notions stemmed from Plato's idea of supernatural 'forms') believed that what made all living things different from inanimate objects was the presence of a spirit which they named the 'anima' or *élan vital*. They divided reality into two parts: this vital force which they insisted was directional and purposeful, and the mechanical, physical world. This abstract universal principle was for the vitalists more real than sensory phenomena. They believed that the passive, inert and unmoving universe was driven to change only through the actions of this *élan vital* (which Galvani himself believed to be electricity). The mechanists (who sided more with Aristotle's rationalism) didn't agree. They viewed matter as passively driven by a mechanical force in a totally determined manner. They denied the existence of any *élan vital*, treating it as so much spiritual hokum, and insisted instead that truth was objective – something which resides in the world outside us and which can be analysed and understood empirically simply by carrying out scientific experiments that alter the world with mechanical forces and measure the results. Truth, they said, is a phenomenon which can only be understood when fully analysed in terms of mechanical laws based on Newtonian physics – the fundamental concepts of mass, energy, space and time. That, claimed the mechanists, is the purpose of science.

Well supported by the philosophical tenets of Descartes from the century before, by 1850 the mechanists had largely won the battle. Galvani's notion of electricity as an *élan vital* was banished to the scrap heap of curious but untenable scientific curiosities and the foundations of our modern biology, firmly based on chemical principles alone, were well set. They have ruled supreme ever since. Anyone who has dared to suggest that electromagnetic principles underlie life processes such as growth, healing, metabolism and regeneration – a notion which suggests a subtle yet pervasive connection between mind and matter – has tended either to be ignored or ostracized from the scientific community.

Electronic Controls of Life?

Nevertheless, even in the twentieth century – that last bastion of mechanistic thinking – there has been a number of researchers who have tried. In the 1920s a Russian-born engineer living in Paris, named Georges Lakhovsky, suggested that the basis of life may lie in 'immaterial vibrations'. He believed that the cells of plants and animals were oscillating circuits – electromagnetic radiators – able, as a wireless set is, to absorb and to emit waves. In 1925 he reported a series of remarkable experiments which supported his notion that health is a matter of equilibrium in cellular oscillation. About the same time an American professor at Texas State University showed in experiments carried out over a period of ten years that plant cells produce electrical emanations. E.J. Lund developed a way of measuring minute electrical potentials in plants and demonstrated that they emit electrical waves and currents. These emanations not only change as does the health of the plant, they appear to direct and regulate plant growth and health. For instance, he found that in the growth of a plant bud (which chemists said was merely directed by plant hormones or *auxins*), electromagnetic radiations from the plant altered *before* any changes in hormone levels could be detected. In 1936 an American scientist named George Crile, a surgeon who founded the Cleveland Clinic in Ohio, wrote a fascinating book called *The Phenomenon of Life*, in which he suggested that, since electrical changes taking place in the cells seem to occur prior to chemical and physical ones, by measuring them in a living organism it should be possible for radio diagnosticians to diagnose the presence of illness long before symptoms appear.

Life Fields

From the theories of Galvani, Crile, Lakhovsky and others about electronic and electromagnetic properties of living things, in the late Sixties two Yale professors, a philosopher named F.S.C. Northrop and a doctor specializing in anatomy, Harold Saxton Burr, suggested that, since living things have electronic properties, they must also be surrounded by electromagnetic fields. And these fields might be the source of organization for life systems. To explore their theories Burr began measuring what he called life fields or L-fields around seeds. He discovered, as he expected, that significant changes in voltage patterns occur even when a single gene in the parent stock is altered. He also found that by measuring the intensity of an L-field of a seed he could predict how healthy the plant grown from it would be and that these fields could easily be diminished by subjecting the seed or plant to chemicals or heat. But with the dominant scientific view that chemical processes were controllers of life – a view which blurs the distinction between living and non-living things greatly – most of Northrop and Burr's research has also been ignored. Contemporary scientific knowledge of how living things are put together and how electricity is generated and transmitted contained no mechanism that would allow electrical currents to flow in any organized manner through living things.

Currents of Healing

When Szent-Györgyi's now classic book, *Introduction to a Sub-molecular Biology,* came along with his idea of proteins as semi-conductors and his notion of 'solid-state mechanisms' (see page 72) as a way of accounting for specific electronic properties found in living systems, among the farsighted scientists whom it inspired was an outstanding American orthopaedic surgeon named Robert O. Becker. In the past twenty-five years Becker has done more than any other living scientist to explore this idea and pave the way for its acceptance. Like other scientists working in the field, Becker (who in 1978 was nominated for a Nobel prize) asked himself a couple of important questions. First, might electronic conduction mechanisms form the basis of control systems in living organisms? In other words, could they be the means by which life processes such as growth and the regeneration of healing take place? And second, if such systems do exist can they be influenced in a clinically useful way by applying appropriate electrical or electromagnetic energy from outside the body?

Electrical Bone Healing

Becker's personal interest and his field of expertise lay in using minute electrical currents to heal damaged tissue – particularly broken bones – in the body. By implanting tiny wires into broken bones and sending minuscule currents through them he has not only been able to speed healing but to restore normal functioning to patients whose broken bones simply would not join, despite their having been treated with conventional methods such as bone grafts – patients who therefore faced the prospect of losing a limb. Becker has become famous worldwide for his high success rate in treating such cases. Indeed, had his work been confined only to the clinical application of electricity for healing, many of his colleagues believe, the Nobel prize for medicine would have been his. It wasn't.

A Second Nervous System

Guided by Szent-Györgyi's vision, Becker postulated a primitive analogue-coded electronic information system in the body which was related to the body's nervous system but which was not necessarily located in the nerves themselves. He reasoned that this system, as Szent-Györgyi had suggested, might use semi-conducting direct currents and that, either by itself or linked to nerve impulses, it might be responsible for regulating growth, healing and other biochemical processes. He repeated some of Burr's experiments on salamanders measuring voltages at nose, tip of tail and other points along the body. But to his amazement he did not find, as Burr had, that there was a *simple* relationship of positive voltage at the tail and negative at the head. Instead he discovered the existence of an elaborate field which followed the order of the nervous system and gave him quite a complex series of readings. He then went on to study *electrical potentials* in other vertebrates and discovered that such a system does appear to exist – an organized crystal-like structure with self-organizing and self-repairing properties based on semi-conductivity. In Becker's words, 'We found that the potentials are organized into an electrical field, represented by lines of force, which roughly parallels the pattern of the nervous system ... Electrical potentials in a conducting medium such as the nerve cell implies there is also a direct current (DC) flow.'

Put simply, what Becker and his colleagues had uncovered was a 'second nervous system', a primitive data or information system, previously unknown to science – in the form of an organized pattern of electrical potentials which roughly parallels the gross anatomical arrangement of the central nervous system and which alters in a predictable fashion when an organism is damaged or repairing itself.

The healing process appears to be a kind of closed-loop negative-feedback cybernetic system in which DC currents linked to the body's nervous system via certain cells direct the healing process. When injury occurs to the body it causes cell damage. This changes the local electrical charge which stimulates DC system input, which on organization creates DC system output, which in turn stimulates cell growth and repair. As healing proceeds, cellular activity diminishes until finally healing ceases and local electrical patterns return to normal. This control system also appears to regulate growth and healing. It can be used to control pain (which is probably why acupuncture is a useful method of pain relief and anaesthesia). It may even explain how hypnosis, psychic phenomena and the directed migration of birds work. It is also rapidly eroding the widespread notion that all life processes must have a chemical basis, and it is introducing into biology notions of cybernetics – the science of communication processes and automatic control processes – and of solid-state physics which deals with electronic processes that occur in organized crystalline-like solids, just as Szent-Györgyi postulated they might in living tissue.

Electrical Mind/Body Links

Becker's findings have wide implications for health and healing. In the area of age-research alone a number of Russian scientists have reported being able to lengthen animal lifespans and to slow down physical degeneration by placing the animals within electrical fields of specific intensity. As yet, no one has begun to apply their work to human age-retardation. But it is sure to come. Meanwhile the discoveries of Becker and a few other scientists working in the same area have led to an increased interest in the potentials of electrical currents for healing, explained how electro-acupuncture gets many of its good results and opened up an awareness of the body as an open system of negative entropy which is not only gaining its organization from chemicals it takes in in foods, but appears also to be nourished by electronic or electromagnetic *information* – particular kinds of which appear to be necessary for high-level health and slowing down physical degeneration.

What is in many ways even more fascinating is the way that Becker and his colleagues have shown that this primitive electronic communications system which he has uncovered appears to be a central means of regulating states of consciousness as well. Sleep, anaesthesia and hypnosis all show common changes in electrical potentials in the brain. And you can bring about similar alterations of consciousness by applying appropriate electrical currents across the brain. This is the basis of electro-anaesthesia. Even more exciting, Becker has discovered that under hypnosis and in certain altered states of consciousness we have the ability to change DC potentials in the system ourselves. And since the same electrical system which regulates pain and healing can be brought under the control of the mind, it could be a powerful tool both for healing and age-retardation as well as for maintaining the body at high levels of health. This may also explain the phenomenon of 'miraculous cures' of illness by 'divine intervention' and much of psychic phenomena. But these new discoveries in electrobiology also have their dark side. And an awareness of these electromagnetic phenomena may be particularly important in protecting yourself from age degeneration.

The Earth's Electromagnetism

Something that is of real concern to Becker is the relationship between the body's solid-state data-transmission system and the kind of ever-changing fluctuations brought about not by the earth's electromagnetic field phenomenon to which we have been subjected throughout human evolution – but by the unnatural electromagnetic environment in which we in the industrialized world now live. Scientists looking at the circadian rhythms of the body and biological cycles of hormone secretions in living things have found that many are the result of rhythmic fluctuations in the earth's electromagnetic field. This field guides the migration of many animals. Alterations to its normal ebb and flow occur naturally as a result of storms on the sun that trigger magnetic storms on the earth. Indeed these things have been related to the occurrence of mental disturbances in many people. But, as Becker says, 'These kinds of natural changes in our electromagnetic environment are small compared with the kind of intense and chaotic electromagnetic phenomena we have created artificially from our twentieth-century lifestyle based on electric power and all that accompanies it. We are now being subjected to electronic pollution which, unless it is taken seriously and controlled, could do untold damage to human life.'

By 1990 incontrovertible evidence had established that there is indeed a direct connection between *non-thermal* electronic parameters – that is, electric or electromagnetic energy that does not produce heat – and living. At the California Institute of Technology, Dr J.L Kirschvink and colleagues recently identified magnetic particles in the human brain identical to those found in birds and other animals which receive electromagnetic impulses from the environment and respond to them via the central nervous system.

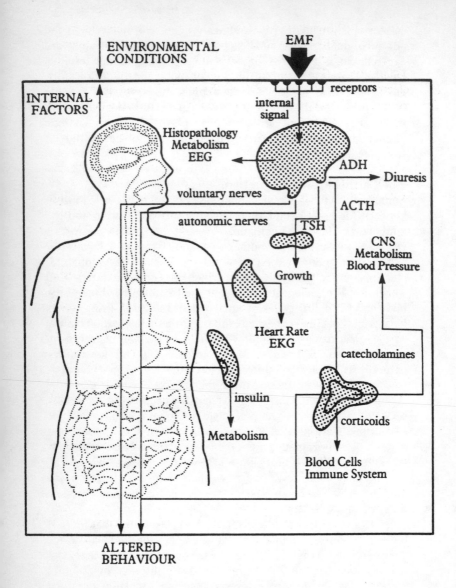

ENVIRONMENTAL
CONDITIONS

EMF

INTERNAL
FACTORS

receptors

internal
signal

Histopathology
Metabolism
EEG

ADH → Diuresis

voluntary nerves

ACTH

autonomic nerves

TSH

CNS
Metabolism
Blood Pressure

Growth

Heart Rate
EKG

catecholamines

insulin

Metabolism

corticoids

Blood Cells
Immune System

ALTERED
BEHAVIOUR

The effects of electromagnetic radiation on the body and brain as yet
go largely unrecognized by orthodox science except in Russia where,
as a health-protection measure, there are stringent controls on
electromagnetic pollution.

Previously Soviet scientists had been the only ones taking it seriously. In Russia there are legal limits governing environmental exposure to electrical power such as that which is emitted by high-voltage cables. Here and in the United States the notion that the electrical atmosphere in which we live affects life and health is not even given lip-service (except in defence departments where it has been investigated as a means of destructive warfare).

Becker in no way wants to eliminate electricity from modern life. But he insists that its environmental effects demand closer study. There have been far too many reports from farmers about inexplicable illness amongst animals and also from people who appear to be suffering the effects of living under high-tension electric pylons. There are even indications that sleeping under an electric blanket may contribute to the development of birth defects in unborn children.

In 1979 British physician F. Stephen Parry reported a statistically significant relationship between suicide and the proximity of patients' homes to electrical power lines. Similarly Dr Barry Wilson at Pacific Northwest Laboratory in the United States in a review of data discovered that depression can be a direct effect of the action of 50–60 Hz magnetic fields on pineal gland functions. Many other researchers have recently presented evidence that exposure to electrical fields can significantly alter body functions as can exposure to low intensity non-thermal microwave radiation. This has been shown in animals to alter important chemical receptors in the brain. A growing area of concern is the widespread use of cellular telephones which many electrobiologists believe could be highly dangerous long-term.

Here, in Becker's own words, are a few guidelines which we need to follow to protect ourselves from illness and degeneration:

- Don't use electric blankets on your bed.
- Don't use microwave ovens. The regulations governing their safety are not stringent enough to protect from leakage.
- Large-screen colour TVs produce strong fields not just in front but at the sides and behind. The bigger the set the stronger the field. These fields can go through walls into adjacent rooms. Always put the set against an *external wall.*
- Video display units on computers and word processors can cause reproductive disorders in women. As a result the state of Ontario in Canada has now adopted regulations for their use which include frequent breaks.

New Views of Healing

An awareness of Becker's findings is not sending us back to looking at reality through the eyes of nineteenth-century vitalism – which is as dualistic a view as the mechanism with which science has been living for the past hundred or more years. But the awareness *is* leading age-researchers and doctors to reject the view of living organisms as either mechanical systems animated by some mysterious *élan vital* or as machines which follow the biochemical laws based on Newtonian science. It is forcing us to revise our long-standing notions of cause and effect in health and disease in favour of an awareness of the body as a harmonious whole whose parts can only be understood through their interactions. Eventually, I believe, it is also going to force even eccentric longevists, committed to the notion that so long as you get your biochemistry right by swallowing massive doses of anti-oxidant nutrients you can dissipate your energies as much as you like and still expect to live for ever, to change their tune. The long-standing methods of life-enhancement and rejuvenation which have come out of the European tradition of natural healing now, more than ever, have an important role to play in making ageless ageing a living reality. Coupled with new discoveries in free radical biochemistry, stress concepts and immunity, they should create a bastion against age-related degeneration which nothing else can even come near.

PART TWO

ELIXIRS OF LIFE

9

The Two Faces of Ageing

JOHAN BJORKSTEN, WHO developed the cross-linking theory of ageing, is probably the most famous age-researcher in the West. What is remarkable about Bjorksten's work – apart from his profound understanding of the ageing process on a cellular level and his ability to construct lucid mathematical proofs of both his own and other scientists' various theories – is the fact that Bjorksten has an integrated understanding of the ageing process, on a molecular level as well as in the body as a whole. It is an understanding which may well be unequalled by anyone else in the world, and an understanding which takes into account the important role that mind and spirit play as well. Bjorksten is also a pragmatist. Instead of getting lost in a mass of biochemical data as some researchers are prone to do, Bjorksten enters his laboratory, as he has done for the last half-century, with one major intention: to find out what works and then to put it into practice. Bjorksten points out that there are really two faces to ageing and each face needs to be approached in a slightly different way.

Bjorksten believes that our *maximum* lifespan is 157 years. He bases this figure on what he has found to be the highest reliably documented age for a man. This then, he says, is the first target for anyone interested in ageless ageing – to reach that age in tolerably good health. If we are not reaching this age it is because we are ageing *prematurely*. Premature ageing is the first face of ageing. Ways and means of counteracting it are available right now to anyone who wants to take the trouble to use them.

The next target is to deal with the second face of ageing: to develop and make use of techniques which will extend lifespan far beyond what now appears to be the human maximum limit – to, say, 200 years or even more. The strategies for wrestling with each face of ageing are quite different. Dealing with ageing's second face means developing ways of removing insoluble accumulations which have come as a result of chemical reactions in the body – for instance dissolving cross-linked proteins. It also means enhancing the speed of repair mechanisms for DNA as well, so that single-strand damage can be restored before mutated cells reproduce. The development of enzymes which are safe to use in the living body and which are capable of removing the broad spectrum of age-related accumulations has been a major goal for Bjorksten – a goal which has often been frustrated by a scarcity of funds for research. He has experimented with chelating (binding) agents and low-molecular-weight enzymes made by certain strains of bacteria such as *Bacillus cerus* - a bacterium present in soil. He has even used free *hydroxyl* radicals as a means of breaking up very dense aggregates which enzymes cannot penetrate. As yet it is too early for us to be able safely to make use of most of these techniques. This second face of ageing still hides too many of its secrets beneath its surface. But with a little effort we can go a long way towards smoothing out the wrinkles from ageing's first face right now.

Magnificent Redundancy

As Bjorksten points out, if an engineer wants to design a factory for trouble-free operation he builds into the system duplicates of all the essential equipment so that a spare will be at hand the moment anything malfunctions. This is known as *redundancy*. As human beings we have been designed the same way – two hands and feet and eyes and kidneys. Our brain is a superb example of redundancy with its 12 billion cells and innumerable pathways which enable us to recall a memory. Brain surgeons are continually amazed by the brain's powers of substitution when part of it has been damaged. Our metabolism too is built upon the principle of redundancy. Every biochemical process necessary for life has several possible paths, all of which work, but often in very different ways. For instance there are at least five pathways for breaking down carbohydrates for energy, and your body can make lecithin in at least three ways.

In order to protect your body from premature ageing and to promote long life, the reactions involved in its metabolic pathways need to be *efficient* and *clean*. They need to take place precisely, with as few by-products and as few hold-ups along the way as possible. When biochemical processes become sluggish, then toxic intermediate products which are formed in excess can build up to a point where they cause damage. Formaldehyde is a perfect example of such an intermediate. It is formed in at least eight normal metabolic reactions. There are two means of avoiding this dangerous build-up. The first comes under the auspices of *natural law* anti-ageing. It consists quite simply of not eating more than your body's chemical processing plant can deal with cleanly and quickly and not taking into your body foods or chemicals which, in effect, can throw monkey-wrenches into the system. (More about what this means in specific terms in the next few chapters.) This in itself will take you a long way towards experiencing a youthful old age and looking good as the years go by. But, insists Bjorksten, ' . . . it is not enough. The bottlenecks in the metabolic pathways must be widened to the largest extent possible to prevent hold-ups and secure smooth passage, even for occasional excess loads, and to maximize safety margins and redundancy.' That is the task of *high-tech* anti-ageing. By bottlenecks, Bjorksten is referring to the enzymes which make biochemical conversions possible.

Precious Catalysts

Enzymes are the essential triggers for the metabolic machinery of every living thing, from daffodil to buffalo. They are complex organic substances which set off chemical transformations of materials – catalysts which bring about chemical changes but are not themselves changed in the process. Without the thousands of enzymes in each living thing there would be no life at all. Enzymes are extraordinarily powerful. For instance, at body temperature, a small amount of pepsin (one of the gastric enzymes we use to digest protein) will break down the white of an egg into small-chain peptides within just a few minutes. The same process can be accomplished in a laboratory only by boiling the egg white for twenty-four hours in a strong acid or alkali solution. The human body has a complex collection of enzymes, each of which has a specific task to perform; and in a healthy body these enzymes are constantly being renewed. In the liver alone there are some 50,000 different enzymes at work, on which your body's life and functions depend. They break down fats, proteins and carbohydrates into their constituent parts, which can then be assimilated into the bloodstream and carried throughout to the cells. So essential is the existence of the thousands of enzymes in our body that when there is a slowing down in the production of them in the digestive system or poor replication of them in the cells, health suffers and the body ages rapidly.

James Batcheller Sumner, who shared a Nobel prize in 1946 for crystallizing the first enzyme, insisted that the 'fortyish' look with its sagging skin, fat around the middle and lack of vitality was attributable to an enzyme shortage that occurs when the body is not efficiently replacing enzymes in its cells. Many highly respected age-researchers now agree with him. They say that an organism grows old when enough metabolic errors accumulate to injure the synthesis of certain enzymes. For instance, the enzymes directly involved in digestion, such as those of the pancreas, seem to play a vital role in preventing age-degeneration and disease. A sufficient supply of pancreatic enzymes appears to be a crucial factor in maintaining immunity to many degenerative diseases, including cancer.

The Fallacy of the Recommended Dose

Enzymes depend for their actions on vitamins and minerals which are essential as activators for them. In order for enzymes to be able to carry out reactions with the precision and cleanliness necessary to protect against premature ageing, the supply of vitamins and minerals in your body must be optimal. It is not enough simply to see that you get the minimum required to avoid overt symptoms of vitamin deficiency.

All vitamins and minerals have multiple actions in the body. This is one of the major reasons they differ dramatically from drugs which are aimed at dealing with specific symptoms. For instance, nicotinic acid – vitamin B3 – is a component of at least fifty-four enzymes, and pyridoxine – vitamin B6 – of almost as many, including those most important for protein metabolism and for making brain chemicals. Nobel laureate Albert Szent-Györgyi (who was honoured for his isolation of vitamin C) says this about the problem of the mechanism of action of vitamins in the body:

I could illuminate this relation by comparing vitamins with lubricants, while comparing your own body with your car. *It is wrong to look upon a vitamin as a substance which just combats specific symptoms. Like a lubricant, the vitamin makes the normal working of your body possible* [my italics]. If there is not enough vitamin the working will be disturbed, leading to all sorts of damages which may accumulate and declare themselves in an early senescence and ill health. In your car, insufficient lubricant will declare itself in the wearing out of pistons and cylinders, with the result that after 40,000 miles your car will run as if it had done 80,000, and you will look at forty as if you were over sixty.

Pick up most books on diet or nutrition and they will give you the official line about 'recommended dosages' of vitamins and minerals necessary, they say, for health. In the case of most nutrients the amounts suggested by such tables are grossly inadequate if your body is to be protected against age-degeneration. These figures have usually been arrived at by slowly decreasing the supply of a specific nutrient in an animal's diet until he shows signs of severe symptoms of some kind. Then, the amount of a vitamin or mineral needed to banish these symptoms is taken to be the 'recommended dose'. What such a practice ignores is the fact that any organism leaches its reserves of a specific nutrient from as much as can be spared in all the enzymic pathways in which this vitamin takes part, causing vital metabolic processes to be reduced. As Bjorksten says:

> Thus all these other processes suffer a drastic reduction of their respective reserves and safety margins. These are reduced to the point where the ability of the body to stand up to overloads in these is sacrificed. Therefore, for maximum longevity in good health, one of the prime requisites is a constantly maintained *optimal* supply of all vitamins . . . Other requirements are: adequate supply of the needed trace elements, but even more important the exclusion of the deleterious elements.

Premature Factors in Ageing

One scientist who has long concerned himself with discovering the ranges of optimal doses of nutrients for protecting the body from degeneration is the late Carl Pfeiffer of Princeton's Brain Bio Center in the United States. Pfeiffer has also looked closely at many of the deleterious elements to which Bjorksten refers, such as the presence of heavy metals like lead and aluminium in the body. Pfeiffer speaks about both when he lists what he considers to be the *premature factors in old age.* And while Pfeiffer's 'premature' factors are by no means exclusive, they give a good idea of what Bjorksten is talking about and are excellent guidelines for what to avoid if you are not to age prematurely.

1. Heavy Metal Intoxication

This is one of the worst factors in premature ageing in industrialized societies where we are continually exposed to lead, mercury, aluminium, cadmium, asbestos, sulphates and phosphates. Even copper – one of the micronutrients necessary in minute quantities for health – acts as a heavy metal when it is present in too great a concentration in the body. Industrial pollutants released into the atmosphere produce acid rains which put aluminium into our drinking water by dissolving it out of clay in the earth. Lead enters our body from industrial emanations, from petrol fumes and when we drink water in houses which have been plumbed with lead pipes. Phosphate, which is a constituent of fizzy soft drinks, couples with white flour, which is very low in usable minerals, to leach calcium from our bones. Silver enters the body from using silver cutlery for eating. Copper in excess can enter the body by drinking water – especially soft water – which comes in copper pipes. It can also build up in the brain if you are deficient in zinc, or from taking 'multiple vitamins and minerals' which include copper but exclude zinc. Both copper in excess and lead can cause hyperactivity in children. Excess copper can make normal people into insomniacs or encourage the development of arthritis as well as of high blood pressure.

Heavy metals are potent cross-linkers. They can also inactivate enzymic functions. And they are poisonous to the body. Bjorksten has looked particularly closely at aluminium, one of the most powerful cross-linkers for proteins, and probably for DNA and RNA – the cell's genetic materials – as well, since these nucleic acids contain several sites to which it can bind. Aluminium appears able to inactivate the sensitive end organs of neurons, disturb intracellular transport of nutrients and to block genetic molecules. It has been found in high concentration in the brains of stroke victims. Yet it is still commonly believed that cooking with aluminium pots and pans, in which acidic foods – such as tomatoes – can dissolve this metal into the foods we eat, is not dangerous. Most so-called authorities still believe that aluminium is not absorbed through the intestines. The avoidance of heavy metal intoxication and the detoxification of any that may be present is an absolute necessity for ageless ageing.

2. Lack of Essential Trace Elements and Vitamins

Vitamins A, E, D and C are amongst those Pfeiffer lists as good candidates for preventing premature ageing and enhancing longevity. Trace elements which Pfeiffer lists amongst those which may provide longevity include sulphur, selenium, magnesium, calcium, potassium, zinc, manganese, molybdenum and iodine. He adds that we need riboflavin (B2) to prevent cataracts, pyridoxine (B6) to prevent arteriosclerosis, chromium for the glucose-tolerance factor to prevent diabetes, and B12 to prevent anaemia and confusion. And we will be looking later at the anti-oxidant nutrients which protect the body from free radical damage and cross-linking. Used as nutritional supplements these nutrients can be enormously helpful in retarding age-degeneration. But never on their own. Thanks to the way the human organism has evolved through hundreds of generations, the *rule of synergy* always applies.

No single nutrient can do anything for age-retardation. As biochemist Michael Colgan says, 'It is the multiple interaction of nutrients, not their single actions, which are the basis of their biological functions. This principle has been only recently emphasized in nutritional science, although top scientists have known it for years.' In the same way that Bjorksten insists we need optimal quantities of nutrients for the smooth running of metabolic pathways, this rule of synergy demands that your body be supplied with all of the more than fifty substances necessary for health and life. Because of the complexity of interlinking metabolic pathways, if even one nutrient is missing you are undermining your chances for vitality, longevity and health. This means we need to eat a wide variety of top-quality little-processed foods, a large portion of them fresh. For most of us in industrialized countries, where fresh foods organically grown on healthy soils are not readily available, it probably also means making use of nutritional supplements.

3. Loss of Calcium from Bones

The loss of calcium from bones, known as osteoporosis, is a common occurrence after the age of thirty; so are low levels of calcium in the body. They used to be considered a 'normal' occurrence in ageing by some scientists. In fact they are the result of such factors as inadequate nutrition, the build-up of aluminium and lead in the bones and brain which replace the calcium that should be there, a diet too high in protein, or just plain inactivity.

Calcium is the most abundant mineral in your body. About 99

per cent of it is deposited in your bones and teeth and the rest is in the soft tissues, circulation and extracellular fluid. Even a moderate calcium deficiency can lead to cramps, joint pains, palpitation, tooth decay, insomnia, impaired tissue repair and excessive irritability of nerves and muscles. It can also slow your blood-clotting and lead to the formation of brittle and porous bones which break easily. Calcium loss is something which must be prevented. You need adequate calcium for ageless ageing. How do you get it? First of all, like the long-lived Hunzas, Vilcabamba Indians and Georgians you get plenty of exercise. Regular physical exercise mineralizes bones and makes you able to make proper use of minerals and trace elements you take in in your foods. You also need to ensure you get adequate zinc, magnesium, calcium and manganese in your diet, which together with optimal amounts of vitamin C can not only keep calcium and other minerals in good supply, but can also offer protection against aluminium and lead. And you need to avoid eating excess protein. As Pfeiffer says, 'Diets high in protein lead to increased urinary calcium excretion. Average calcium loss with such diets can amount to 30 per cent of the calcium intake. The affluent American is apt to eat a high protein diet and many obese individuals use a protein diet to lose weight *and calcium and bone.*' The best mineral supplements are either *chelated* – that is linked to proteins for good absorption – or *orotates*. Ordinary or 'elemental' mineral supplements are much less well absorbed by the body. As with all nutritional supplements, care is needed, since mineral calcium salts can, if taken without adequate magnesium, promote stone formation.

4. Loss of Vital Hormones

A number of important hormones decline with age. They include the sex hormones testosterone and oestrogen, thyroid, insulin and thymosin, which is related to immune functioning. Taking steps to stop this decline when it is occurring can effectively slow down the rate at which you are ageing. It can even help rejuvenate your body. Pfeiffer relates how in 1980 when the use of thyroid substance was introduced, ' . . . this proved to be a miracle anti-ageing drug. The patients' heavy facial wrinkles disappeared, dimwittedness turned to laughter, hearts speeded up and body-swelling gave way to firm muscle and energy.' Of course this kind of improvement only occurs in people who are iodine or thyroid-deficient. And as Pfeiffer says, for some people, ' . . . even the iodine of kelp or seafood is enough to restart the synthesis of the thyroid hormone'. So important are the minute quantities of trace elements we need for protection from age-degeneration.

Most hormones are made from amino acids – the building blocks of protein – in the presence of certain vitamins and minerals. As people get older the ability of their digestive systems to break down the proteins from the foods they eat into their constituent amino acids, from which hormones and enzymes and collagen and other body proteins can be built, often declines. Sometimes this decline is the result of inadequate hydrochloric acid in the stomach or pancreatic enzymes in the gut. It can also frequently be corrected by nutritional supplements. Inadequate production of vital hormones may also be due to lack of specific trace minerals – for instance iodine in the case of thyroid hormone, and chromium which is necessary for insulin. Many of the most famous of the natural anti-ageing treatments, such as cell therapy, owe a great deal of their effectiveness to the way in which they appear to reactivate hormone production.

These are the major areas of premature ageing, according to Pfeiffer: premature degeneration can be the result of lack of vitamins or essential minerals, lack of exercise and of mental stimulation, lack of hormones or contamination by heavy metals. Together they share a couple of important things in common. First, all of them are preventable provided we become aware of what is happening and take steps to stop it from happening. Second, either directly or indirectly all of them cause the problems of metabolic bottlenecks of which Bjorksten speaks, and highlight the necessity of preventing them. Your body must be provided with optimal quantities of vitamins and minerals to do this.

The Orthomolecular Approach

Twice Nobel laureate Linus Pauling, and many other eminent scientists, have been saying the same thing for years, often to the distress of less informed nutritionists and doctors who still believe vitamins and minerals are only substances necessary in minute quantities to protect the body from gross nutritional diseases such as scurvy and beriberi. Pauling coined the word *orthomolecular* to describe the treatment and the prevention of disease by providing an individual organism with optimal quantities of specific vitamins, minerals and other nutrients in order that its metabolic processes take place smoothly and cleanly in the way Bjorksten insists that they must if we are to prevent premature ageing. Orthomolecular means molecularly straight or correct. The orthomolecular approach to ageless ageing is aimed at providing the optimum molecular environment – specially the optimum concentrations of substances normally present in the human body. So far removed from this goal are the typical lists of 'recommended doses' of nutrients and the kind of common medical advice that you should eat a 'well-balanced diet' (which usually means the 'meat-two-veg' routine), that they can be considered virtually useless in any programme for ageless ageing. When it comes to devising a serious programme for preventing premature degeneration, only an ortho-molecular approach will do.

Le Compte's Amazing Law

One physician for whom this approach forms the basis of all his work is the Belgian ageing expert Herman Le Compte. Le Compte is the Robin Hood of age-retardation. For years in his clinic in Belgium he has been treating the wealthy and mighty and teaching them the skills of age-retardation as well as the poor and needy and charging for his treatment in direct proportion to a client's ability to pay. As a result of some forty years as a clinician, during which time he was studying the ageing process and working to slow it down in himself and his patients, Le Compte came to formulate a law which is undoubtedly the most important guideline currently used to understand premature ageing and how to prevent it. It is called simply *the first law of Le Compte* and it goes like this: *Ageing proceeds more rapidly where the deficiencies are greater and more numerous.* We'll take a closer look at the implications of Le Compte's law in a moment. But the story of Le Compte's discovery of it is too good to pass up.

The African Connection

When Le Compte finished his medical studies, the prospect of starting up a practice in Belgium – what everyone expected of him – somehow didn't appeal to his adventurous spirit. So he and his young wife decided instead to go to West Africa where, after a short period as an assistant to a large hospital and after a few months of running a leper centre, he was sent to take charge of a brand-new hospital which served 50,000 patients and had 300 ward beds. Within a month of its opening he was treating up to 300 outpatients a day as well as paying house calls on others in remote villages.

Working eighteen hours a day, seven days a week, Le Compte had no help except three European nurses and a dozen Congolese who were hard workers but who could neither read nor write. His operating room had neither electric lights nor running water and he had to carry out even major surgery under local anaesthetics, for medical supplies were scarce. In three years he performed more than 3,000 operations, supervised some 2,500 births and dealt with sicknesses ranging from malaria to blackwater fever. And, despite the fact that he had no x-ray machinery, no cardiac monitors, no resuscitation equipment, and no laboratory, in all that time he only lost two of his surgery cases.

Drugs were as scarce as the proverbial hen's teeth and limited to local anaesthetics and penicillin. But the one thing Le Compte was never short of was vitamins. Because doctors in Europe used very little of the vitamins which were provided for them and because their surplus medical supplies were collected every few months by Boy Scouts who sent off unwanted medication to the 'poor Africans', Le Compte's storerooms were piled high with them – hundreds and thousands of bottles and jars and boxes of every kind of vitamin imaginable. 'Vitamins were considered useless,' says Le Compte, 'so they were all given away. Since I had nothing else I started to administer massive doses of all types of vitamins to my patients. I would keep a patient in hospital for a few weeks before a major operation to give him a chance to rest and gather his strength. During this time he would receive mega-multi-vitamin injections. Then, as now, my methods were empirical. I had little to guide me but my diagnostic instincts.'

His results were amazing. The recovery rate of patients treated before surgery in this way showed Le Compte that something quite extraordinary happened to the human body when you provided it with very large quantities of these natural substances – substances which he had been taught in medical school were only useful for preventing a few diseases of malnutrition. Not only that, on megadoses patients' resistance to illness and to degeneration after surgery was very high indeed. One rule Le Compte went by as director of the hospital was that he never refused an aged patient. In fact more than half of his surgery was performed on old people who, because of their poverty, had been refused help at hospitals in other regions and countries – the Portuguese Congo and the French Congo, mostly.

Le Compte noticed from his contact with these people that not all

Africans aged equally quickly. By means of sociological investigations he discovered that the difference in the rate of ageing had little to do with hygiene, housing, clothing or infections. It rested instead on how people were fed. The poor Africans were always badly nourished. They aged most rapidly. Those who were better fed aged more slowly.

Slow and Fast Agers

After three years of backbreaking work, leaving home before dawn each day and returning home late at night too exhausted to do anything but collapse into bed, Le Compte himself suffered a major heart attack at the age of twenty-eight. For three months he lay in bed unable to move. Then he was sent back to Europe where he faced a long period of recuperation. Fascinated by his discoveries in the Congo and by the process of ageing itself, he used his convalescent time to research intensively everything that he could get his hands on related to ageing and degeneration. It was then that he developed the simple but profound maxim which bears his name: *Ageing proceeds most rapidly where the deficiencies are greatest and most numerous.*

As with many fundamental scientific laws, it may appear so simple as to be self-evident and yet it is an essential foundation for any ageless-ageing programme. As a result of this basic statement, many important research projects have been started all over the world. Bjorksten himself has even published a detailed mathematical proof of Le Compte's first law. A close corollary to this law – one particularly important for ageless ageing – is this: *Ageing is maximally retarded where a maximum of potentially limiting strictures in the metabolic processes are widened.*

Oiling the Valves

Probably the most accurate way of analysing human metabolism is by viewing it as a network of interconnected pipelines where the maintenance of the necessary minimum flow in many critical areas depends on multiple interconnected valves and structures. In biochemical terms these valves or structures are enzyme-catalysed processes where the amount of processing depends largely on the availability of enzymes at appropriate multiple points. And this in turn depends mostly on how available are the materials for synthesizing the enzymes – vitamins, minerals and essential acids. Again in Bjorksten's words, 'Such a high level of the metabolic enzymes is maintained by a correspondingly high level of all the relevant vitamins, essential trace elements, and anything else that could become a limiting factor of any vital step in the normal metabolism.' In practical terms what this means is that, as Pauling and other scientists who advocate an orthomolecular approach to health and age retardation insist, if you want to prevent the premature ageing (which is so common in our society as to have become the 'norm') then you need to begin now to provide your body with *optimal* amounts of all the nutrients it needs for carrying out its myriad metabolic processes smoothly, cleanly and without bottlenecks. That is quite a challenge. For most of us, meeting it involves not only improving our diet but also eating less, taking nutritional supplements and even ensuring that we get enough exercise to see that we prevent loss of essential nutrients. Let's begin by looking at the kind of changes in eating habits which can lead you closer to this orthomolecular state which forms the foundation of ageless ageing.

10
Eat Less and Live More

'MAN LIVES ON one quarter of what he eats. On the other three quarters his doctor lives.' This observation carved permanently into an Egyptian pyramid more than 5,000 years ago should be chiselled into the brain of anybody serious about ageless ageing. Eat less and you will live longer is the simplest yet the most potent piece of advice you can follow. In 1973 E. D. Schienker, heading a research team at Michigan State University, published the results of an interesting investigation of a group of ninety-seven women, middle-aged and older, whose histories he had followed since 1948. Originally, each woman had provided the research team with a list of foods and quantities eaten during one day as well as a health and nutritional history. At that time all these women were rated in good, fair or poor health following the qualitative index of ageing set out by the *American Journal of Public Health*. In 1972, those still living were again examined. Researchers found that women who looked younger than their years ate fewer calories. Also, fewer of their calories came from fats and they managed to consume substantially more vitamins B1, A and C than their older-looking counterparts.

Not only is avoiding obesity a major means of preparing for a good-looking and healthy old age, the avoidance of excessive food intake is important because, as you may remember from Chapter 4, eating more than your body actually needs is a major cause of oxy-stress to your system – free radical damage and cross-linking. When animals are underfed yet provided with optimum quantities of all the essential nutrients in their diet they not only live longer, they tend to remain free of chronic infections and degenerative diseases including cancer, arteriosclerosis and arthritis. Cut your calories but increase the quality of the foods you eat and you will dramatically *decelerate* the rate at which you are ageing.

Calorie Restriction for Life Extension

Back in the Thirties a researcher called Clive McCay at Cornell University carried out a series of experiments in which he severely restricted calories in rats but supplied them with vitamin and mineral supplements from the time of weaning. He discovered that these animals lived as much as two times as long as a control group which were allowed to eat as much as they wanted. Not only that, their longer lives were far healthier.

McCay fed his experimental rats every day, starting from weaning, 60 per cent of the calorie intake of his control group. He then supplemented their diet with enough vitamins and minerals to make up for the 40 per cent deficit of these nutrients. By day 1,000 of the experiment, all of the normally fed rats were dead – yet most of the underfed animals were not only alive and well, they were sexually active and showed little sign of ageing or degeneration. McCay's work was later validated by other investigators in a number of laboratories. Morris Ross at the Institute for Cancer Research in Philadelphia, for instance, was able to extend the maximum lifespan of rats by 50–60 per cent using similar methods. In human terms this would correspond to our being able to live around 170 years. Meanwhile other researchers found they could also extend an animal's lifespan by 'intermittent fasting' – fasting them every second day, every third day or every fourth day. This method brought about a 20–30 per cent extension to an animal's life. And, as with McCay's calorie-restricted animals, not only was their lifespan increased, the rate at which they aged was slowed. This was determined by what are known as *biomarkers of ageing*.

The All-Important Biomarkers

Biomarkers are measurements designed to determine how old an animal or a human being is, not chronologically, but functionally and biochemically. You can have a chronological age of seventy-five yet your skin may be as smooth as someone twenty years younger, your heart and lungs may have the fitness of someone much younger and your immune system may work as well as a sixty-year-old's. In this case your *biomarkers* would indicate that you are much younger physiologically than your chronological age implies. Biomarkers include the degree of skin dryness, the greying of hair, level of blood cholesterol, patterns of liver enzymes, the incidence and the time of onset of cataracts and so forth. When researchers have tested calorie-restricted animals they have found that by all known biomarkers they are significantly younger than their chrono-logical age indicates they should be. These animals are also highly resistant to degenerative diseases including cancer, heart disease and kidney disease. For instance, in one study where 50 per cent of the well-fed group of mice developed cancer a mere 13 per cent of the calorie-controlled group did, while in another carried out on rats in Australia these figures were 64 per cent and 15 per cent respectively. Similar results were shown with other diseases as well.

Such findings caused a great stir amongst those concerned with age-retardation. Yet for quite a while they seemed to have little relevance in retarding human ageing. For calorie-restriction from weaning is hardly something we can carry out acceptably on our children. First of all, a small percentage of these calorie-restricted animals die very early and no one could take such a risk with a human baby. Second, there is always the chance that calorie-restriction might cause some kind of brain damage in a developing child. So McCay's findings and those of other researchers working in the same way were relegated to that place on the bookshelves of science which holds the curiosities of laboratory research. Then, a dynamic American age-researcher at the UCLA (University of California at Los Angeles) Medical School began to play about with calorie-restricted diets and to design his own laboratory experiments which were variations on the McCay theme. His name is Roy Walford. He is a hardheaded sceptical research scientist of the highest order with an all-encompassing fascination with finding means not only of halting premature ageing but of increasing *maximum lifespan*.

A Workable Alternative

Walford reasoned that if you could start to restrict calories not from weaning but from middle age – all the while replacing any nutrients lost with supplements – then perhaps you could avoid the undesirable 'side-effects' of trying to do it from birth but still extend life. Trouble is, nobody had yet been able to do this by adult-initiated caloric restriction. The reason why, Walford reasoned, might be that they had made the changeover from normal diet to restricted one too rapidly. Together with his colleague Richard Weindruch he decided to try it more gradually. It worked. Walford and Weindruch were not only able to retard the ageing rate of these animals and to lengthen their maximum lifespan, they were even able to bring about some degree of immunological rejuvenation.

This particularly intrigued Walford because, as you may remember from Chapter 5, immune response is a major biomarker of ageing. He says:

> One good biomarker test measures the response of critical agents of the immune system – white blood cells or lymphocytes – to a substance called phyto-hemagglutinin (PHA for short). PHA causes a lymphocyte to produce fresh DNA (the hereditary gene material in each cell) and divide into two new cells. The ability to respond to PHA declines with age. Dr Weindruch and I found that the lymphocytes of 16-month-old mice, who had been restricted since 12 months of age, responded to PHA at the same level as 6–8-month-old mice. (Natural lifespan in mice is 2 to 3 years, so 12 months is well into young adulthood.) Evidentially, the rejuvenation does not involve *all* bodily systems, since the maximum lifespan of mice restricted as above is extended by only about 20 per cent. But the results – displaying actual rejuvenation of at least one parameter of ageing – are encouraging.

In fact, Walford is being very modest about his findings, which are almost revolutionary in a world where orthodox science has for fifty years insisted that rejuvenation of any kind is little more than a pipe-dream.

In common with animals whose diet had been restricted from weaning, Walford and Weindruch's mice also showed significant resistance to illness and degeneration. About 50 per cent of his fully fed mice developed cancer while only 13 per cent of the restricted mice did. The incidence of kidney disease, vascular disease and heart disease at 800 days old amongst the fully fed group was 100 per cent, 63 per cent and 96 per cent respectively while in their leaner counterparts the figures were a mere 25, 10 and 26 per cent. Also the restricted animals did not develop increased blood cholesterol as they got older. Their fat cells remained significantly more responsive to hormones (a decrease in responsiveness to hormones also tends to occur with age) and the auto-antibodies which are believed to be an underlying cause of senile dementia were greatly reduced. The findings of these two scientists have by now been well substantiated by other researchers such as those working at the Gerontology Research Center in Baltimore.

It is now generally accepted that their findings can be translated into human applications and that there is a high degree of probability that, started in adulthood, such dietary restrictions will bring the same benefits to people. For, as we have seen, ageing, like growth and development, is a *general* process, one of the most general of all biological phenomena. And biologists usually agree that such general processes are fundamentally the same within all mammals. They know that such a general anti-ageing tool as caloric restriction which works on mice and rats is likely to work for humans too. The prospects offered by such findings are very exciting indeed to anyone concerned about initiating an ageless-ageing lifestyle. For what Weindruch and Walford uncovered was a method of age-retardation, life extension and prevention of degeneration which was not only effective but safe, simple and available to any with enough initiative and motivation to put it into practice.

Undernutrition without Malnutrition

Walford is quick to point out that his methods have nothing to do with going on slimming diets. Far from it. Neither are they some kind of crankiness, as they might seem to uninformed scientist and layman alike. They are based on well-established and accepted scientific facts. Also, undernutrition is not malnutrition. It is a way of nourishing your body on fewer calories yet ensuring you get a full supply of essential vitamins, minerals, fatty acids and so forth. What this means in practical terms is that as human beings we need *gradually* to restrict our calorie intake to about 60 per cent of what we would eat if, like his mice, we let ourselves eat as much as we wanted – about 1,800 calories a day for the average man and 1,300 for the average woman. And this caloric restriction should be achieved gradually over a period of five to seven years. Walford believes that you can also get the same results using intermittent fasting – in other words fasting on water for two days of the week – which would increase your daily restricted intake of calories on the other days to 2,520 for men and 1,820 for women. Slowly, such a restriction will lead to a 20–25 per cent reduction in your body weight. And there's good news for people who have all their lives fought the battle of the bulge because of a lowered metabolic rate which prevents them from eating as much as their thin cousins can without gaining weight. According to Walford these kind of people practising undernutrition without malnutrition may be able to live longer still, for their decreased metabolic rate and the lower body temperature characteristic of their body type are two factors which can increase lifespan.

Supremely Nourishing Foods

It is only possible to achieve 'undernutrition without malnutrition' by choosing your foods very carefully (more about that in the next chapter) and by eliminating all of the overprocessed, nutritionally 'empty' foods which make up the greater part of most people's menus – from white sugar and white flour to margarines containing hydrogenated oils, soft drinks and potato crisps. Walford suggests a way of eating in which people in midlife – between thirty and fifty – get only 10–15 per cent of their calories in *fats* (the average Briton or American now takes in some 40 per cent or more of his calories in fats), 20 to 25 per cent of their calories in the form of *protein* and the remainder in *complex carbohydrates* such as grains, pulses, fruits and vegetables. Such a low-calorie-high-potency regime will need to be rich in fresh vegetables, preferably eaten raw to preserve as many of their nutrients as possible; and it is easier to achieve by combining grains, pulses, vegetables and fruits for your proteins rather than eating meat. Most meat contains too much fat and all meat is low in fibre. *High fibre* is another important characteristic of any ageless-ageing way of eating. It not only helps safeguard you against excess cholesterol formation, diverticulitis and cancer of the bowel, it also helps your body detoxify itself of many toxic substances which you take in from your environment and which are powerful free radical formers and cross-linkers.

The final essential ingredient in this new approach to age-retardation is a good supply of extra nutrients from supplements of vitamins and minerals, essential fatty acids and possibly amino acids. Particularly important are the anti-oxidant nutrients, vitamins C and E, the mineral selenium and the sulphur amino acids cysteine and methionine (see Chapter 19 for guidelines) because they act as free radical scavengers. (Walford refers to free radicals as 'great white sharks in the biochemical sea' because of their ability to do untold damage on a cellular level.) But the other vitamins and minerals are important also. For, as we saw in the last chapter, all essential nutrients are synergistic – they work together – and, because of the complexity of the web of metabolic pathways in our bodies, a nutrient without all its related nutrients is of no use against age-degeneration. Computer analyses of attempts to establish wholefood diets without taking nutritional supplements point up common deficiencies. In descending order they are: zinc, vitamin E, copper, magnesium, iron, niacin, vitamin B12, pantothenic acid, calcium, riboflavin, folic acid, vitamin A, vitamin B6, thiamine and vitamin C. But a number of studies show that four of these nutrients are commonly deficient in the average Western diet – vitamin C, vitamin A, calcium and iron, while zinc, chromium, manganese and potassium follow close behind.

Putting it into Practice

Walford advises anyone interested in pursuing this new dietary approach to age-retardation to begin by going through a health check-up with their doctor and having as many tests of biomarker functions taken as are available. They can include measurement of blood pressure, blood cholesterol and triglycerides, treadmill tests for heart function, a glucose-tolerance test to detect blood-sugar disorders, and tests for lung and kidney functions. One of the simplest of all medical tests – a lung function test known as the *forced pulmonary expiratory volume* – is one of the best human biomarkers of all for indicating physiological, as opposed to chronological, age. It measures the amount of air you are able to expel in a specific length of time (usually a second) and gives a good indication of both the elastic recoil of your lungs and the integrity of your breathing passages. Having these checks done at the beginning of such a change in nutritional habits will do two things. First it will ensure that you are in good health and let your doctor know what you are planning. Second it will give you some hard data against which you will be able to measure your progress. People who have already begun to follow this kind of nutritional lifestyle (Walford among them) report that these biomarkers usually begin altering for the better very rapidly.

What's It Like?

To most people the idea of restricting the number of calories they consume and leaving the sticky buns and chocolate out of their lives seems like some kind of terrible deprivation – an action which can only be carried out by a gargantuan effort of the will. In fact this is only the view of someone who has not yet experienced the enormous rewards that come with dietary temperance. My greatest health-fault has always been a tendency to eat far too much because I am such a hedonist by nature and because I learned early on from my grandmother (who raised me as a very young child) that if anything went wrong or you felt tired or tense or confused, FOOD was the answer. Happily, since for many years the foods I have overindulged in have been top quality, I have suffered no serious health consequences yet. But since I have begun my own form of high-potency-low-calorie eating I can honestly say that the rewards far outweigh what at the beginning I thought would be the sacrifices. I not only look better, feel better and have more energy than ever, I actually enjoy food more than I ever have before. The dishes I prepare have become beautifully light symphonies of colour and texture and taste. Like periodic fasting (see Chapter 15), such a way of eating keeps your mind clear and your senses heightened. It has enabled me to get greater enjoyment out of almost everything I do.

There are other bonuses in store from such a lifestyle too. Animal studies show that it should markedly increase your resistance to infection. Arthritic changes in the spine, the greying of hair and many of the other age signs should also be significantly delayed. Animals on such a regime are more active and more energetic. They also retain sexual interest and energy long after their fully fed brothers have fallen by the wayside. Let the last word on the subject be left to Walford himself: 'Appropriate dietary restriction will give you better vision, hearing, mental function, an improved sense of physical well-being, retained sexuality, and increased disease resistance in relation to your chronological or birthday age.' Here he quotes the Greek poet Hesiod who, some 2,700 years ago, wrote:

Fools not to know that half exceeds the whole, how blest the sparing meal and temperate bowl.

11
The Seedbed of Ageing

NOT ONLY IS the quantity of food you eat a central factor in how rapidly you age, so is its quality – and I am not only talking about how many vitamins it contains. Even ten years ago such a statement might have been considered crankish. Food was simply fuel for the body and so long as you got what was considered the right quantity of calories, protein, and fats, plus a few vitamins, that was all you needed to worry about. Food was believed to have little to do with health unless, like the starving Africans, you didn't get enough of it.

Now we know differently. Almost daily reports appear in the scientific literature and the popular press linking processed fats with arteriosclerosis or stressing the importance of fresh vegetables and fruits and fibre in the avoidance of stroke and cancer. The medical profession and the general public are keenly aware that there are many things wrong with the average British or American diet. We know now that most of us should eat less fat and meat and sugar, less white flour and coffee. We are also told that we would be healthier if we got more fibre and ate more pulses and whole grains, even if we don't always understand why. But what few people are yet aware of (probably because much of the research has been done in Europe and published in languages other than English) is that the state and *quality* of the foods you eat is one of the most important issues in determining how well you remain and how rapidly you age. The state of our foods is determined by such considerations as freshness, the condition and health of the soil on which they have been grown and both whether and how they have been cooked or processed.

Nurturing the Cells
Food is more than just nutrients. The state and quality of what you

eat also determines the health of your capillaries and the condition of the *mesenchyme* – connective tissue, blood and blood system and the smooth muscles through which nutrients *and* oxygen must pass to nurture cells, glands and organs. This microscopic tissue element – the mesenchyme – carries the 'nutritional stream' to all parts of your body. The Swiss expert in the use of nutrition for healing and for retarding degeneration, Max Bircher-Benner, always referred to it as *vegetatives Betriebsstück* – the *seedbed*. Giving it this name is an excellent way of understanding its importance. For the mesenchyme is very much like a seedbed – a medium in which your organs and glands, like flowers, have to live. And any gardener will tell you how important it is to the health and beauty of flowers that the seedbed is not allowed to deteriorate. When it does they fade, wither and sicken. If the seedbed of the body is right, if it facilitates an easy passage of oxygen and nutrients and the rapid elimination of cellular wastes, then your cells' metabolic processes are carried out as they should be: *efficiently* and *cleanly*. Then you also get a high degree of protection from oxy-stress, free radical damage and cross-linking. If not, then the foods you eat – no matter how delicious or how much vitamin this or that they may contain – can slowly and persistently increase the rate at which you age.

What's Missing in Modern Nutrition?

Like much of modern science, most nutrition tends to be highly reductionist. Reductionism, you may remember from Chapter 7, is the world view which asserts that an effective understanding of any complex system can be gained by investigating the properties of its isolated parts. That is exactly the mistake made not only by nutritionists and food scientists themselves but also by most of the food industry as well. It is a mistake by which our health suffers greatly. The science of nutrition is based on the notion that the function of a vitamin or mineral or protein is encapsulated in its chemical structure. It assumes that man needs certain quantities of these nutrients as well as some protein, fat, carbohydrate and so forth in order to avoid gross nutritional deficiencies such as beriberi, pellagra and scurvy, and it doesn't concern itself greatly with how he gets them. But it gives little thought to the importance of the complexity of how they are combined in natural fresh foods.

In truth, the function of a vitamin or protein or any other nutrient can only be expressed by the interaction of this nutrient with its biochemical and physiological milieu. And unless you are reasonably knowledgeable about this milieu, its function cannot be understood. The body's biochemical milieu, like fresh foods grown on healthy soils, is highly complex. It includes vitamins, minerals and other accessory factors and there is much evidence that a shortage or an excess of one vitamin interferes with utilization of another. Once you begin to split off a nutrient from the milieu in which it occurs, even if later you combine it again with all of the known factors with which it was originally linked, you greatly reduce its health-promoting potential. (This is a mistake many pill-popping longevists make when they assume they can eat anything they like so long as they take massive quantities of anti-oxidant nutrients.)

Structural Information for Ageless Ageing

As Russian biochemist I.I. Brekhman would say, we significantly alter the *structural information* which comes to us from the natural foods to which our bodies have become accustomed through our evolution. Brekhman and his colleague M.G. Kublanov have studied this issue at length, examining scores of natural and artificial chemicals and foods from the point of view of the structural information for high-level health which they contain. He says:

> Foods and drugs can be regarded as factors of chemical regulation of homeostasis. Since any regulation in the organism is an informative process the molecules of bio-logically active substances are chemical transmitters of information. Besides specific informative substances such as DNA, pheromones, endorphins, neurohormones, any com-pounds of complex composition and molecular structure can be 'informatively active'.

Brekhman has shown that drugs or highly processed foods which are relatively simple, both in their chemical structure and in the low level of structural information they impart to the organism using them, have little to offer either in terms of strengthening the organism's adaptive energy or in contributing to homeostasis. But vegetables, fruits – particularly when they are eaten fresh and raw – whole grains, pulses and so forth are complex natural compounds which carry a high degree of biological information necessary for wellness to the living organism. And, as you may also remember from Chapter 7, this kind of biological information appears to be very important if we are to maintain the high degree of order or negative entropy necessary to resist ageing and degeneration.

Yet this is something of which most nutritionists and food technologists are still ignorant. Over 70 per cent of the foods we eat in Europe and North America continue to be factory processed. Modern food technology still disassembles the molecules of wheat or oats or corn and oil-bearing seeds and then modifies them in inventive ways to make our ready-in-a-minute meals and packaged and frozen products. Manufacturers also routinely add almost 200 chemicals to bolster the texture, taste, and appearance of foods engineered from modified starches, proteins, carbohydrates and fats, and there are several thousand more chemicals close at hand which can be thrown in for special purposes.

The American biochemist Roger Williams expresses our need for structural information in the maintenance of a high degree of negative entropy slightly differently when he says that the body extracts *trophic factors* from the molecular balances of the entire food for high-level health. We have great need of the trophic factors in natural fresh foods – the quality of structural information they contain. For only *it* can provide the right kind of seedbed for our cells and organs to make ageless ageing a reality. Even many of the positive effects of high-tech anti-ageing tools such as supplements of the anti-oxidant nutrients or free amino acids, which we will be looking at in Chapter 19, can be wasted if this internal milieu – through which they must pass to do their work – at a molecular level does not facilitate this happening.

The European Experience
To my knowledge most of the study of what kind of diet can do this comes out of Austria, Germany, Switzerland and Scandinavia. This is probably why the topic is so little understood in English-speaking countries like Britain and the United States. In continental Europe there is a long tradition of healing and age-retardation using natural foods – a high proportion of them uncooked. European scientists have also carried out elaborate clinical and laboratory studies to determine how, on a cellular level, fresh foods are able to work wonders for the health of human beings. Their clinical experience and their laboratory findings can contribute greatly to natural law anti-ageing. And as we will see, many of their findings – things about how raw foods increase the microelectrical potentials of cells

and so forth – are directly relevant to the growing awareness of the body as a *negentropic* open system and probably also of the role that electromagnetic phenomena appear to play in growth, health and regeneration.

The tradition of using natural foods for healing is a long and interesting one involving the use of simple, often organically grown foods. Healthy soil is needed to impart the right kind of biological information for health to the plants grown on it. Many of these foods are used in their uncooked state for the treatment of serious chronic illness from cancer and arthritis to high blood pressure, arteriosclerosis, migraine and diabetes. In the finest European clinics for natural healing, a diet of such foods is combined with exercise, good stress management and simple treatments with air, water and sunlight. They are used to treat emotional disturbances, resistant obesity and addictions as well as chronic illnesses. The story of how the tradition developed, its phenomenal successes and how it is now being used is a fascinating one but far too long to tell here. My daughter Susannah and I have explored it in some depth in another book, *Raw Energy*. (The book also contains a number of recipes and nutritional guidelines.) But there are a couple of aspects of it which are particularly important to ageless ageing.

Rah Rah Raw

The foods which European physicians at those clinics commonly use to perform what to the uninformed can seem like miracle transformations in their patients are nothing special. They are the common-or-garden foods we see in our greengrocers and whole-food emporiums: fresh vegetables and fruits of all sorts, whole grains such as wheat and brown rice, and barley and oats, pulses and beans such as lentils, split peas, beans, and so forth. Those that are cooked are cooked simply but deliciously. The proportion of cooked to uncooked foods in a person's diet which these physicians employ while treating a patient is proportional to the seriousness of the illness being treated. The more serious it is, the greater proportion of the foods will be raw. An all-raw diet is used to treat cancer, to induce safe and easy rapid weight loss, to treat diabetes and so forth. Then, as the patient improves, the physician gradually reduces the quantity of uncooked foods – fruits and vegetables, seeds and nuts and flaked grains, plus yoghurt, perhaps, or cheese – to somewhere between 50 and 75 per cent. Once a high level of well-being is restored to the patient then he is encouraged to maintain himself permanently on a diet in which at least 50 per cent of the foods eaten are raw. Such a way of eating is the most powerful tool for natural law anti-ageing you will find anywhere. It helps create a seedbed of the highest order as well as improving the efficiency with which your cells use oxygen. It also strengthens cell walls and improves cell metabolism. And it protects your body from a build-up of the toxic wastes we have been looking at which can cause the molecular damage of ageing.

Why a High-Raw Diet for Ageless Ageing?
The first, most obvious, reason is that fresh uncooked foods are higher in almost all of the anti-oxidant nutrients important in protecting your body from oxy-stress as well as in the other accessory nutrients which make it possible for them to do their work. It is well-established scientific fact that storing, heating and processing destroy vitamins and cause mineral loss. And as Walford insists, if we are to make use of calorie-reduced eating as a tool for ageless ageing, we need as much nutritional value from our foods as possible. But this only scratches the surface of the high-raw phenomenon.

What has recently come to light is the fact that cooking not only destroys nutrients. Four kinds of damage to amino acids can occur as a result of heating and processing protein foods:

- Under high heat some food proteins can become resistant to digestion so that the availability of all amino acids is reduced.
- Lysine is lost when you heat proteins especially in the presence of reducing sugars – as in the pasteurization of milk.
- When protein is exposed to treatment with alkali as it is in many food-manufacturing processes then lysine and cysteine (one of the natural anti-oxidant nutrients) residues can be eliminated and toxic products such as lysinolalanine are formed.
- When oxidizing chemicals such as sodium dioxide are used in food processing considerable methionine from the protein is lost. Methionine is one of the natural anti-oxidant aminos of which it is important to get plenty as a protection against cross-linkage and peroxidation in the cells.

Another fact about cooking which has only recently come to light, and which is probably relevant to why raw foods are so important for ageless ageing, is that cooking creates chemicals which are mutagenic and *carcinogenic.* Carcinogenic means cancer-producing, while mutagenicity is the ability to produce changes in gene patterns which can be transferred to future generations. Researchers such as T. Sugimura and others have discovered that the burnt and browned matter which results from heating protein during cooking is highly mutagenic. And a number of chemicals isolated from heated protein have been shown to be cancer-causing when they are fed to animals. Also, the browning-reaction products that come from caramelizing sugars and from the interactions of amino acids and sugars during the cooking of foods (such as the brown crusts on bread and toast) contain a wide variety of DNA-damaging substances.

The amount of this burnt browned material which is taken in the normal western diet can be several grammes a day. Even coffee, which contains a considerable amount of burnt material, is a source of several mutagens. One cup of coffee contains about 250mg of the natural mutagen chlorogenic acid. Caffeine itself inhibits the cells' DNA-repair system and can increase the production of cancer tumours in animals. And there is now preliminary epidemiological evidence that heavy coffee-drinking is associated with ovarian cancer as well as cancer of the colon, bladder and pancreas. Fats – particularly unsaturated oils such as those we cook with – have also been shown to change during heating and processing. Not only is much of their nutritional value lost, they too can produce mutagenic and carcinogenic compounds.

More than the Sum of its Parts

A number of European scientists who have investigated the high-raw healing phenomenon believe that there are other important substances such as the essential oils in plants, the chlorophyll, the bioflavonoids and the saponins, with health-enhancing properties. These too can be changed or destroyed by heat. Although ignored by orthodox nutrition, such substances are probably also part of the structural information biologically necessary to support high-level health and to slow degeneration. Also, unlike the average western diet, a high-raw way of eating does not tax the body with excessive acidity and it is low in salt – particularly important when our high salt intake has been indicted as a possible cause of high blood pressure and vascular disease. Some experts on the relationship between a high-raw diet and health believe that the reason why orthodox nutrition has not yet twigged to the value of fresh natural

foods is precisely because of the reductionist nature of the science. Ralph Bircher – biochemist son of Bircher-Benner – has spent the past fifty years compiling laboratory and clinical research in this area, has edited a scientific journal in Europe for more than a the
generation and has written almost a dozen technical books on the subject. He says:

> It is not the vitamins, nor the mineral salts in raw vegetable foods which do it, nor chlorophyll, nor the quality of the proteins, nor essential oils, nor excess of alkalines, nor fibre, nor the fact that this diet is low in sodium. The problem is complex and much more interesting than that. Heating and even wilting destroys many qualities the significance of which is not yet known and mankind will possibly never know it completely. But new analytic work of recent years has given interesting insight.

High-Raw Protects Immunity
Some of the work to which Bircher is referring was done by scientists such as Paul Kouchakoff at the Institute of Clinical Chemistry in Lausanne, who discovered that there are significant differences in the way the body responds to cooked foods and to raw foods. Kouchakoff found that a phenomenon which he called *digestive leucocytosis*, which was believed to take place whenever we eat food, doesn't actually occur if the food eaten is raw. In digestive leucocytosis, some kind of message triggers the release of leucocytes – white blood cells. These cells swarm out to the intestine walls – especially to the colon – as if to defend a front-line attack on the body. This was assumed to be a normal physiological phenomenon until Kouchakoff's discovery. He also found that it does not occur if you only *begin* your meal with something raw. Raw foods appear not to challenge the immune reactions in the way cooked foods do – leaving immune functions free to deal with day-to-day biochemical housekeeping. Kouchakoff's findings have been confirmed by other researchers as well.

Raw foods also contain natural enzymes which are destroyed when food is cooked. Orthodox nutrition pays no attention to these enzymes in the belief that they are rapidly destroyed by digestive processes as soon as we eat them and therefore can have no beneficial effects on the body. But researchers such as Kaspar Tropp in Würzburg and Nobel laureate A.I. Virtanen in Finland have shown that this is simply not true. Virtanen (who incidentally was Johan Bjorksten's teacher) found that many of these enzymes are broken down in the mouth as a result of chewing and their substrates react chemically with substances in saliva to produce new chemical compounds which appear to be beneficial to the health of animals and man. Tropp discovered that the human body knows how to protect many of these enzymes and escort them through the digestive tract so they reach the colon intact. There they attract and bind whatever oxygen may be present, thus removing the aerobic condition which can result in putrefaction, fermentations, intestinal toxaemia and dysbacteria or dysbiosis – a condition to which almost no attention has been paid so far in Britain and North America but which appears to have far-reaching consequences for human health.

Dysbiosis – an Insidious Menace

Dysbacteria or dysbiosis strictly means colonic dysfunction as a result of 'altered colonic flora'. The large intestine contains a colony or flora consisting of many forms of bacteria including various strains of *E. coli*, lactobacilli and so forth. In the colon are also smaller quantities of yeasts such as *Candida albicans* and some bacteria which can cause harm. The enzymes in raw foods appear to stimulate the production of the helpful bacterial flora such as the lactobacilli and *E. coli* which synthesize vitamins – particularly the B complex. When the bacteria present in the large bowel are abnormal, then the body can suffer from insufficiency of some of these nutrients. This is a common occurrence in people who suffer from food allergies. When the flora is abnormal, as it is in dysbiosis, then the gastrointestinal mucous membrane becomes abnormally permeable, allowing the absorption of toxins from the bowel. These wastes can enter the circulation and be carried throughout the body to disrupt cell metabolism and cause toxic effects. In North America recently there has been great concern over the widespread incidence of high colon concentrations of *Candida albicans* yeast. It has been associated with a number of common illnesses from arthritis to chronic depression and fatigue.

Cell Power for Ageless Ageing

Even more interesting are the effects which raw foods have been shown to have on the body's circulatory system, the mesenchyme or seedbed and the cells themselves. A central issue in protecting the body from degeneration is ensuring that there is a constant interchange of energy, substance and information between the capillaries – the very ends of the circulatory system – and the tissue cells. This goes on simultaneously at something like a billion points in every part of your body. Its efficiency depends to a large degree on the electrobiological events such as those we were looking at in Chapter 8 which make exchange possible. Scientists such as Hans Eppinger at the University of Vienna have found that a diet high in raw foods significantly improves intra-extra cellular exchange, micro circulation and waste elimination from the cells. Ralph Bircher describes this process rather well:

> The nutritive substances of the blood and the waste sub-stances of the cells have to pass through two fine membranes and a narrow dividing interstice. In a dead body such an interchange would be ruled by nature's law of levelling contrasts, the principle called 'diffusion', but during life the cells overcome diffusion. They tend to create the exact opposite of levelling, i.e. antagonistic contrasts and tensions of a chemical, physical and electrical nature, by attracting from the blood what they need and rejecting other material.
>
> The stronger these antagonisms are the better, for in them life finds the power of defence against disorder and the power of healing illness. On the other side, ill-health is expressed by a partial loss of this 'selective' capacity of the cells, by undue and diffused exchange of minerals – salts penetrating the cell walls for instance – also by a lowering of the tensions, by distortion and spasms of the capillaries, by a sticky coating of the blood platelets and by a sort of 'marsh' resulting in the dividing interstices between the membranes by waste products being scattered around the cells. Cell life slows down. This is an insidious aspect of ill-health, a condition which may exist long before clinical symptoms appear.

What Bircher is describing in slightly different terms is what Bjorksten is concerned with when he says that, unless metabolic pathways are kept open, biochemical processes become sluggish and toxic intermediate products are formed in excess building up to a point where they cause damage. A high-raw diet protects from this happening, which is one of the main reasons it can be so useful in ageless ageing. It restores the selective capacity of cells and ensures that nutrients carried through the bloodstream via the capillaries are available for clean and efficient cell use. In fact a substantial intake of raw foods was the only thing that Eppinger and his co-workers found which could do this in people already undergoing the effects of degeneration. Again in Bircher's words, 'Under the influence of a raw vegetable diet the life-giving antagonistic tensions grew and capillaries were slowly restored to their vigorous efficient state. You see how raw vegetable food works. It is an unspecific, general treatment, tending to restore the organizing centre in every cell in the organism.'

Light Quanta and Cell Order

Eppinger's discovery that raw foods have regenerative power and an ability to restore order, as well as to encourage clean and efficient metabolic processes in organisms which have lost them, still can't fully explain precisely how and why this happens. Bircher-Benner said that fresh foods are the *sine qua non* of natural health and healing because they carry to the organism eating them 'complex sunlight energies which have been stored in the vegetable kingdom during its construction of living matter, in the form of *light quanta*. This means that our blood, our organs, our tissues and our central nervous system are not being nourished by calories alone, as was hitherto assumed, but by light quanta – very small but highly charged energy waves which show their rich diversity in the colours of the rainbow.' Because in the Thirties what Bircher-Benner referred to as 'light quanta' (which he claimed we acquired through the electronic construction of living material) couldn't be measured the way we can measure calories obtained from combustion, his conclusion was not understood by nutritional science, which was intent on devising tables of vitamins and on dismissing whatever was not explainable in chemical terms alone. So the famous Swiss physician was accused of 'mysticism' despite the quite exceptional results that application of his theories brought to patients. In fact they still do, at the same Zürich clinic, which bears his name but is now owned by the Swiss government. Yet still much about raw food's healing, organizing and rejuvenating properties remains shrouded in mystery.

Electron Clouds and Changing Shapes

Now, however, thanks to developments in submolecular biology and quantum physics, what once appeared 'mysticism' is beginning to be explainable in terms of scientific theory. The handful of scientists who from one point of view or another have tried to penetrate the mystery of life energy and how it is maintained within a living system – many of them Nobel laureates such as Erwin Schrödinger and Albert Szent-Györgyi – have come up with explanations very close to Bircher-Benner's own. Szent-Györgyi has said, 'An electron going around is a little current. What drives life is ... a little electric current kept up by sunshine. All the complexities of intermediary metabolism are but lacework around this basic fact.'

What he means is, we know now, that while a classic chemical reaction in a living system – called *bivalent oxido-reduction* (which is what chemistry concerns itself with) – involves a rearrangement of molecular structure, there also exist *monovalent electron transfers*. These are electrons going it alone which do not necessarily involve such rearrangements. They belong to the world which Becker and scientists working in the field of electrobiology are now beginning to unravel. Bircher-Benner's 'sunlight quanta' which he believed to be the healing force behind the high-raw phenomenon – a force destroyed when foods were heated or processed or when they wilted – also appear to have a place within this world. For currents such as these – single electrons cascading down and giving up their energy piecemeal – as Szent-Györgyi says 'can do anything but cannot be expressed in classic chemical terms. A wandering electron belongs to the changing shapes. . , of those electron clouds which belong to the submolecular, dominated by quantum mechanics.' It is a world about which orthodox nutrition and biochemistry know nothing as yet. And it may be several years before it is charted. But you needn't wait until then to make use of the remarkable age-retarding benefits of high-raw eating. That can begin right now.

12
Slimming Revolution

ONE OF THE great worries many people have about beginning to follow an ageless-ageing way of eating centres around their being overweight or their having had to be constantly fighting the battle of the bulge. They are afraid they could never adjust to a low-calorie-high-potency diet because for them the ritual of slimming has always consisted of constant self-abnegation and been a kind of continual battle with guilt and overindulgence. For others it has been a source of constant frustration or impossibility.

Thin for What?
In the western world we have developed an obsession about changing the shape of our bodies, especially trying to make them thinner. Yet making a body thinner is not always the best thing to do – either for its health or its good looks. A thin body is a wimpish body. It is a body depleted of energy and of power. When you are *lean* you are strong, you can have sleek muscles, good tone, and you can feast heartily on wholesome, natural foods and stay that way. You are also highly resistant to illness and early ageing as the years pass and you feel comfortable and at ease in your body. It is a very different experience from the anxiety over thinness which dis-empowers so many men and women. Leanness brings a sense of power with it – a sense of being in control of your own life that is a far cry from the inadequacy many women feel as they continue to struggle against weight gain with conventional slimming diets. I believe it is time we forgot about thin and chose instead to *go lean*. This calls for revolution.

To revolutionize means to change completely and fundamentally – your body and your life. It is not a word chosen lightly but because it most accurately describes the powerful positive transformation that takes place in how you look and feel when you throw out convenience foods which are loaded with hidden sugar or junk fats, and begin to feed heartily on wholesome low-fat complex carbo-hydrate foods, drink large quantities of pure water and increase your muscle mass through slow, steady exercise. (See my 1994 book *Lean Revolution* for more details.)

The word *lean* means 'muscular . . . containing little or no fat.' Being lean is as different from being thin as an ageless-ageing way of eating is from all of the quick-fix slimming diets you may have tried over the years which have slowly but inexorably eroded your energy and increased the sense of disenchantment with your body.

Go Lean

When you have lost enough weight, you will be thin. That is the goal of slimming diets. To be thin is commonly understood to mean having a *low body weight*. But in time a thin body becomes a soft body – a body without tone. It is a body prone to fatigue, early ageing and degeneration. It is also a disempowered body – one that needs to be watched carefully lest it eat something forbidden and change shape again. A thin body can have a high proportion of body fat. To be lean means to have a *low* percentage of body fat. A lean body is always smaller in size than a thin body of the same weight. Go lean and you gain enormously in energy, stamina and general health. You can also end up looking years younger. And where you once had to watch every calorie you consumed to avoid gaining weight, you will be able to eat without worrying about calories.

A rugby player who is six foot one can weigh as much as one hundred kilos, yet be lean – if his muscle to fat ratio is very high. He may have to eat as many as 4,000 calories a day to look and feel his best. His brother who is the same height weighs only 75 kilos. He would be considered thin according to the weight tables from insurance companies. Yet he may *not* be lean – not if he boasts very little muscle and carries a lot of fat. Say he also leads a sedentary life and eats convenience foods. As a result he has to be very careful how much he eats. If he takes in more than 1,800 calories a day his waistline starts to spread dangerously. It works the same with women. A thin woman, 5′6″ tall, weighs 57 kilos and wears a size 10 dress. But her body is soft since lots of her weight is fat tissue. The same woman, when she becomes lean, will weigh 60 kilos yet only wear a size 8.

Ready . . . Steady . . .

Once you commit yourself to an ageless-ageing way of living all sorts of good things start to happen. You discover you are free to eat with pleasure and enthusiasm as much as your body wants. Soon you find yourself living in a way that supports your health in the highest possible degree and brings you lots of energy, self-confidence and a sense that you are strong enough to meet whatever challenges life has in store for you.

There is one important question to answer. How did we get into the situation where almost half the people in the western world are fat? Widespread overweight is a relatively new phenomenon. Obesity, adult-onset diabetes, kidney stones, hypertension, coronary heart diseases and cancer of the bowel, together with many other chronic degenerative ailments, belongs to a group of illnesses now known as *Diseases of Western Civilization*. These conditions are hard to treat – so hard that despite all the sophisticated drugs and leading-edge techniques of modern medicine, we have been unable to halt their spread. For unlike the microbe-generated infectious diseases like typhoid and tuberculosis, western diseases are *lifestyle-caused*. Thanks to pioneering works from scientists such as Sir Robert McCarrison – who did the first epidemiological studies on the relationship between diet and health – and Drs Weston Price, Denis Burkitt and Hugh Trowell, it is now widely accepted that overweight and other degenerative conditions have developed as a direct result of the massive changes that have taken place over the last 150 years in how we live – especially in the way we eat.

Let's Go Back a Bit

A lot has happened to our foods in the last century to produce this state of affairs. First, they are *grown* differently from the way our ancestors, for thousands of years, grew theirs. We grow food on chemically fertilized soils in which the organic matter has been degraded or destroyed. Eating foods this way leads to a depletion and imbalance in the minerals and trace elements available to our bodies, both of which we need in good quantities to support complex metabolic processes on which health depends. Second, our foods are now highly *processed*. Raw foodstuffs, instead of being made into meals in home kitchens as they were in our grandparents' time, are sent to food manufacturers where they are fragmented – literally broken apart physically and chemically – then put through complex processes to alter them out of all recognition. Third, our foods are *shipped* over long distances and *stored* for long periods of time, both of which lowers their nutritional value. These modern practices destroy food's wholesomeness – a property very hard to measure except in terms of the degenerative effects that eating such foods has on our bodies. Destroy a food's wholesomeness and you destroy a food's ability to support the highest levels of health. And once the health-giving integrity of any food has gone, it has gone for good. It can never be compensated for by vitamin and mineral supplements or by eating cereals to which extra fibre and vitamins have been added.

Our great-grandparents – whether they were Africans, Indians, Orientals or Europeans – regardless of the staple foods they ate – rice, wheat, rye, barley, corn, cassava, yams or what-have-you – had two important things in common. Their meals were mostly prepared from foods of vegetable origin, and the foods they ate were little processed. They were *eaten whole, as closely as possible to their natural state*.

Such foods form the basis of an ageless-ageing lifestyle. This kind of eating helps prevent the development of obesity and other degenerative conditions – even if you happen to have inherited a tendency towards them. The even more exciting news is that studies carried out at leading universities and published in highly respected medical journals such as *The Lancet* and *The New England Journal of Medicine*, as well as clinical results from centres for health education and lifestyle medicine, now show that returning to this way of eating can restore normal weight even to people who are very overweight. It can also free them from much suffering caused by degenerative conditions such as high blood pressure, arteriosclerosis, diabetes, diverticulitis and other western diseases.

Food for Degeneration

The typical western diet is based on 'foods of commerce' – the stuff you can buy at the local corner shop and in run-of-the-mill supermarkets. These foods are very different from the simple foods that human beings have eaten throughout history and to which our bodies have become genetically adapted. Our ancestors did not eat massive quantities of white bread, white sugar, junk fats, and pre-packaged, pre-cooked foods like we do. They ate simple, ordinary, wholesome foods – as much of them as they could get. Their diet was *low* in fat, *high* in complex carbohydrates and only *moderate* in protein. Modern convenience foods on which we now feed are high in fat and depleted of natural fibre. They consist of highly refined carbohydrates like white bread and packaged cereals, spiked with lots of sugar and junk fats – that is oils which have been separated out from the foods in which they occur in nature, then chemically altered by solvents and heat processing. We now consume masses of animal protein riddled with fat – milk, cheese, meat, eggs, fish and poultry. Even the leanest beef, pork, or lamb, is more than 50 per cent fat. Our ancestors never consumed massive quantities of protein or high concentrations of fat – not in all history. As a result our bodies are ill-equipped to handle them. With a few rare exceptions such as the Eskimo and the Masai, in all primitive cultures – Chinese, Greek, Indian, European, African, and Egyptian – meat was used as a condiment or was eaten only on feast days – never every day. It did not form the main part of a meal.

There is one more major change that has taken place. Today we also swallow a kaleidoscope of chemical colorants, flavourings, additives and 'enhancers', not to mention pesticides, herbicides and fungicides, which our ancestors never imagined in their wildest dreams. We slurp down chemical pollutants with each sip of our diet cola and every bite of our pre-cooked meals. Such is the western diet. So next time you upbraid yourself for what you perceive to be your lack of will power as you reach for yet another biscuit and feel guilty about it, let the guilt go. It does not belong to you. The denatured, degraded, food we eat bears the lion's share of blame for the fat state we find ourselves in, as well as for how hard it is in our culture to stay lean and to remain healthy.

Ask Any Rat

It is not just human beings who respond to processed foods in this way either. Studies show that when you feed rats on foods of commerce – what is commonly called a cafeteria diet – most of them get fat too. The more highly refined and processed the food you eat, the hungrier you can become. There are many reasons for this. Because such foods are bereft of some essential nutrients, your body in its natural desire for them eats more and more. Also, continuing to eat foods 'constructed' from the same raw materials – things like milk, flour, corn oil and sugar – stresses your body's enzymes – all of which are food-specific. Because there is a particular enzyme needed to break down a particular food, this can deplete your system of those enzymes and create food sensitivities

– commonly and often wrongly called food allergies – so that every time you eat something containing milk or flour you crave more. This is part of the bizarre but widespread phenomenon of chemical and food addiction. Another important reason for food craving is that the convenience foods are full of junk fats and sugar. The more you eat of either the more you want. After a couple of packaged biscuits, or a sloppy hamburger or one of those chic and expensive packets of chicken drenched in wine sauce you crave more and more. Some foods are even sprayed with so-called flavour enhancers which encourage greed. Tinned dog foods fall into this category, which is why dogs seem ravenous when they devour them. Foods that have been chemically grown, sprayed, treated and highly manipulated like this can never really satisfy hunger because they are nutritionally inadequate and chemically distorted. Whilst we can overlook this fact with our mind each time we feel a hamburger craving coming on, it is a truth our bodies know very well at the deepest levels.

Many overweight people blame themselves for compulsive eating and worry about their cravings for carbohydrates which are caused by eating a high proportion of foods from which the fibre has been removed. Refining and processing foods strips our foods of their natural fibre and in changing their physical form makes them absorbed very quickly into the intestine. This is especially true of the average breakfast cereals and most of our bread and biscuits, cookies and sweets. It is why you get a slump of energy and hunger at 11 each day after eating them. Such foods give only a temporary feeling of having eaten enough. Very soon your stomach is back again complaining of emptiness and demanding more.

Go Primitive

Dietary fibre is an integral part of every vegetable food as it appears in nature. Fibre plays a central role both in weight loss and in the successful maintenance of normal weight. The naturally high-fibre diet of our ancestors had a low caloric density. People eating this way reach satiety far quicker than those munching away on the products of the western food industry with their very *high* caloric density, since these are devoid of fibre and stuffed with junk fats and hidden sugars. Eighty-five per cent of the calories we eat in the western world – animal products, refined cereals, sugar, oils and fats – now come from foods that lack fibre. The average person on a western diet gets only 10–25 grams of fibre a day. The diet our ancestors ate and the more primitive diets of developing countries contained between 35 and 60 grams. So important is fibre in whole plant foods that these facts alone would be enough to account for our spreading waistlines and rampant degenerative conditions. The bulky and moisture-rich foods our ancestors ate – and which are still eaten in the few primitive cultures that remain on the planet – are the foods from which ageless ageing's menus should be prepared. Eat them and they make their full journey through your digestive tract while skilfully clearing away wastes and toxins and decreasing the number of calories absorbed by the intestine.

Typical Western Diet	*Ageless Ageing*
25–35% carbohydrate (simple)	50–75% carbohydrate (complex)
25% protein	15–20% protein
40–45% fat	20–25% fat

Comfort Foods

Ageless-ageing foods are archetypal *comfort* foods. They are the kind of foods that make you feel deliciously satisfied. Rich wholesome breads, legumes, fresh vegetable stews, crunchy cereals and luscious natural sweets. They are foods in which the integrity of their components – natural proteins, fatty acids, fibre, minerals and vitamins – has been preserved. You will find they satisfy hunger as no other foods can, since they are the kind of foods to which your body has been genetically adapted for hundreds of thousands of years. If you can get them in their organic form so much the better. If not, buy them as fresh as you can and incorporate special nutrient-rich items into your diet such as sprouted seeds and grains, seaweed or spirulina, chlorella or green barley.

In a world where much confusion abounds over how much of this and that you should or shouldn't eat, the simple ageless-ageing diet is nothing short of revolutionary. For many, starting to eat this way is rather like coming home again. You begin to re-experience all the rich textures of real foods, with their wonderful aromas, colours and textures – all those things that our widespread foods of commerce have lost and are continually trying to compensate for with the addition of chemical flavourings and colourings and bright seductive packaging. You may even find, as I have, that for the first time in years you enjoy cooking and food preparation again. For these natural raw materials – the crunchy grains, the colourful fresh vegetables and succulent fruits, the seeds and beans and nuts – can create meals that are as delicious as they are health-giving. I call it Sensuous Austerity.

13

Eat for Your Life

IF WE MAKE Walford's undernutrition without malnutrition the basis of an anti-ageing lifestyle, then how do we go about achieving this orthomolecular state? What kind of foods do we need to eat and what attributes of these foods will be particularly important in forming the foundation on which we can build with anti-oxidant nutrients and other substances that can be useful for ageless ageing? Canadian expert on the orthomolecular approach Abram Hoffer has been treating people with anti-oxidant nutrients for more than a generation. But before he ever gives a patient nutritional supplements he insists that they get themselves into a new way of eating – a way of eating based on four principles:

1. Foods eaten should be whole foods, not fractions of foods which are the result of refining and processing.
2. Foods need to be as fresh as possible and as close to a living state as possible. They should be allowed as little time as possible for deterioration which comes as a result of oxidation. When they are cooked it should be as lightly as possible since cooking increases the carcinogenic properties of foods.
3. All foods should be non-toxic. They should not contain synthetic flavours, colours, preservatives or other additives used cosmetically to 'enhance' the food.
4. The diet should be varied, for down through evolution the human body has adapted to a wide range of foods which offer a broad spectrum of nutrients.

Add to Hoffer's list of requirements for a healthy diet one more:

5. The diet must be low in calories. (How low depends on whether

you are male or female and how high a level of strenuous physical activity you have in your life. A top athlete, for instance, will need many more calories than an office worker but for most people the calorie count will hover between 1,200 and 1,800 calories a day.)

and you have guidelines for an anti-ageing nutritional lifestyle which can't be beaten.

Eating for Ageless Ageing
Following these guidelines will automatically provide you with anti-ageing nutrition of the highest order – a way of eating which is low in fat, high in fibre, low in calories, eliminates all chemically processed foods, and it is of necessity low in meat (meat tends to be far too high in fat) and rich in a full complement of essential nutrients. It is a diet rich in the structural information necessary to maintain a high degree of order or negative entropy in your body and therefore to protect it from degeneration. Provided your foods are fresh enough, and from 50 to 75 per cent of them are eaten raw, this way of eating should also carry with it whatever as yet undefined electromagnetic properties – what Bircher-Benner called 'sunlight quanta' – appear to give fresh foods their ability to retard degeneration and promote a high level of health in living systems. Such a nutritional lifestyle has three other attributes which are particularly important for ageless ageing as well: it is low in protein, high in fibre and an excellent source of *usable* essential fatty acids. Let's look more closely at all three and why they are important.

The Longest-Living People
Almost all of the world's cultures studied by scientists such as Sir Robert McCarrison and Weston Price which have had a very low incidence of degenerative illnesses, as well as all of the long-lived cultures – the Hunzas, the Georgians, the Vilcabamba Indians studied by Alexander Leaf – lived on a low-calorie diet. And it was a diet rich in fresh uncooked foods. Considering the effect that such a diet has on promoting healing in an organism and on increasing vitality, it is not far-fetched to assume that it is also likely to be the optimal diet for us to use in promoting human longevity. But there is another important characteristic which the diets of long-lived cultures have in common as well: unlike the normal western way of eating, all of their diets are also low in protein. There are strong

indications that any diet designed to retard age-degeneration and to prevent degenerative illness should follow a similar pattern. In cultures which have the lowest life expectancy in the world, the Laplanders, Greenlanders and Eskimos (for whom it is only thirty to forty years) live on diets high in animal protein.

The Dangers of Too Much Protein

So insidious and destructive are the effects of the high-protein diet, and so extensive is the research which demonstrates that excess protein hastens early ageing, that it is difficult to believe the 'lots-of-protein-is-good-for-you' myth still survives. A diet which supplies more protein than your body needs can cause severe deficiencies of many essential vitamins, including vitamin B6 and niacin. Excess protein also actually leaches important minerals such as calcium, iron, zinc, phosphorus and magnesium from the body. And when your body metabolizes protein, complex by-products are formed, some of which, such as ammonia, can be highly toxic to the system, encouraging free radical damage and cross-linking, and stressing your body's adaptive energy. Eating more protein than you need creates deposits of these toxic residues in the tissues leading to over-acidity, autotoxaemia, an accumulation of purines, and dysbacteria or dysbiosis of the colon, all of which can contribute to degenerative illnesses – from gum disease to arthritis and arteriosclerosis, heart disease, cancer and even schizophrenia. Many animal studies have now shown conclusively that while a high-protein diet brings about early rapid growth, it also results in early and rapid ageing and disease.

Beware of Amyloid

Ralph Bircher and Henning Karstrom – a Swedish scientist well known for his work with nutritional methods of health promotion and healing – both stress the danger of a build-up of amyloid deposits, which occur on a high-protein diet. Amyloid is a fatty-waxy compound which is the result of serious and extensive cross-linkage. Associated with age-degeneration, amyloid builds up in the tissues of people on a very high-protein diet – particularly one which contains a lot of meat. Professor of physiological pathology at Frankfurt University, Dr P. Schwartz, one of the world experts on amyloid deposits and their implications, refers to it as 'the most important and perhaps decisive cause of decline with age'. Amyloid in the tissues interferes with the transport of nutrients and oxygen between bloodstream and cells and with the elimination of wastes, as well as lowering immune functions. It creates a physiochemical environment which not only stifles proper cell metabolism but can damage genetic material and cell membranes. Its build-up in the body causes tissue and cell degeneration and leads to premature ageing. If you care about preserving the youthful integrity of your body it is certainly something you need to avoid.

How Much Protein Is Enough?

This is a question that can provoke heated argument, even in scientific circles. At the beginning of the century the idea that 'the more protein you eat, the better' developed. Recommendations for health made by Voit and Rubner were for 120–160g a day. Chittenden however showed that high-level health and peak athletic performances could be achieved on less than half that amount. And other studies such as those of Hipsley and Oomen indicate that good health is possible on as little as 15–20g a day. Ralph Bircher, who has studied the question thoroughly for fifty years, places the figure around 50–60g, which he says is probably on the high side and 'allows a good margin for error'. In Britain and the United States, recommendations usually hover somewhere between 60 and 100g a day, but an increasing number of scientists now insist that this is still excessively high. Expert on the relationship between diet and ageing Dr Myron Winick of the Institute of Human Nutrition at Columbia University School of Medicine says that for maximum protection against ageing and degenerative diseases the 'recommended daily intake for healthy adult men and women of almost any age is 56g and 46g respectively'. And even that recommendation offers a 'high margin of safety'. People on a low-calorie diet rich in a variety of vegetable foods, however, are likely to need even less protein. For it is not just quantity that matters, but quality. And the quality of protein in a mixed vegetable diet which supplies all eight essential amino acids in easily assimilable form is very high indeed.

The Meat Question

The long-standing notion that you have to eat meat or eggs to get enough protein is simply untrue. As Carl Pfeiffer, co-author of *Total Nutrition*, says, 'There is a general belief that only meat gives us protein and that vegetables could never be the equal. This is quite erroneous. It is a matter of calorie density: a helping of broccoli has a very high protein value in proportion to the calories consumed. There is also the advantage that the calories are in a high-fibre form.' Meat is also very high in fat yet low in fibre and essential nutrients apart from protein (even the *leanest* steak boasts over 50 per cent of its calories in fat). It is virtually impossible to follow an ageless-ageing way of eating and eat much meat. The long-lived peoples of the world have all eaten meat but only occasionally – say once a week and only in very small quantities. Most people find that as they increase the quantity of fresh raw vegetables and fruits in their diet and eliminate coffee and other stimulants, they no longer have much desire for meat. If you like it, by all means eat it – but not too often and not in large quantities. The best meats are the game meats such as partridge, pheasant, wild duck, venison and so forth. Fish is a good source of essential fatty acids and a good flesh food for health. But it too is a very concentrated source of protein. Enjoy it in smaller quantities. Both meat and fish are low in fibre and high fibre is an important constituent of eating for ageless ageing.

Fibre Power against Degeneration
The importance of the high-raw diet in promoting health and protecting the body from degeneration is right now in the same position that fibre was twenty-five years ago. And, just as it has taken fifteen years for the value of fibre for health to be recognized –so is it likely to be with fresh foods. Twenty-five years ago no one but old-maid schoolteachers and a few eccentric scientists concerned themselves with fibre. The rest of the scientific world aggressively dismissed any hint that fibre bulk or roughage in the diet would be important in reducing excess weight or protecting the body from illness. Wholegrain bread, they insisted, was no better for you than white bread. Theirs was a sentiment which received strong support from vocal food manufacturers, organizations intent on defending the virtues of white bread and sticky buns. Fibre, after all, was something unnecessary. It was the part of your food which, unlike the nutrients, was not assimilated into the body. Twenty years back if you mentioned 'roughage' in your diet to your GP he dismissed you as yet another annoying 'crank'. In a decade, however, all of this changed dramatically, thanks to some pioneering scientific research into the relationship between a low-fibre diet and the development of degenerative diseases, as well as lots of popular publicity. Now 'How much fibre do you get in your diet?' is

one of the first questions the average GP asks his or her patient. Meanwhile millions of people are sprinkling extra bran on their breakfast cereals or their baked beans, and most people think they know all about fibre. But do they?

In truth the fibre story is just beginning to reveal its mysteries. Did you know for instance that wheat bran is not the perfect form of fibre, as some journalists and manufacturers of cereal products would have us believe? That for some people it can be an intestinal irritant, and as such is actually constipating rather than laxative? Are you aware that supplementing your diet with high levels of bran can result in anaemia and the loss of several important minerals from your tissues? Did you know that lesser-known kinds of fibre appear to be far more useful for slimmers than bran and also as a help in preventing degenerative illnesses such as cardiovascular disease and diabetes? Or that some recently investigated forms of fibre can lower blood cholesterol and low-density lipoprotein (LDL) levels in the blood? (High LDL levels are associated with coronary disease.) At this point the fibre story is far from ended but the latest research into fibre, its importance in health and its usefulness in preventing and treating many abnormal conditions – from diabetes, gall-stones and obesity to intestinal stasis and heart disease – is so exciting it needs to be told.

What Is Fibre?

Dietary fibre is a biological unit, not a chemical entity such as a vitamin or mineral. We get it in our diet by eating plant foods, whole grains, beans, seeds and pulses, fresh raw vegetables and fruits. From simple sugars plants make a number of carbohydrate polymers. Some, the starches which serve as energy stores for the plant, are almost completely digested and absorbed in the small intestine when we eat these plant foods. Others, the fibrous or viscous *polysaccharides* and *lignins* which lend plants their structure and form, we cannot digest. Instead they pass through to the colon intact where they are fermented to some degree before being eliminated from the body as waste. These indigestible poly-saccharides, which in the plant make up its cell walls, are known collectively as dietary fibre or fibres. Individually plant fibres have a number of different characteristics and qualities, and the chemical and physical properties of dietary fibre differ greatly from plant to plant. They are also influenced by the age of the plant and the conditions in which it was grown. So far there are at least six known kinds of fibre, which shows up in everything from porridge oats to strawberries. And as yet still far too little is known about the inherent characteristics of each type – although what is known is quite fascinating, for the differences in physiological actions of these six classes of fibre can be as varied as those between spring water and gin. Here they are:

Cellulose
This is the most common fibre in bran and is what most people think of when the word is mentioned. It is one of the structural fibres. Its main physiological action when you eat it is to bind water which is why it increases faecal bulk and is helpful to some people in treating constipation. You'll find cellulose not only in bran but also in fruits and vegetables, wholemeal bread and beans. It even occurs in nuts and seeds. Not only does cellulose prevent colonic stasis, many fibre experts believe that it may also dilute and flush out cancer-causing and degeneration-encouraging toxins from the intestinal tract. It may also help level out glucose in the blood and curb weight gain. On the ageless-ageing regime you will have no need to supplement your diet with extra bran or any other kind of fibre because this way of eating naturally restores the high degree of natural fibre necessary for health which has been lost by the way we have been nourishing ourselves for the past hundred years in industrialized societies.

Hemicellulose
Its name sounds as if it should mean 'half-cellulose'. In fact hemicellulose has its own character entirely but it usually occurs together with cellulose in natural foods and it shares some of its characteristics. It also helps to relieve constipation, aid weight reduction and chase carcinogens from the bowel.

Pectin
So different in texture and character is pectin from other forms of fibre that it is hard to believe it is classified in the same group of substances. Unlike cellulose and hemicellulose it does not bind water. Instead, it is water-soluble. It has no influence on stools and can do little to deter constipation. However, pectin appears to be an excellent substance for lowering cholesterol and may also help eliminate bile acids from the intestines, thus short-circuiting the development of colon cancer and gall-stones. Common sources of

pectin are fruits such as apples, oranges and grapefruit, grapes and berries. Even bran contains a bit of pectin. Because of pectin's ability to bind cations (positively charged ions) and organic materials such as bile acids, it is also used as a natural chelating (binding) agent to take up unwanted heavy metals such as aluminium in the system and to eliminate them from the body. This is a very important role in terms of protecting the body from age-degeneration. You may remember that heavy metals are potent cross-linkers and very dangerous to the functioning of brain and body. That is why if anyone has heavy metal poisoning pectin is usually given along with vitamin C and other natural substances as a nutritional chelating agent to remove the heavy metals.

Gums and Mucilages

These are the sticky fibres which food manufacturers make good use of as thickening agents in ketchups and making biscuits. They are not components of cell walls in plants as are many forms of fibre. Instead they perform the important task of repairing injured tissue in plants. They are widely used in cosmetics and are currently being investigated as nutritional supplements in an attempt to improve the quality of collagen in the skin and circulatory system. The gums such as locust-bean, karaya gum, guar gum, oat gum and others can lower cholesterol significantly. Guar gum, which is found in good quantity in the cluster bean, has proved itself particularly helpful in the treatment and prevention of diabetes because of its ability to stabilize blood sugar – something of increasing concern as you age.

Lignin

This is the woody fibre which you find in cereals, raspberries, strawberries, Brussels sprouts, cabbage, spinach, kale, parsley and tomatoes. It too is able to eliminate cholesterol and bile acids from the intestines and there is some indication that it may prevent the formation of gall-stones.

Because the ageless-ageing way of eating is high in all types of fibre, and because much of the fibre is uncooked and in its natural state, it offers help against biological degeneration on several different levels at once. It keeps the intestines clean and it helps detoxify the body of heavy metals and poisonous wastes (some of the fibres present in seaweeds and kelps are even able to clear radiation from the system). And eating in this high-raw wholefood way you need never again give a thought to sprinkling flaky bran on to your baked beans.

The Essential Fatty Acids

As important as the fibre which ageless-ageing nutrition offers is the perfect complement of unprocessed and unadulterated essential fatty acids (EFAs) it supplies. For many years lipids or fats were all but ignored by nutrition, for until relatively recently science understood very little about these fascinating chemical substances. As we get older, our body tends to lose its ability to make proper use of them. Fatty acids are the chemical building blocks from which oils and fats are made. They consist of molecules which are mostly chains of carbon atoms. Some, such as those present in butter, contain hydrogen on their open links as well as carbon atoms, and are known as *saturated fats*. Others are called *unsaturated*. Instead of being connected to hydrogen atoms their chains link back to each other in double bonds. Two of these unsaturated fatty acids – linoleic acid and alpha-linolenic acid – are absolutely necessary for life and health and are known as essential fatty acids or EFAs. Your body can neither manufacture these EFAs nor can it convert from one to the other. The first family of EFAs, called the omega 6 group of acids, includes linoleic acid and its biologically active derivative, gamma-linolenic acid – GLA – as well as a couple of other fatty acids which are conversions from these two. The second family, called the omega 3 group, includes the parent alpha-linolenic acid and its biologically active derivatives eicosapentaenoic acid – EPA – and docosahexaenoic acid – DHA – which exist in green leaves and in good quantity in oily fish such as mackerel, *wild* salmon, sardines and trout. These EFAs need to be supplied in small quantity through the foods we eat – primarily via the oils in vegetables and seeds, and from animal foods which contain them, such as fish and game.

EFAs have a number of important functions for ageless ageing and lasting good looks. For instance, they are the building blocks of cell membranes and of the intercellular cement. When properly supplied they encourage proper cellular exchange of nutrients and oxygen. From a more cosmetic point of view, they help to ensure that the skin's moisture retention is optimal, thus protecting it both from dehydration and from some of the premature signs of ageing. They also help protect blood from clotting too rapidly and therefore appear helpful in improving one's resistance to heart disease. They play important roles in the health of the eyes, brain, inner ear, adrenal and sex glands too. And EPAs are essential for the production of prostaglandins in the body. These are hormone-like substances (scientists have now delineated the functions of about thirty different prostaglandins) which perform such functions as ensuring the proper function of T-cells in the immune system – important in preventing premature ageing – and keeping skin soft and smooth and hair and nails strong, and helping to prevent susceptibility to heart disease, inflammatory disorders and even depression. Some prostaglandins affect the release of compounds from nerve cells which transmit nerve impulses, still others keep blood platelets from clotting together.

Conversion for Youthful Well-Being

In order to make use of both EFA families (which we should take in through the foods we eat) two things are important. First, like the ageless-ageing eating plan, your diet needs to be one which is not rich in saturated fats from meats and dairy products nor in fats which have been highly processed, such as most margarines and vegetable oils you can buy on supermarket shelves, not to mention the many processed bakery goods which are full of these hidden highly processed fats. Processed fats can actually block the proper assimilation of EFAs, even when they are present in adequate quantities in the foods you eat. Second, your body needs to be able to convert the EFAs in your diet into their biologically active forms GLA, EPA and DHA – a conversion which can only take place if there is adequate vitamin C, B6, B3, zinc and magnesium in your system. For it is only after these biochemical conversions have been made that your body can make use of the many positive attributes EFAs offer for health, good looks and age-retardation. Generally EPA and DHA are made in the body from alpha-linolenic acid in the foods you eat. But as the body ages the ability to make conversion diminishes. This is where specific supplements of GLA, EPA and DHA can play an important role in an ageless-ageing lifestyle.

EFA Deficiencies are Widespread

There is also considerable evidence that even in some young people these conversions are not efficiently made or that they are blocked by poor dietary habits so that insufficient quantities of GLA, EPA and DHA are available in the body to prevent degeneration. In other words it appears that many apparently healthy people are deficient in EFAs. The consequences of such a deficiency, as shown by animal experiments, include a number of symptoms, from hair loss, dry scaly skin and poor tissue structure which can make a face lose its firm contours rapidly, to irritability, lethargy, a susceptibility to infections, painful swollen joints and premenstrual tension. In recent years a number of interesting clinical research projects have shown that supplementing the diet of such people with very small quantities of one or both EFA groups can have remarkable results in improving a great variety of conditions from eczema and simple dry skin to menstrual difficulties – simply by giving four to six capsules of 500mg per day of an EFAs preparation which includes the biologically active forms DHA, GLA and EPA. Most longevists add these supplements to their formulas. Such supplementation is also proving a helpful means of lowering blood cholesterol levels and restoring the right balance of blood lipids in men prone to heart disease, and in strengthening the immune system, because of the action of the prostaglandins derived from them. GLA, usually given in the form of evening primrose oil which is probably its richest natural source, has also shown itself to be effective in controlling rheumatoid arthritis in a substantial number of sufferers.

Getting the Most from EFAs

The ageless-ageing way of eating makes sure that you get the most out of what EFAs have to offer for age-retardation. It does this, somewhat paradoxically perhaps, by cutting down your overall level of fat intake from all sources, for you need only the smallest amounts of these important essential fatty acids – it is just that they have to be in a form in which your body can make use of them and free of the conversion problems caused by the presence of trans-fatty acids (the unusable form which occurs in heated and processed oils) in your system, which block them. And the ageless-ageing approach eliminates hydrogenated oils in margarines, commercial mayonnaises and highly processed foods such as cakes, breads and biscuits, all of which contain them. This helps prevent conversion problems. It also provides you with a good source of unadulterated EFA from seeds and nuts, grains, and fish (mackerel and other oily fish are particularly high in the biologically active forms of EFA) and also with the co-factors needed for their conversion into prostaglandins and other active *metabolites* in the body. However, many people who have been living on an average diet for years and have developed conversion problems as a result can gain help, at least at the beginning, from nutritional supplements of these nutrients. But one of the best things about ageless-ageing eating is that for most people the basic changes in food intake itself and the improvement in food quality are enough to restore normal metabolism relatively quickly. Meanwhile use only extra virgin olive oil and cold-processed organic flax oil as your sources of oil, eat two meals a week of cold-water fish – wild salmon, trout, mackerel, sardines – and eliminate saturated fats from your diet.

14
Sensuous Austerity

IF ALL THIS talk about fibre and fat and protein has led you to think that following an ageless-ageing way of eating means gritting your teeth and doing what is good for you but expecting to hate every moment of it, there is good news to come. For the hedonistic splendour of good ageless-ageing cuisine couldn't be further away from the heavy stodge you get in some so-called health-food restaurants. The variety of colours, textures, tastes and culinary experiences which delicious natural foods offer to anyone with an interest in food preparation and a love of fine cuisine at the very least equals the best traditional cooking. Many of the most beautiful meals will be found on the ageless-ageing table. And there is another advantage to the low-calorie-high-raw way of eating as well: thanks to the effect of eating these fresh foods rich in 'life force' and to the fact that you are living on far fewer calories than you were used to before, your taste-buds, sense of smell and aesthetic awareness of food become dramatically heightened so that the appreciation of all that you eat can be greater than ever before.

This has certainly been my experience and the experience of many others I know who have tried it. From being someone who used to love fresh cream and rich sauces I've become infinitely more appreciative of the fine flavours implicit in ageless-ageing cuisine. And I love it. Not only because I look younger, feel better all round and have infinitely more energy than before, but because the experience of eating itself has become so much more delightful. Most of us eat far too much and we dull our senses and our appreciation of food in the process. Even the most subtle of Beethoven's late quartets begins to dull the senses when you have too much of it. So can too much food, even if it is the very best. Ageless-ageing cuisine revives them.

One Main Meal

Not only do most of us eat too much, we also eat too often. And while growing children thrive on three hearty meals a day, most adults do far better on one – preferably eaten at midday but taken in the evening instead if you can't manage it then. Two light meals or wholesome snacks a day to go with your main meal create a way of eating which doesn't tax your body's enzymic systems and keeps you feeling light and clear headed while nourishing you well. There are several good books with recipes which fit nicely into the low-calorie-high-raw way of eating. One of my favourites is a real treasure-house from the Bircher-Benner clinic itself written by Bircher-Benner's daughter Ruth Bircher. It is called *Eating Your Way to Health*. It contains hundreds of recipes for main dishes, salads, sweets, breakfasts and suppers which are delightful and simple to prepare. Another I like is the *A Good Cook. . .Ten Talents* by Frank J. Hurd & Rosalie Hurd, a Seventh Day Adventist cook book. *Raw Energy*, which my daughter Susannah and I wrote, also has a large selection of recipes, and so does my own *Lean Revolution* which sets out 'undernutrition without malnutrition' as a total lifestyle. After a few months of ageless-ageing eating you will find you no longer have to count calories, and if you have been an on-off-on-again slimmer you are also probably going to feel really *satisfied* for the first time in years, since eating wholesome *real* foods brings a real sense of fullness to the body and banishes for ever 'slimmer's hunger'. You will know from internal signals how much is enough and when you have stepped over the bounds.

Your main meal, like all your meals, should begin with something raw in order to avoid digestive leucocytosis and the immune challenge which it brings. This can be a piece of fruit or a raw salad or some crudités. Follow it with whatever you have chosen for a main dish – perhaps a casserole of pulses or vegetables or a small piece of fish or game, or even a rich and festive large salad made from a myriad of vegetables and sprouted grains and seeds topped with chopped hard-boiled eggs. This can be accompanied by a baked potato or some brown rice or couscous or bulgar wheat. There are also some wonderful home made peasant soups based on fresh vegetables, grains and legumes, which are a meal in themselves and are great taken with a beautiful salad. I make them using Low Salt Marigold Swiss Vegetable Bouillon Powder as a stock (it is a delicious vegetable product which contains no additives and can be used for seasoning salad dressings, sauces, casseroles and soups). If your main dish has been cooked then have a side salad with it. If not then you might have some mixed vegetables lightly steamed or wok-fried in a small amount of butter or olive oil. There are also some wonderful low-calorie sweets. One of my favourites is 'Apple Bread Pudding' (in *Lean Revolution*). Or you can serve some fresh fruit. The varieties of what you can prepare for a main meal are just about endless. Here are a few suggestions for main-meal menus for a week:

Day 1
RAW DISHES: melon; cauliflower and tomatoes mixed with red peppers and lettuce salad topped with yoghurt-herb dressing.
COOKED DISHES: Chinese steamed fish; wok-fried beans and peas; brown rice.

Day 2
RAW DISHES: lamb's lettuce, celeriac and wild-herb salad topped with chopped egg dressing; fresh pears and plumped raisins.
COOKED DISHES: cream of oatmeal soup with cashews; steamed baby carrots and basil; young peas with mint.

Day 3
RAW DISHES: mushrooms, watercress and chicory salad topped with Italian herb dressing; 'Apple Bread Pudding'.
COOKED DISHES: 'Luscious Lentil Soup'; wholegrain bread.

Day 4
RAW DISHES: 'Sunburst' platter of avocado, beetroot, cos lettuce, mushrooms, tomatoes, celery and peppers served with raw houmous dressing.
COOKED DISHES: carrot and coriander soup; or venison burgers; Scottish oatcakes; strawberry whip dessert.

Day 5
RAW DISHES: 'Jungle Slaw' salad made from cabbage, tender green beans, carrots, spring onions, red or yellow pepper and raw, unsalted peanuts served with citrus dressing.
COOKED DISHES: baked beans; black bread.

Day 6
RAW DISHES: gazpacho; pineapple salad stuffed with orange, mango, papaya and strawberries and topped with coconut.
COOKED DISHES: vegetable tart.

Day 7
RAW DISHES: 'Sandstone Loaf' made from carrots, lemon juice, almonds, pumpkin seeds, tahini and herbs; apple and ginger salad; home made blackberry sorbet.
COOKED DISHES: bran muffins and almond cheese.

Small Meals
The two small meals of the day can consist of fresh fruit, some natural yoghurt, a slice or two of wholegrain bread spread with some low-calorie herb cheese or – best of all – fruit muesli. If you have never tasted real muesli (and it bears no resemblance to the flaky sweet stuff you can buy on the shelves of supermarkets) you have a real treat ahead of you. Fruit muesli was the invention of Swiss physician Max Bircher-Benner who devised it as the perfect light meal. It is a delicious and easy-to-digest completely uncooked dish which can contain all of the essential vitamins and minerals, and which is an excellent source of high-quality complete proteins and essential fatty acids. It can provide you with sustaining energy but will never lie heavily in your stomach. And it can be made low in calories.

Real muesli (often called Birchermuesli after its inventor) is not a grain based but a fruit-based dish with only a very small quantity of top-quality freshly rolled wholegrain flakes in it. It is usually made with apples and oats but there are so many varieties which you can make, calling on whatever fresh or dried fruits and whatever kinds of grains, nuts and seeds you have available, that you could quite literally eat it twice a day all the year round and never get tired of it. Children absolutely adore Birchermuesli both as a complete breakfast and as a sweet after a main meal. A small bowl of muesli in the morning will keep you going all the way to lunch with none of the 'elevenses slump' that has many people reaching for a cup of coffee, and a pastry or a chocolate bar. It is also an excellent food to eat in the evening since it is so easy to digest that it never interferes with sleep. I do a lot of travelling and for many years I dreaded having to stay in hotels because the food available in so many hotel dining-rooms is so poor. I have got into the habit of carrying with me a small 'muesli bag' with a hand grater in it plus some grain flakes and minced nuts and a small bowl so I can make my own breakfast or supper whenever I want and not be forced to eat what I don't want just because there is nothing else. Here is the basic recipe:

Birchermuesli
For each person you'll need:

1 level tablespoon rolled oats soaked in 4 tablespoons water
1 heaped tablespoon raisins or sultanas
1 tablespoon lemon juice
3 tablespoons natural unsweetened yoghurt
1 large apple
½ banana
1 teaspoon raw honey (if desired)
1 tablespoon minced hazelnuts and almonds or other mixed seeds and nuts
1 pinch cinnamon (if desired)

The preparation can be done in the same bowl from which you will eat if you are only making enough for yourself or in a large bowl for the whole family.

Soak the rolled oats and raisins in water, preferably overnight. This begins to break down the starch present in the grains and turn it into natural sugar so it is easily assimilated. If you have no time to soak the grains then simply mix with the water (you will need slightly less water in this case) and carry on immediately.

Wash the apple(s) and remove core and stem but don't peel. Then, using a stainless-steel hand grater or a food processor, grate the apple into the mixture and, stirring, add lemon juice to protect it from discolouring.

Cut the banana into small cubes, add to the mixture with the honey (if desired) and mix with yoghurt. Sprinkle the top with the minced nuts and a little cinnamon if you like.

Instead of rolled oats you can use other cereal flakes such as wheat, rice, barley, millet or buckwheat. These are available from wholefood shops. I find I don't usually add honey to my muesli because it is so beautifully sweet already, thanks to the soaked grains and fruit. You can substitute a good unsulphured black molasses for the honey (it is rich in minerals). You can also make muesli with soft fruit such as strawberries or raspberries, loganberries, red and black currants, blackberries or blueberries as well as with apricots, cherries, peaches, plums or greengages. Or you can mix your fruits together. Also you can make the muesli from dried fruit which has been soaked for twelve hours (or overnight) in spring water. But make sure you get sun-dried, not sulphur-dried fruits to which no glucose has been added (it is commonly added to figs, for instance) or you can end up with a gastrointestinal upset.

Seasoning and Spices

Salt is unnecessary when you begin to prepare foods with all of the wonderful culinary herbs that are available. And the list of seductive possibilities seems almost endless: caraway, fennel, dill, chervil, parsley, lovage – the *Umbelliferae*; summer savory, marjoram, the mints, rosemary, and thyme – the labiates, which have a strong aroma and are particularly useful for seasoning; the *Liliaceae* such as garlic, onions, chives and leeks; and three of my favourites, basil and tarragon and horseradish. Herbs have a special role to play in any ageless-ageing regime. They contain pharmacologically active substances such as volatile oils, tannins, bitter factors, secretins, balsams, resins, mucilages, glycosides and organic vegetable acids, each of which can contribute to overall health in a different way. The tannins, for instance, which occur in many common kitchen herbs, are astringent and have an anti-inflammatory action on the digestive system. They help inhibit fermentation and decomposition. The secretins stimulate the secretion of pancreatic enzymes – particularly important for the complete breakdown of proteins in foods to make them available for bodily use. Organic acids have an antibiotic action and are helpful in the digestion of fats and the bitter factors which are found in good quantity in rosemary, marjoram and fennel. They also act as a tonic to the smooth muscles of the gut and boost secretion of digestive enzymes. Use herbs lavishly in your meals and you will find you can create the most remarkable combinations of subtle flavours and aromas.

Drink Yourself Younger

Coffee, although not completely forbidden on any serious programme of ageless ageing, is not something to drink daily. The occasional cup after dinner is not likely to do much harm. More than that and you are really undermining your potential for age-retardation not only because it contains mutagenic and carcinogenic compounds which cause oxy-stress and free radical damage but also because regular coffee tends to make cadmium (one of the heavy metals) build up in your system and can interfere with proper pancreatic functioning. It also leaches calcium from the bones. Tea is OK in moderation – no more than a cup or two a day – but there are other drinks which are not only good for you, they can be highly enjoyable as well.

Alcohol is another substance you want to go easy on. Not only is it very high in calories yet practically worthless in terms of the nutrients it supplies, it also causes your liver to produce one of the most potent cross-linkers known – acetaldehyde. A glass or two of wine can be easily accommodated within the low-calorie limits. More than that as a daily intake is likely seriously to undermine your effort. And make sure it is good wine. The run-of-the-mill, non-organic bottle of wine is full of toxic substances which your cells can do without.

You'll find some delicious mixtures of herbs in ready-made tea bags if you comb through a few delicatessens and healthfood stores. Some of my favourites have names like Cinnamon, Rose, Almond Sunset, Creamy French Vanilla, and Red Zinger. They are great to drink for pleasure and refreshment the way most people drink coffee and ordinary tea. But there are others which are quite wonderful simply because they affect the body in specific ways. Lemon verbena, for instance, is a refreshing sedative, camomile soothes the digestive tract, and both horsetail and solidago (goldenrod) are excellent natural diuretics. The teas I like best just before bed are orange blossom, which you make by boiling a few blossoms for 2–3 minutes in two cups of water, red bergamot and lemon peel, all of which are natural sedatives. This last tea comes from an Italian tradition. You make it by peeling the outer yellow skin off a lemon (which has been washed well) with a potato peeler. Pour boiling water over this and let steep for 5 minutes. Then strain and drink.

Make Way for a New Lifestyle

Eating for ageless ageing leads most people to a totally new way of living. You become more alert and more active. You will probably sleep less yet far better than before. This is because your whole system will be far clearer of toxicity than before and you will need less time for tissue repair and restoration than you do on a normal diet. You will also probably find that you are better able to deal with stress than ever. The low-calorie-high-raw way of eating provides you with high levels of potassium and rapidly restores the sodium-potassium balance in most people. This leads to increased resistance to fatigue and a greater feeling of calm stability, day in, day out. It may also set you slightly apart from your gravy-eating, hard-drinking friends and may even have them feeling slightly suspicious of you in the beginning. But it has been my experience that as soon as they find you are not trying to sell them anything – that you have a live and let live attitude to whatever they do – they show a similar respect for your new lifestyle. In fact, the people who have been the most resistant to what you are doing and the most opinionated are very often the ones who are first to become intrigued about what an ageless-ageing lifestyle might offer them. And they are usually the ones with the energy and interest to carry it out.

15
The Fast Way to Rejuvenescence

FEW THINGS SEEM as strange to the average person as the notion of going without food for several days. Just mention the idea in a group of people and wait for the reactions: 'But my dear, it's so dangerous! Don't be ridiculous, no one can fast for more than a few hours: I remember the day I skipped lunch and I felt terrible'; or 'I could never find the willpower.' In fact, almost all of the popular notions about fasting are untrue. Having personally followed more than three dozen fasts of varying lengths from one day to as long as three weeks, and having read everything I could lay my hands on about the subject over the past twenty years, I know first-hand that fasting can be one of the most rewarding experiences most people can have. There is also a mass of evidence from animal studies that regular short fasts – fasts of a day or two at a time – can slow ageing and prolong life. Periodic and controlled fasting is a superb way of detoxifying your body of cross-linkers and of reducing oxy-stress. And from an aesthetic point of view, such fasts can make you look great. They smooth out fine lines on your skin, make your eyes crystal clear and leave your face glowing with colour. Used wisely, fasting can be a highly successful technique for ageless ageing.

What is Fasting?
The word is used to describe total or partial abstinence from food for any one of a variety of reasons. There are religious fasts: Jesus went into the desert where he fasted for forty days to purify his body and prepare it to receive the Holy Spirit. In nature you find physiological fasts such as the hibernation or seasonal abstinence of specific animals or people when they feel they just can't eat. Some people fast to lose weight, of course (not a good use of fasting, however), and then there are therapeutic fasts for the purpose of

restoring and maintaining optimal health. None of these reasons for fasting is new. All of them have been practised since the beginnings of history. Pythagoras fasted for forty days before sitting his exams and then insisted that his students fast also before they could be taught by him. Ancient Egyptians used fasting as a tool for treating syphilis, and Hippocrates prescribed fasting for his patients during critical periods of illness. In the sixteenth century the famous Swiss physician Paracelsus insisted that 'Of all the remedies available, fasting is the greatest one.'

In the past century many thousands of therapeutic fasts have been conducted and recorded at such centres as Otto Buchinger's Bad Pyrmont in Germany. As a result a vast quantity of information has been collected about fasting, in Europe and America after the turn of the century, and more recently in Russia where scientists have found it to be a useful method for healing mental symptoms. Yet the orthodox medical profession remains largely ignorant of the value of fasting both for health and age-retardation. Meanwhile the average man in the street continues to regard with awe somebody who goes without food for even a day. So there are a lot of unanswered questions: Just what can fasting do? Why should anyone consider it as part of a lifestyle for ageless ageing? How safe is it? What are the pitfalls and how do you avoid them? Let's investigate the remarkable benefits of fasting as an anti-ageing tool. First let's look at the regenerative effects fasts have been shown to have on animals and humans. Then we'll explore what happens on a long fast – a fast of more than two or three days – which is something that on no account should be done except under medical supervision, preferably in a clinic atmosphere. Finally we'll examine short fasts of a few days and how for healthy people they can form an exciting and enjoyable (yes, *enjoyable*; most people who look on fasting with distaste have never experienced its physical benefits and the heightened state of mental and emotional clarity it can bring) vacation from the kind of habitual eating most of us find ourselves doing.

Rejuvenescence Starts Here

Rejuvenescence is an old-fashioned word which means 'the acquiring of fresh vitality and the renewal of youthful characteristics in the cells and tissues of the body'. It is a word which was used frequently early on in the twentieth century by clinicians and researchers investigating and making use of fasting as a natural technique for healing and for enhancing health. Like fasting itself, in the face of allopathic medicine, the word has rather fallen from use. But it is an excellent word to describe the remarkably revitalizing effect of going without food for periods of a few days (which most people can safely carry out at home on their own provided, of course, that their doctor approves) and several weeks – something that should under no circumstances be done unless you are in a controlled environment under medical supervision. If you want to look in depth at the physiological effects of fasting you have to look back to the time in which it was seriously studied.

The Invincible Worm

In the first decade or two of the twentieth century C.M. Child at the University of Chicago carried out lengthy studies of the effect of fasting on animal life. He took a group of flatworms which had become old and infirm and fasted them for months until they were reduced greatly in size. When he began to feed them again and they re-grew to normal size he found they were functioning as young animals again. Similar studies were carried out on earthworms by a British researcher about the same time. He fed these creatures their usual foods but one of the worms he isolated from the rest and fasted at periodic intervals. In every other way the life and diet of all the worms were the same. This isolated worm lived on while nineteen generations of worms in the colony lived and died. In 1915 Child published a book called *Senescence and Rejuvenescence* in which he describes the effect of fasting on lower forms of life. He says, 'Partial starvation inhibits senescence. The starveling is brought back from an advanced age to the beginning of post-embryonic life; it is almost reborn.'

Interesting though these results are, they were performed on very low forms of life which, unlike human beings and other mammals, have an ability for regeneration lacking in more complex organisms. However a number of studies have also been done on mammals which also highlight the relationship between fasting and age-retardation. For instance, scientists at the Gerontology Research Center in Baltimore, Maryland, discovered that when rats are fed every other day they live sixty-three weeks longer than those allowed to eat all they want. They also remain more active later in life than their well-fed cage mates. Rejuvenescence effects have been often reported by people who have fasted and by fasting researchers. When researcher A.J. Carlson at the University of

Chicago fasted a forty-year-old man for fourteen days, he reported that at the end of the fast his tissues were physiologically in a similar condition to those of a seventeen-year-old. When Gandhi, an enthusiastic periodic faster, was examined in May of 1933 on the tenth day of a fast his physicians reported that 'despite his sixty-four years, from a physiological point of view the Indian leader was as healthy as a man of forty'. Otto Buchinger, who is generally considered *the* European expert on fasting, has conducted thousands of fasts in the treatment of many age-related diseases and has demonstrated that fasting can be an effective technique for healing – from high blood pressure and arthritis to rheumatism, early diabetes, angina, early arteriosclerosis, vascular ailments, menopausal symptoms, allergies and nerve disorders, to mention only a few.

Nature's Wrinkle-Banisher

The aesthetic benefits of fasting as an improver of good looks and a rejuvenator of skin are well known. That is why (often in modified form such as a juice fast) fasting is the cornerstone of treatment at most of the famous spas in Europe where people spend a fortnight and return home afterwards looking ten years younger. Lines and wrinkles on the face become softened even after a fast of a few days, and blotches, pimples and discolorations disappear. Skin texture and colour also improve and eyes become bright and clear. The elimination of wastes and toxic substances from the body which a fast brings about clears the skin and the eyes and can give the flesh a new softness which our polluted atmosphere and poor eating habits take out. It also helps restore elasticity to the muscles. People who hadn't seen me during my first fast were amazed at how it had changed me physically. Not knowing that I had been fasting, they came up with some rather amusing hypotheses to explain the improvement. The most common was that I must have fallen in love. (That, alas, is one of the things which fasting *cannot* do for you.)

Changes from the Word Go

Drastic changes take place in your body right from the first missed meal. Almost immediately wastes stored in your tissues are thrown off – sometimes at an incredible rate. This can lead (and usually does) to a coating of the tongue and teeth with an unpleasant tasting stuff and in some people even to a headache or a feeling of being unwell which lasts for perhaps a few hours or as long as a day. For this reason fasting experts generally insist that their patients follow a special diet composed of raw fruits, juices and vegetables for a day or two before beginning a medically supervised long fast, to start clearing the system somewhat and avoid too drastic an elimination of waste products all at once. Twelve hours after you begin your fast your body starts to use whatever glucose it has stored in the liver. This supply lasts less than a day. Then body chemistry begins to change. Abstinence from food forces the body to produce and circulate *ketone bodies* – normal products of fat metabolism which can be oxidized to produce energy. Elevated levels of ketones occur since fat in the body is being rapidly metabolized. There are two points during an extended fast during which *acetone* excreted through the urine and the skin reaches a peak – usually on the fourth and fifth day and then again on the ninth or tenth. This gives some fasters a scent of acetone on the surface of the skin and can make your system very acidic, which is why many experts in fasting insist that it is better to fast on fresh vegetable and fresh (non-citrus) fruit juices whose alkalinity can balance any excess acidity.

American researchers have found that your body adjusts itself to the fasting state by utilizing these ketones as fuel for brain and nerve cells. A mild state of ketosis on a fast is fine. If it becomes too severe it can be damaging, particularly if the patient already suffers from kidney or heart trouble or is pregnant. But in these conditions fasting is not advisable anyway. Fasting also tends to lower blood pressure, which is useful in the treatment of hypertensive patients. From the beginning of a fast there is also often a slight increase in temperature which lasts only a few days and which most fasting experts attribute to the rapid burning of stored toxins. Sometimes on about the thirteenth day the level of ketones in the blood serum rises drastically to as much as ten times above the previous level, while alkali reserves fall, and temporary disturbances can take place in the fat, cholesterol, sugar and diastase levels in the blood. Often on these days the faster feels slightly unwell. Doctors working with fasting have termed these periods the 'crisis of acidity'. They stress that it is a natural occurrence in the fast, nothing more than symptoms of the body's readjustment. These symptoms disappear quickly and don't occur again throughout the rest of the fast, but they can be a cause of great concern to the uninformed and only serve to underline the necessity for careful medical supervision on a long fast.

Cleansing the Depths

The healing, rejuvenating and regenerating effects of a fast come from its ability to eliminate toxic waste products from the body – sometimes wastes which have been stored in the cells and tissues for almost a lifetime. For a long time critics of fasting insisted that these wastes were the invention of overactive minds and that they didn't really exist. Now laboratory tests are even able to measure the fact that things such as *xanthoprotein* and *indican* are eliminated rapidly during a fast. Wastes which accumulate as a result of the build-up of metabolic by-products and from exposure to environmental pollution from foods and water, as well as from excess stress, are prime movers both in lowering vitality and in the development of degenerative diseases and ageing, because they cause auto-intoxication of the system. Most of the metabolic toxins which play a decisive role in the origin of disease and premature ageing come from protein metabolism, although carbohydrate metabolism also produces some, such as pyruvic acid and a form of lactic acid, as does fat metabolism.

An organism can only stay healthy and youthful so long as it is able efficiently to detoxify itself of its metabolic intermediary products, waste products or *autotoxins* as they are sometimes called. On an extended fast the material which is burnt first from the body for energy comes from superfluous fat and unwanted matter. Some experts in fasting believe that one of the reasons it is so useful in retarding the rate at which the body ages is that it may be able to break down and use as fuel cross-linked proteins which make it possible then for your body to build new collagen and new cells. Fasting may well be nature's own tool for breaking down and clearing out morbid cross-linked proteins – something which gerontologists such as Bjorksten and others have been searching for years to find a chemical way of doing.

The Fast High

The experience of fasting is a highly subjective one. Many fasters claim that their concentration is improved and that they are better able to carry out creative tasks like painting or writing. (I will often do a fast of a week or two before beginning to work on a book.) Naturally fasters lose weight. How much varies tremendously. Weight loss is greater in people who are most overweight. It usually varies between 4½lb to as much as 10lb a week. The average is about 7lb. You lose weight more rapidly at the beginning of a fast.

Most fasters sleep less than usual and feel better for it – although this is usually not true of patients who previously suffered from insomnia. They often sleep more – sometimes as much as eighteen hours a day in the beginning. A few people, particularly those who have been chronically ill, experience a feeling of weakness and tiredness and seem to need a lot of time simply to lie around and do nothing. However there are also many cases recorded where just the opposite is true. The once famous heavyweight fighter Harry Wills always used fasts during his training period before a big fight because he claimed they gave him strength, and both American and Swedish athletes have been known to carry out long walks – of two weeks or more – while fasting. Experts on fasting say that usually patients who are weaker at the beginning of the fast will tend to gain strength rapidly from the beginning of the period of abstinence. Sexual desire is usually reduced during a fast although in some instances people have reported an increase in sexual activity. In any case it returns almost immediately after the fast is broken – often with renewed vigour.

Keep Moving

Fasting for more than a day or two tends to lower your metabolic rate so that you can begin to feel rather sluggish and lazy. It is important that you don't let this happen, by making sure you get plenty of exercise such as long walks in the open air. I often use a bouncer – one of those mini-trampolines which you can tuck behind the sofa in the sitting-room when you are not using it – when I am fasting. Bouncing, or rebounding as it is sometimes called, is a pleasurable way of exercising, either gently or hard. (I like watching films on a video or listening to music while I am exercising.) This kind of exercise encourages good lymphatic drainage and as such helps to get rid of the sludge that your body is burning up in its tissues and then to eliminate it. Long fasts also tend to lower body temperature. You will need to wear warmer clothing than you ordinarily would while on a fast.

Many uninformed people worry a lot about vitamin and mineral losses on a fast. While it is true that vitamins and mineral stores do get drawn on during a fast, almost all physicians with much experience in fasting are quick to reassure you that it is nothing to worry about in a healthy person, for any loss is quickly replenished when you start eating again. In fact the fasting organism is exceptionally efficient. You use less of everything when you abstain from foods.

Fasting and Mental Health

American physician and fasting expert Alan Cott believes, as do most doctors with a long experience of fasting their patients, that a long fast can be a powerful force for restoring mental health. He has fasted about 300 chronically ill schizophrenics – the kind of people who tend to end up in the back wards of mental hospitals – and found that after twenty-five and thirty-two days without food about 65 per cent of them improved enough to leave hospital and return to life with some degree of being able to function in society. Of these people, the ones who after their fast stayed on a well-balanced vegetarian diet were least likely to experience any relapse. At the University of Athens, scientists have recently discovered that fasting blocks the brain's uptake of the neurotransmitter dopamine. This may be one of the reasons why it can be useful in the treatment of mental illness, for many medications given to control schizophrenia do the same thing.

British and Russian scientists have found that fasting raises the level of *serotonin* – another neurotransmitter which is important in bringing relaxation to the body and mind and in harmonizing mood. Russian scientists such as Yuri Nikolayev have also had considerable success in rehabilitating mental patients. Cott quotes Nikolayev, who believes that fasting 'purifies every cell in the body. I am sure that 99 per cent of sick people suffer because of improper nourishment. People simply do not understand that they litter their bodies with many unnatural foods and... because of this ... poisonous substances are collected in the body. If you are interested in being in good mental and physical health and in increasing your vitality, start to work today *with* nature, not against her.' Nikolayev believes, as does Cott, that fasting helps the body mobilize itself against many ills. And also that when you temporarily stop putting food into the body it gives it a chance to catch up with elimination, forcing it to draw off stored toxins from the tissues and then to excrete them. Finally, he believes that the practice biochemically rebalances the whole system. Both the elimination of toxic wastes and this rebalancing act are probably responsible for the way fasting brings a sense of being uplifted emotionally and very clear mentally.

Crystal Consciousness

The first time I fasted (about twenty-five years ago), I did a three week fast under the guidance of a doctor friend. I was going through a particularly difficult period of my life where there were serious decisions to be made and I felt somehow I didn't have the clarity to make them. My friend suggested that if I fasted for several days it might clear my mind so that I would be able to know better how I really felt. When I began the fast I had no idea how long it would last. The first three days passed quickly with the occasional pang of hunger, which I ignored. In fact, they were not *hunger pangs* at all, I learned later, but *appetite demands*, for when you are used to eating all the time (I have a real passion for food and have always tended to use it for comfort as much as for nourishment) and suddenly there is no food to be had, you feel hungry. But after the first three days this 'hunger' passed and never returned again during the whole length of the fast – much to my amazement. I felt well physically and I had lots of strength. However I found I needed to exercise every day or I tended to become sluggish, so I took long walks in the country. As the fast continued I found I felt more clear mentally and more emotionally centred – in fact more balanced than I had ever felt in my whole life. I would awaken in the morning feeling full of joy. The world looked beautiful to me in a calm and quiet way. All the creatures I saw, from the spider on my bedroom window to the neighbour's dog, seemed marvellous, the way a coloured picture book looks to you when you are still six years old.

During the three weeks I was fasting I was working (something fasting experts advise you not to do) but I tried to spend as much time as I could alone and resting. My friend, the doctor, advised me not to allow myself to be with any people with whom I didn't feel at ease. 'If anyone tries to lay his problems on you,' he said, 'politely excuse yourself by saying you are fasting and can't be disturbed, and get away from him.' I did. A few acquaintances were offended at my insistence that I remain calm and not get involved in their troubles, but my real friends understood and encouraged me. They noticed that each day my skin became smoother and my complexion brighter, and my eyes clearer, and were almost as pleased about the changes as I was. Two of them even began fasts themselves after seeing what mine had done for me.

But no matter how pleasing the physical effects of my first fast, what were most important of all to me were its psychological ones. My head became clearer and clearer. After the first few days my vision was so sharpened it was as if I was looking at the world through a crystal glass. It is difficult to describe the changes that took place in my thinking and my emotions during the fast. I can only say that the world looked different. I realized that there was so much beauty around me which I ordinarily miss in my hurry from one task to another. Fasting made me stop and think, stop and feel. I found delight in the simplest of things – just sitting under a tree, or washing vegetables, or combing my hair. Everything seemed important. I felt I wanted to do everything with awareness. I also gained a sense of distance from my own problems which enabled me to make the decisions facing me calmly and quietly. As a result, since then, whenever I feel myself hung up over something or whenever I feel I am not seeing things clearly I will often quietly fast for a day or two until I feel clear again. To some people this may seem an eccentricity, but not, I suspect, to anyone who has actually tried fasting.

It is the End that Matters
Something that almost nobody understands except doctors proficient in fasting their patients, and people who themselves have undergone long fasts – is that the way a fast is broken is as important as the fast itself in bringing about lasting benefits. When you go without food for a week, or even a few weeks, your digestive system has a complete rest. One of the results of this is that digestive secretions slow down and eventually stop altogether. Also your body becomes highly sensitive to whatever you put in it. With what and with how much food you break your fast matters a lot. Break it sensibly on small quantities of raw food and you will find that a week or two later you will continue to feel as well and as clear as you did during your period of abstinence, but even stronger. Break it carelessly by eating too much or the wrong kind of thing and you can throw your organism into complete chaos, a chaos which can result in mental and emotional confusion, fatigue, and even serious illness.

Most experts believe that the best way to break a long fast on which you have had nothing but water is by eating a couple of apples throughout the morning and then taking a glass of fresh vegetable juice or wholesome home made vegetable soup which contains no flour. Then the next day you can begin the 'build-up' programme which takes you back to normal eating *gradually* over a period of about a week: prunes or figs soaked overnight in water for breakfast, a fresh raw salad with a little yoghurt dressing for lunch and some fresh fruit with, perhaps, a piece of crispbread or a sugarless oatcake spread with about a third of an ounce of butter. On about the fourth or fifth day after breaking a fast you can have

Birchermuesli for breakfast, and soup and salad for lunch and dinner, and by the end of the week you can eat your first fish or meat if you want them. This slow transition back to normal eating is absolutely essential in fasting. In fact, control over the breaking of a fast is one of two essential reasons why fasting for more than a few days at a time must be done under medical supervision. The other reason is that fasting, although a perfectly healthy and beneficial practice when carried out by the rules, is also quite an extraordinary state. It is *not* a game. And, until you are absolutely sure of how it works and have yourself experienced a number of fasts of different lengths, you need the support of a doctor or a trained professional who can guide you and reassure you. This is particularly important in the face of the kind of well-meaning but really very destructive 'advice' you tend to get from people who have never fasted and generally know nothing about it. Comments like, 'You mustn't fast, it weakens the heart and you could have a heart attack' or even, 'Oh you poor darling, you must be *starving*, do have just a little something with us' can be very detrimental to the inexperienced faster. The friendly medical practitioner who monitors your progress and reassures you that all is well helps counteract all this beautifully.

It is also important that while fasting your state of mind is a positive one and that you are at peace. A genuine willingness to fast and an optimistic attitude towards it are essential for therapeutic fasting. As Otto Buchinger (the European physician who is considered a world expert on fasting) says:

> The mental attitude of the patient is of fundamental importance in the direction of the metabolic processes of the whole body. (This is the reason why it is necessary to explain to the patient the nature of the cure before it is undertaken and to guide him psychically during the cure.) Hunger brings about an inward position of coercion and protest. This in turn leads, via the central nervous system, to a dysfunction of the capillary circulation as well as to disturbances of the organs.

Do-It-Yourself Fasting

For many people a short fast – a fast of from a couple of days to a week or more – carried out once a year (preferably in spring when the earth's regenerative powers are rising strongly) can be an excellent way of periodically eliminating any stored wastes, regenerating new tissue, clearing your mind, balancing emotions and making you look five or ten years younger very quickly. But it must be done either at a spa or clinic where fasting is well understood and regularly carried out, or under the wise care of a physician oriented towards natural methods of healing and age-retardation. Although fasters claim that complications are rare, if they do occur they need to be dealt with professionally. Fasts of from one to three days are different. The general medical consensus (which includes the opinions of a great number of doctors for whom the very idea of fasting is anathema) is that, so long as you are in good health, this kind of short-term self-chosen abstinence can only do you good (particularly in our overly indulgent world) provided you go about it in the right way and provided your doctor approves.

If you can, prepare for your fast by eating only raw fruits and vegetables the day before you begin. Then spend from one to three days on fresh spring (not tap) water. Drink herbal teas if you like but adamantly no tea or coffee. Be sure to get plenty of rest. Fasting is an ideal time to spend most of the day in bed with a good book every once in a while but make sure you also get whatever exercise is normal for you during your abstinence. If you get any symptoms such as a headache from going without food for a day or two this is a sign that your body is rapidly detoxifying itself. Rest if you can until it passes – for it usually does within a few hours. Your tongue can also be coated with white or yellow fur. This too is a sign of rapid elimination. After a few weeks of eating in a low-calorie-high-potency way you will find soon that you no longer get any symptoms at all except a kind of 'lightening' of mind and body and perhaps increased energy during the days of your fast.

Return to your everyday eating habits slowly. Your body needs time to readjust. Some longevists fast for a day or two a week all year round to decrease the number of calories they take in, to give their system a rest from food and having to deal with it, to eliminate wastes built up and to clear their minds. It is something which I have tried for periods and I must admit I thrive on it. While everybody else is making noises about how much willpower you must have to do this every week, you keep trying to tell them the truth and they never believe you: there isn't much willpower needed. The sense of reward which comes with regular fasts such as this and the uplift they bring far exceed any qualm about giving up a meal or two. Fasting like this can also make you so much more aware of the delicious textures, tastes and colours of food when you resume eating. For me, however, a short fast will never replace the quite exceptional pleasure of a longer fasting 'cure'. It is something that, having discovered its benefits a quarter of a century ago, I think I will never want to be without doing once a year. But whether you choose a short fast on your own or a long fast under supervision, one thing is sure: any technique as powerful as fasting needs to be treated with the utmost respect and never entered into lightly.

16
Spring-Cleaning for Youth

NO MATTER HOW sparse and how good your diet or how many anti-oxidants you take, no matter how conscientiously you deal with stress and how enthusiastically you exercise – all of which are central to ageless ageing – it can be helpful periodically to spring-clean your body from within. Controlled fasts are not the only way of doing this. In fact I have come to believe that they are not even the *best* way. The natural law approach to age retardation and the long tradition on which it is based also offer a number of other simple methods. Some – such as a spring-clean semi-fast or the sauna – are helpful when used every few weeks, while others, such as techniques for improving lymphatic drainage, can be used to advantage every few days or even more often. The whole purpose of spring-cleaning is to stimulate your body's eliminative capabilities so that any sluggishness in the blood and lymph circulation and any stasis in the tissues is cleared away. Then whatever toxicity may be present – heavy metals and cross-linkers for instance – can be broken down and eliminated via the skin and lungs, bladder and colon before it can cause degenerative damage and premature ageing to your body.

Toxicity and Ageing
As we've seen, apart from inadequate nutrition, the primary cause of premature ageing – and all the fatigue, cell damage and disease which accompany it – is a build-up of waste products which are toxic to the system. They result in poor circulation to and from the cells and in a stagnation of cellular fluids. A continuous interchange takes place between your body's trillions of cells and their surrounding interstitial fluids. This is where nutrients and oxygen are exchanged for waste products from the cells. Wastes are then

picked up by minute lymphatic tubules or ducts and sent through the lymph vessels to be detoxified. It is an exchange regulated by subtle electrochemical processes. Living cells will only thrive when both nutrients and oxygen are well supplied and toxic wastes are concurrently removed and eliminated from the body. The methods for encouraging this are extraordinarily simple yet their effects can be remarkably profound. Many are also immediately experienced in terms of improved good looks and vitality and a new-found sense of calm well-being. Let's look at the Long Weekend Spring-Clean Diet to start with.

Long Weekend Spring-Clean

This is a method I like to use when for one reason or another (such as after Christmas celebrations or living in hotels) I have not been able to eat the same kind of foods I do at home, or when I am feeling tired and need a lift. It takes three days to carry out. Ideally you should eat all raw foods the day before you begin but this is not always possible. It is an ideal way to regenerate yourself over a long quiet weekend.

On rising, or at 9 a.m., each day you begin with a cup of herb tea – not too hot. You can sweeten it with a little honey if you like.

Day 1

9 a.m.	Herb tea
11 a.m.	8oz fresh fruit (not citrus) or vegetable juice
1 p.m.	1 cup potassium broth
4 p.m.	Herb tea
7 p.m.	8oz fresh fruit (not citrus) or vegetable juice
9 p.m.	1 cup potassium broth

Day 2

9 a.m.	Herb tea plus half an apple – be sure to chew it thoroughly
11 a.m.	Fresh fruit or vegetable juice
1 p.m.	Cup of potassium broth
4 p.m.	Herb tea
7 p.m.	Cup of potassium broth
9 p.m.	Fresh fruit or vegetable juice

Day 3

9 a.m.	A dish of prunes which have been soaked overnight in water
11 a.m.	Fresh fruit or vegetable juice
1 p.m.	Salad of raw vegetables with a little yoghurt dressing
4 p.m.	An apple
7 p.m.	Fresh fruit or vegetable juice
9 p.m.	Cup of potassium broth

During the Weekend Spring-Clean you can drink as much spring water as you like. It is important that you take a brisk walk in the open air for at least half an hour each day. You can continue to work if you like but it is especially pleasant to carry out over a long weekend when you have time to yourself. You must not smoke, or drink alcohol, tea or coffee. Herb teas are available from healthfood stores. So is potassium broth which is made from fresh vegetables and herbs and contains no additives. The best you make yourself simply by boiling masses of fresh vegetables. Alternatively you can buy it in little cubes over which you pour boiling water, or in a powder form which I prefer. The best I have found is called Low Salt Marigold Swiss Vegetable Bouillon. You can make your own fresh vegetable or fruit and vegetable juices (half apple and half carrot is a particularly delicious and effective combination to use) provided you have a centrifuge juice extractor. Otherwise look for those processed by low heat to preserve their natural enzymes and nutrients. They too are available in health-food stores. The Biotta juices from Germany are the best. Daily baths are a must during the Long Weekend regime and you will probably find you need to brush your teeth more often than usual since your body will be rapidly eliminating wastes and both teeth and tongue can become coated when this occurs. *Skin-brushing* is excellent for hastening the eliminative processes. Do exercise regularly. Do not take a sauna during the Long Weekend Spring-Clean however. On the fourth day simply return to your normal low-calorie-high-potency way of eating, with particular emphasis on raw foods for a day or two.

Skin-Brushing Works Wonders

Skin-brushing is an old and well-proven European technique for getting rid of toxic wastes from the body, both because it stimulates lymphatic drainage and because it increases the quantity of waste which is eliminated directly through the surface of the skin (a staggering one third of our wastes can be eliminated this way). I first learned the technique more than fifteen years ago. It was taught to me by a West Country physician named Phillip Kilsby who used it in conjunction with a high-raw diet as part of a programme for healing many kinds of illness – from migraine and arthritis to high blood pressure and depression. When he first told me how effective it was in eliminating wastes and toxins from the body I did not believe him. He suggested a little experiment by which I could prove to myself just how effective it was at eliminating rubbish through the surface of the skin. He said, 'Take a washcloth or flannel and wet it then wring it out well. Now brush your skin dry using the directions below. When you have finished rub the flannel over the surface you have brushed all over just once. Then hang the flannel up and don't use it again until tomorrow when you perform exactly the same routine. After three or four days smell the flannel.' That was all the proof needed!

You can either use skin-brushing on its own or together with the Weekend Spring-Clean. I use it regularly, year round, several times a week. Many of the natural techniques for detoxifying the body are more effective if your body is not allowed to become accustomed to them by doing them every day. Skin brushing, for instance, can be done steadily for three weeks with a week's break before resuming it again. After even a week of skin-brushing you will also notice an improvement in the look and feel of your skin. After a few weeks it even seems to improve muscle tone although I have never been able to figure out why this should happen.

Here's How

You will need a natural vegetable-bristle brush (the long-handled kind is best) but a hemp glove will also do. Such brushes and gloves can be found in most health-food shops or good chemists.

The brush should be kept dry. It is best to brush first thing in the morning before you shower. Brush the entire skin surface, except for your face. Begin with your feet, including the soles, then move up your legs, front and back, with firm sweeping strokes. Brush from your hands up your arms and across your shoulders, then brush your back and buttocks. On your front, brush a little more gently – your neck, chest and abdomen. In the abdominal area use a clockwise circular motion. To begin with brush fairly gently, increasing the firmness of the strokes as your body becomes more accustomed to it.

After brushing take a shower. If you are brave you can alternate with warm and cold water (always beginning with warm and ending with cold). This is an excellent way of getting the circulation going and speeding up elimination.

Stimulating Lymphatic Drainage

Skin-brushing is not only effective as a natural law tool for detoxification because it stimulates the release of wastes through your skin's surface. It also encourages better lymphatic drainage – something which is vitally important to (as Bjorksten says) making sure metabolic processes run *cleanly* and *efficiently*. Your body's lymph system is, amongst other things, a kind of metabolic rubbish dump. It helps the body rid itself of dead cells, toxins, metabolic wastes, pathogenic bacteria, foreign substances and other assorted junk the cells cast off. Unlike the circulatory system, in which the circulation of blood is controlled by the pumping of the heart, the lymphatic system has no such pump. The plasma which has seeped through capillary walls gathers in the tissues and then slowly enters the lymphatic channels. These are tiny vessels with one-way valves in them for carrying lymph, along with whatever small bits of foreign matter, wastes and bacteria it has gathered, through the lymph nodes and eventually back into the bloodstream.

The normal contractions and relaxation of your muscles and the force of gravity on the body keep the lymph flowing. They act to pump the lymph back through its channels and eliminate these wastes. Regular vigorous exercise encourages this elimination. It brings about a general flushing of the wastes from tissue fluid and then helps them be carried away through the lymphatic tree of vessels until eventually they empty into the subclavian veins beneath the collarbone and are eliminated from the body through the actions of all the excretory organs – the skin, lungs, kidneys and colon. In Europe some of the finest natural treatments for healing involve a kind of massage dubbed 'lymphatic drainage' which helps the body do this. It is not only used to treat serious chronic illness and fatigue but even as a beauty treatment for women on the face. Skin-brushing stimulates the tissues beneath the skin, encouraging efficient lymphatic drainage. It is an extraordinarily efficient technique for cleansing the lymphatic system and for clearing away waste materials from the cells all over the body as well as those which as in the case of cellulite in women have become trapped in interstitial spaces where they are held by hardened connective tissue and where they build up to create pockets of water, toxins and fat that make the skin look like *peau d'orange*. Skin-brushing is something any woman with cellulite should do twice a day.

The Breath of Youth

Chinese medicine (which I spent three years studying and working with) has a long tradition of natural-law ageless ageing. And a great deal of it centres around the use of the breath. This is something to which we give little attention in the west and it is strange to think that specific breathing techniques are so ignored when, as we have seen in Chapter 3, the body's use of oxygen is *the* central determinant of the rate at which we age. Despite the negative effects of oxygen described earlier, every one of our cells needs a continual supply of oxygen. It is this oxygen that feeds our brain, sparks metabolism and calms nerves. One of the reasons why regular aerobic exercise is so beneficial in slowing down the rate at which you age and warding off degenerative diseases is because it improves your use of oxygen. So can learning to breathe fully. It can also improve your mood, increase your resistance to colds and illness, and improve sleep as well. Full breathing is also an important tool for encouraging waste elimination. It is a kind of spring-cleaning process that can go on all year round, every day of your life.

Few people breathe fully. Most of us, particularly if we have sedentary jobs, *breathe high* – that is we breathe quickly and shallowly, concentrating the inhalations in the upper chest area, which is the part of the lungs which holds the smallest quantity of air. Not only does this kind of breathing inhibit oxygen intake, it can also encourage the lungs to atrophy and to lose much of their natural elasticity – something which is a common occurrence as people get older. Other people, who allow the air to flow deeper into their lungs are *mid-breathers* – an improvement over breathing high because it encourages the ribcage to move and brings more oxygen into the lungs for body use. But to make the best use of oxygen for ageless ageing it's important to develop the habit of taking *total breaths* so they become your normal way of breathing.

The Total Breath

This is not something which you can learn overnight, for there is nothing more unconscious and habitual than the way we breathe and that takes time and a little persistent effort to change. In breathing totally, all of your breathing apparatus comes into play – the chest and ribs are lifted, but not by themselves. The intercostal muscles expand the ribs outward to create a large space in which your lungs can inflate to their maximum. Finally the diaphragm moves down, pulling the lower ribs outward, which lets even the very bottom of your lungs fill up completely with air. With total breathing a much higher proportion of your lung power is used, as are most of your chest, rib and stomach muscles. Practise it lying down for five minutes a couple of times a day – perhaps just on awakening or just before going to sleep – and gradually it will become an automatic way of breathing which will not only help in ageless ageing but will also improve your resistance to fatigue, improve the glow of your skin and help protect you from minor illness.

Here's How

1. Lying flat on your back with a small pillow beneath your neck, place one hand on your abdomen and rest the other on one side of your ribcage. Now inhale slowly through your nose while imagining that you are sending your breath to a place about 2 inches below your navel. Your tummy will start to well outwards, rather like a balloon. This has the effect of filling the lower part of your lungs with fresh air.

2. As the in-breath continues, let it fill the rest of your stomach and then expand your ribcage outwards to the side as well as the mid-section of your chest. You can feel this side expansion by keeping your hand against one side of your ribcage and making sure it moves outward.

3. Now let the fresh breath fill the upper part of your chest area as well, watching it as it expands outward and to the side. (The whole process of inhalation should take about 5 seconds altogether.)

4. Hold your breath for another 5 seconds. (In time you will find you can hold it for much longer, which gives your lungs a good opportunity to absorb all the oxygen available to them.)

5. Now exhale following the same process you did in inhaling: first, contract your lower abdomen gently to move the air upwards,

then, as the lower lungs deflate, you should feel the ribcage contracting again, followed by the upper chest. This process too should take about 5 seconds.

6. Rest for a second or two before beginning the whole cycle again.

Whereas detoxification by improved breathing can be used every day of your life to advantage, the final technique for spring-cleaning – self-induced fever – is best used only periodically. But then it can work wonders.

Feverpower

Like many old wives' tales the adage 'sweat it out' is beginning to look like good advice. For generations medicine has tried to suppress fever, believing it to be a state detrimental to the body. Latest findings show that fever can not only significantly strengthen your body's defence system, it appears to be a critical component in immune function. As such, so the new findings indicate, when it occurs naturally, for instance as a response to infection, it should not be completely eliminated by drugs the way we have been wont to do. Fever weakens the force of invading enemies and is a potent positive force for fighting infections. Some scientists now believe that, because of its many immune-supporting characteristics, even when fever is artificially induced in a healthy body by saunas, Turkish baths or vigorous aerobic exercise it can act as a powerful prophylactic to ageing, it can increase vitality and it can help provide you with a high level of well-being.

This approach to fever is anything but new. Ancient Greek physicians considered fever a beneficial sign of vitality in an organism. They believed that disease was the result of an imbalance between the four humours – blood, phlegm, yellow bile and black bile – and they considered fever a means of burning off the bad humours and clearing the body of them. To this end they employed sudorific (sweat-producing) herbs, steam and hot baths to treat fevers in their patients. Such practices went on well into the seventeenth century when the famous British physician Thomas Sydenham commented that 'Fever is Nature's engine which she brings into the field to remove her enemy.' Then in the middle of the last century, with the discovery of antipyretic (temperature-lowering) drugs such as aspirin, doctors began to insist on reducing fevers when they occurred. Drugs such as aspirin not only lower bodily temperature, they also eliminate many aches and pains associated with fever, thanks to their analgesic properties. This makes patients feel temporarily better. So gradually both doctor and patient began to lean heavily on the use of these drugs to suppress fever, and fever came to be considered a negative thing – something to be eliminated as rapidly and effectively as possible.

Recently researchers such as Matthew J. Kluger, a professor of physiology at the University of Michigan Medical School, have begun to examine the phenomenon of fever afresh and to ask questions such as: Just what happens when the body is plunged into a feverous state? Why did evolution develop the phenomenon of temperature-raising fever in its creatures? What is the purpose of this remarkable response? What Kluger and others have discovered is that fever's occurrence is not a sign that something is wrong with your body's temperature control system. Instead, a superbly modulated, deliberately chosen temperature has been created, at which several important physiological and biochemical events occur to heal the body.

Fever's Bounty

Among their known benefits (and there are probably many as yet unknown), even slight elevations in temperature not only increase white-cell concentrations, they make the body's defence army of white blood cells more mobile so they can reach any site of infection quicker. There is also considerable evidence that fever makes them more effective in engulfing and destroying invading micro-organisms. Indeed it appears to make many other immune functions more effective too. For instance interferon, one of the body's natural anti-viral, anti-cancer (and therefore probably anti-ageing as well) chemicals, about which we have heard so much in the news lately, has been shown to be more effective at elevated temperatures. Of course illness is not the only way that many of the beneficial effects of fever can be brought about. EP stands for *endogenous pyrogen* which is a low-weight protein produced by leucocytes to help destroy infection in the body. After a good workout of aerobic exercise, substances appear in the blood which have identical characteristics to EP.

Naturopaths have long insisted that fever is an important force for healing the body. They claim that controlled overheating of the body also increases the rate of metabolic processes as a whole and stimulates the functioning of the endocrine system. Since Hippocrates – some 2,400 years ago – doctors have been using artificial methods of inducing fever, for instance giving the herb *Echinacea* or putting people into sweat baths or steam baths and applying hot compresses, to improve their vitality or stimulate the body's natural healing processes. The new fever research has begun to explain why many of their time-tested methods work. It is also beginning to lend credence to the beliefs of the Turks and Russians that periodic steam baths are strengthening to health and vitality, and to those of the Scandinavians, who have used saunas as a means of both stimulating immune response and spring-cleaning the body from within – two useful tools for ageless ageing.

Words of Warning

Despite new findings that fever is of benefit to the body, there is every indication that it needs to be treated with respect and that your physician is the best guide to dealing with any illness. For extreme fever can have a damaging effect on a body. And there are some people in whom the benefits of fever may well be outweighed by the risks involved. For instance, in a pregnant woman a high fever could potentially damage her unborn child, and young children with very high fever can be subject to convulsions. Also, fevers in very old people have to be carefully watched because of possible damage they could do to the heart. But for most of us the new findings indicate that it could be potentially harmful not to allow a fever to work its natural course. When Kluger and other researchers have given aspirin to infected animals the animals have shown a significant increase in deaths.

Fever as a Prophylactic

Provided you are fit, aerobic exercise such as cycling, running, walking very briskly, swimming, rowing or dancing is probably the best way of all to benefit from small elevations in temperature. Saunas too can be helpful provided you are in good health, don't overdo them and follow the basic guidelines. A sauna helps make your joints more supple while it soothes your muscles and refreshes the mind. It is also an excellent adjunct to any serious anti-cellulite programme for a woman. And early spring, when one's body is suffering from too much heavy winter food and clothing, too little fresh air and exercise, is an excellent time to make use of it. Here are the guide lines:

- Give yourself lots of time. It will do most for you if you take it leisurely so you have time for several sessions in the heat, with short rests in between and a rest of at least thirty minutes – preferably an hour – after you are through.

- Never take a sauna until at least two hours after a meal and never take a sauna during a juice fast. (It is an excellent idea to use the sauna the day before a juice fast or special eliminating diet begins, however.)

- Never take a sauna if you have the symptoms of an illness.

- Wear little or nothing in the sauna – a towel wrapped around you is more than enough. The more you wear, the less effective will the heat treatment be.

- Take off any jewellery and your watch. They become very hot.

- Stay in the sauna room for only 5–10 minutes at a stretch. Then plunge into cold water or take a cold shower and rest before going back in.

- Don't water the stones during your first session and be sparing with the moisture you put on afterwards.

- Lie down in the sauna room if you can or sit quietly. Once you are used to the heat you can move to a higher bench.

- Take at least a half-hour rest at the end to let your body readjust to the normal temperature of the room. This is just as important as the sauna itself to make sure you reap all the benefits.

- Don't towel-dry yourself afterwards. Instead let the air dry your skin naturally. Then you can have a shower.

Not only can heat applied to the surface of the body be useful as a spring-cleaning tool, it also has a role to play in skin-care. Steaming your face over a pan of hot water into which you've tossed a handful of herbs such as camomile or peppermint can do for skin what the sauna does for the whole body. It will leave it deep-cleaned, fresh and glowing. Let's look now at what can be done using high-tech biochemistry to slow the ageing process.

17
Anti-Oxidants – Keys to Ageless Ageing

SINCE THE 1950s gerontologists have reported success in retarding ageing and promoting longevity using chemical substances, both natural and artificial, which protect living systems from oxidation and free radical damage – anti-oxidant chemicals and free radical scavengers. They are usually grouped together under the label 'anti-oxidants'. Using anti-oxidants, researchers have been able significantly to extend the life of laboratory animals as well as to prevent, or at least to postpone, much of the degeneration of illnesses such as cancer and lung diseases which are usually associated with ageing. Anti-oxidant chemicals slow down destructive peroxidation of lipids in your body by allowing themselves to be oxidized, thereby trapping unstable oxygen molecules in the process before they can destructively react with lipids. They then turn into relatively stable and harmless compounds which can be easily eliminated or metabolized. Free radical scavengers work in much the same way. By reacting harmlessly with highly active free radical molecular species, they deactivate these free radicals before they can do harm to cell membranes and DNA and RNA, and before they can cause dangerous cross-linking to the body's many other proteins. In practice, most substances which protect from peroxidation are also able to deactivate free radicals. Together with the low-calorie-high-potency way of eating, these anti-oxidants can create a massive bastion of defence against ageing and degeneration in your body. That is why they are a vital part of any serious programme for ageless ageing.

Home-Grown and Lab-Made Anti-Agers
Anti-oxidants come in two varieties: natural and artificial. The natural anti-oxidants are simple nutritional elements which occur

naturally in the foods we eat. These include ascorbic acid, vitamins A, E, beta-carotene and the other carotenoids, many of the B complex vitamins, zinc, selenium, L-glutathione and the sulphur-based amino acids such as L-cysteine and L-methionine. The artificial anti-oxidants such as BHA and BHT appear on the labels of many processed foods – they are chemicals used to retard spoilage.

The Power of Synergy

In the last few years anti-oxidant nutrients have begun to receive a lot of attention. You will find long lists of them in books and articles on age-retardation and on the backs of bottles in health-food stores and pharmacies. The trouble is that much of the interest in them as age-retarders has come from a fragmented kind of thinking based on the assumption that if you take one or two – say vitamin C and vitamin E – then you should be able to take advantage of their anti-ageing properties. In fact, anti-oxidants work together and no single anti-oxidant can do much for ageless ageing unless it is well supported not only by the other anti-oxidants but also by all the other forty or fifty nutrients essential for maintaining life. For it is not the single actions of these nutrients but their multiple interactions which make them biologically efficient in detoxifying your body and protecting it from degeneration.

Experts in free radical metabolism Elmer M. Cranton and James P. Frackelton give some idea of just how complex and interrelated the body's natural anti-oxidant defence system is in relation to the anti-oxidant nutrients:

'Vitamin E (tocopherol), vitamin C (ascorbate), selenium in glutathione peroxidase, the amino acid cysteine in reduced glutathione, riboflavin and niacin are all interrelated in a recycling process which provides on-going neutralization of free radicals. If each one of these nutrients is present in adequate amounts, they can all be restored to their active anti-oxidant forms after reacting with free radicals.' This principle is too often ignored in anti-ageing programmes. It mustn't be. For as Le Compte's first law states, *ageing proceeds more rapidly where the deficiencies are greater and more numerous.*

Clinical Applications of Anti-Oxidant Nutrients

So potent are the anti-oxidant nutrients in protecting the body against illness that high doses of them are now beginning to be used in both the prevention and treatment of many serious illnesses, from cancer to ischaemic heart disease. In addition to their ability to protect from oxidation destruction, they appear to have many other health-promoting properties as well, such as an ability to improve immune functions. They are also anti-inflammatory agents. In the words of another expert in the field, E. Crary:

> High but well tolerated doses of the nutritional anti-oxidants selenium and vitamins E and C (400–1,000mcg, 400–1,200mcg, 1g respectively) have significant immunostimulant, anti-inflammatory and anti-carcinogenic effects which are well documented in the existing biometrical literature. In addition, these anti-oxidants help to protect the structural integrity of ischaemic or hypoxic (oxygen-starved) tissues and may have useful anti-thrombotic actions as well. Supplementation with high-dose nutritional anti-oxidants may eventually gain a broad role in the prevention, treatment or palliation of cancer, cardiovascular disease, infection, inflammatory disorders and certain diabetic conditions.

He then adds:

> While there is little evidence at present that high doses of manganese, copper or beta-carotene will produce special benefit, it is wise to assure adequate intakes of these nutrients, which play anti-oxidant roles. The apparent ability of beta-carotene to reduce lung-cancer risk in smokers merits special mention in this regard.

With all of this in mind, let's take a closer look at some of these natural anti-oxidant protectors and the kind of wonders they can work to keep you looking good and to protect your body from degeneration. The first is ascorbic acid, so important it really deserves a chapter to itself.

Vitamin C – the Non-Vitamin?

Ascorbic acid or vitamin C was first isolated in 1928 by Nobel prizewinner Albert Szent-Györgyi. He extracted it from orange juice, cabbage juice and adrenal glands of animals and he called it hexuronic acid because of its chemical structure. A lack of it in the diet was found to be responsible for the development of scurvy and it was later dubbed vitamin C. Since then it has been the subject of much enthusiasm and even more controversy despite the fact that it has quite conclusively been shown that ascorbic acid helps prevent arthritis, that it helps cure the common cold, that it can slow down the growth of cancer cells, and that it can even help protect the body from airborne and waterborne pollution. High levels of ascorbic acid are essential in protecting from the kind of free radical oxidation damage which is central to age-degeneration.

Many researchers, amongst them Szent-Györgyi himself, believe that vitamin C has been badly misunderstood. They claim that it is not a vitamin at all but a substance which encourages energy transfer in the cells. Szent-Györgyi believes that vitamin C is capable of creating heightened electron exchanges and thereby raising the level of vitality in the cells and tissues. If this is true – and, thanks to current findings in electrobiology (see Chapter 8) it seems very likely – then its actions on the body in many ways parallel those of a high-raw diet, raising electrical potentials in the cells, increasing cellular exchange and stimulating cell metabolism. Certainly ascorbic acid is a powerful anti-oxidant with particular protective properties for proteins of all sorts – from essential hormones to enzymes, collagen and even nucleic acids. It even offers significant protection against radiation. And, among vitamin C's most important anti-ageing properties is its ability to detoxify the body of both organic and inorganic poisons (including the heavy metals such as mercury, lead and cadmium), arsenic and benzene. It can even clear away toxicity caused by such agents as spider and snake poisons, bacterial toxins and many industrial pollutants and contaminants.

Szent-Györgyi has insisted that once we come to understand how vitamin C really functions in the body we will probably learn many other biological secrets as well, such as why cancer cells reproduce and how to stop them doing so. Many ascorbic-acid researchers have reported that this substance, vitamin or not, helps maintain physiological homeostasis throughout the system. Irwin Stone, one of the world experts on the vitamin and author of *The Healing Factor*, says, 'On a molecular basis, the whole living process is nothing more than an orderly flow and transfer of electrons. Therefore, having an abundance of a substance like ascorbic acid present in living matter makes this orderly flow and transfer of electrons proceed with greater ease and facility. It acts substantially like an oil for the machinery of life.'

Protecting Homeostasis

Vitamin C has been found to perform many important functions in the body. Because it is a reducing agent it acts as an anti-oxidant, disarming highly reactive oxygen molecules and free radicals before they can do damage to membranes, tissues and cells. It also promotes the formation of red blood cells, helps prevent internal bleeding which leads to bruising and broken veins, and is of central importance to the proper functioning of the controlling centres of the body, such as the pituitary gland, brain, adrenal cortex and even the eyes. It has also been found to speed the healing of wounds and burns, since it facilitates the formation of connective tissue in the scar. Vitamin C (along with zinc and the bioflavonoids) is also an essential substance for the synthesis of collagen in your body. A truly adequate amount of it (more about adequacy later) strengthens intercellular cement, helps keep muscles firm and helps protect skin from sagging and wrinkling.

Vitamin C has well-demonstrated antibacterial and antiviral actions. In part this is because as an anti-oxidant it offers cells and body tissues protection against colds and other viral infections. In part it is due to more direct actions which it has on the immune system. For instance, vitamin C is essential in good quantity if leucocytes are to function at optimum capacity in their efforts to engulf and destroy invading bacteria. But studies have shown that this is not possible, even on a daily intake of 250mg of the vitamin – already more than most official tables recommend as necessary for 'health'. Vitamin C also protects your body from the cross-linking damage that is perpetrated by acetaldehyde – a toxic substance found in raised amounts in people who drink large quantities of alcohol or smoke many cigarettes. This is one of the reasons why it is a well-tried and proven remedy for detoxifying the body from alcohol and why it banishes many of the symptoms of hangover, particularly when taken with a little fruit sugar.

The Missing Enzyme

Irwin Stone spent most of his professional life studying the biological functions and activity of ascorbic acid and putting them to therapeutic use. He believed also that it had been misclassified when it was dubbed a vitamin. It is instead, he says, an important metabolite, and an ancient genetic mutation has led to our being one of the few animals (in company with apes, guinea-pigs, Indian fruit bats, rainbow trout and the coho salmon) who do not produce the substance naturally within their own bodies. In all the other mammals there is a chain of enzymes involved in the production of vitamin C from glucose in the liver. The amount of ascorbic acid an animal produces at any particular time is directly related to the animal's environmental condition. For instance, when subjected to conditions of stress, cold, illness or a polluted environment, more ascorbic acid is naturally produced than in normal, low-stress conditions when the animal is well fed, peaceful and not faced with high-risk situations.

Man and the few animals who do not produce this substance naturally are not so fortunate. Not only are we entirely dependent on our diet for an adequate supply, but the concentration of ascorbic acid in our blood falls dramatically just when we need it most – when we are under any kind of stress – making us more susceptible to infection, age-degeneration and fatigue. The reason we are unable to manufacture this metabolite in the body is that in this chain of enzyme-controlled reactions in the liver which produces it, we are missing the last enzyme of the series – a little gem called L-gulonolactone oxidase. This, Stone and others believe, is a result of a genetic mutation which occurred several million years ago and which eliminated this important enzyme from our biochemical make-up.

Beyond Deficiencies
Scurvy is the deficiency disease associated with insufficient vitamin C. The symptoms of severe ascorbic deficiency were first recognized in the eighteenth century when James Lind carried out controlled therapeutic trials on sailors suffering from scurvy and discovered that a simple daily prophylactic dose of 1oz of lemon or lime juice per seaman would prevent the dreaded disease which was costing the Royal Navy hundreds of thousands of men. It was an important discovery, for scurvy is a very nasty illness: first the complexion changes and the skin becomes sallow or muddy. Then vitality is lost so you tire easily and suffer from breathlessness, with a desire to sleep most of the time. There can also be pains in the joints and limbs, particularly the legs. The gums become sore and bleed easily and reddish spots appear on the skin. Sometimes the eyelids become purple or swollen, nose-bleeds occur, and blood is passed in the urine. As the gums become increasingly spongy the teeth start to fall out, the jawbone begins to rot and the bones become so brittle that they easily break. Finally death comes either through a

secondary infection such as pneumonia or from collapse at even the mildest of exertions.

Optimum Levels of Vitamin C

The usual way of determining adequate amounts of vitamin C has been to ask the question, 'How much of the vitamin will prevent scurvy?' The official answer that comes back is between 45 and 60mg a day, because in most adults such an amount will prevent the *overt manifestations* of scurvy. Since science has been largely blinkered by the notion that ascorbic acid is a vitamin and therefore performs only one function – that of preventing gross symptoms of scurvy – it has tended to ignore another question, which for most people is even more important: 'How much vitamin C do we need to live at *optimum* health and vitality and to retard the degenerative processes associated with ageing?'

This is a question which Linus Pauling, twice a Nobel laureate, has long investigated. He has come to the conclusion that while a few milligrams of ascorbic acid each day will prevent the symptoms of acute scurvy, we need much larger amounts if we want to live in the best possible health, to prevent age-degeneration in the body and to promote longevity. Just exactly how much depends, as always, on biochemical individuality. But most people, he believes, probably need between 1 and 5 grams a day to remain optimally healthy. Some may actually be able to get along with as little as 250mg while others may find they require up to forty times this much – 10g or more a day. For when less than truly adequate amounts of ascorbic acid are taken, although symptoms of acute scurvy can be prevented, many people nevertheless develop chronic symptoms of 'subclinical' deficiencies which include lack of mental alertness, bleeding gums, borderline anaemia, irritability, and a strong susceptibility to infections and age-related degeneration. And requirements of the vitamin in an effective programme of supplementation for ageless ageing are likely to be even higher – probably between 10 and 15g a day for most people – although many ageing experts take much more.

Daily doses of this size and larger have been shown to have quite remarkable effects on human beings. Susceptibilities to colds or 'flu usually disappear. Injuries, broken bones and bruises heal rapidly. Even cancers and tumours have been regressed, and the lifespans of animals have been significantly prolonged on high daily doses of ascorbic acid. Many researchers, including Stone, claim that such doses will delay wrinkling and other visible signs of ageing as well as prolonging youthful vitality.

Of Apes and Men

Current recommendations for daily intake of vitamin C are about 60mg a day. For an 11-stone man this is proportionally less than 1mg for each kilogram of body weight. When you compare this requirement with the Nutrient Requirement of Laboratory Animals from the Committee on Animal Nutrition it seems very low indeed. Drawing on their recommendation of 55mg per kilogram of body weight for monkeys, one would expect proportionally it to be almost 4g (4,000mg) for a man. The average adult gorilla living in the wild (who like us cannot produce his own ascorbic acid) consumes in excess of 4,500mg of the substance every day, while animals who are able to synthesize it in the liver tend to produce even higher quantities of it – about 70mg per kilogram of body weight. Under stress of any kind or when they are ill, this production more than triples. Pauling and others have often pointed out that since civilized man is continually under stress, an 11-stone man can need somewhere near 15,000mg of the vitamin a day to maintain a high level of well being and protection from degeneration. One of the reasons why a high-raw diet of fresh foods can be so useful in slowing down degeneration and even in rejuvenating the body biochemically and physiologically may be because, compared to the average overprocessed and overcooked foods most people eat, it is quite rich in natural vitamin C. But even a high-raw diet cannot supply that much.

Ascorbic Acid Scares

If you intend to take 10g or more of ascorbic acid a day, is it safe? After all, there has been a lot of negative publicity about vitamin C. Some claim not only that it is not effective in preventing or curing the common cold, but even that it may cause a deficiency of vitamin B12 and/or kidney stones. Dismissals of ascorbic acid's many health-promoting properties tend to come from professionals who have little or no experience in using it either for prevention or therapy. Most criticism of high-dose usage comes from early studies done to validate Pauling's original findings that the vitamin has antiviral and antibacterial properties. A number of these studies were carried out in which subjects were given supplements of vitamin C in low doses – amounts in the fifties and hundreds of milligrams a day. These studies showed no increase in their subjects' ability to resist infection nor did they give any indication that extra vitamin C helps speed the healing of colds. And their findings received a lot of press coverage and brought forth not a few expressions of disdain from physicians who had never used the vitamin. What the publicity did not make clear is that the amounts of the vitamin which had been tested had been far too low to be effective – sometimes as much as fifty times less than those Pauling, Stone, Ewan Cameron, Robert Cathcart and the other experts were using for the same purpose.

Other worries began in 1974, when two doctors, Victor Herbert and Elizabeth Jacobs, published an experiment suggesting that large doses of vitamin C could destroy vitamin B12 in foods and lead to a B12 deficiency in the body. This too brought a lot of publicity in its wake. But when the methods these researchers used for analysis were examined, it became obvious that their findings could not be considered reliable. For their experiments had been carried out in the presence of oxygen, which is involved in the reaction that destroys B12. This is highly unlikely to occur in a living organism, where the proportion of oxygen in its digestive system is very low indeed.

Finally there has been the worry that large doses of ascorbic acid might cause kidney stones. Since some ascorbic acid is converted in the body to oxalic acid, a few professionals have expressed fear that someone who takes both a lot of vitamin C and calcium could produce calcium oxalate urinary stones. But there have been no actual reports of this. Quite the contrary. Many studies have shown that a high intake of vitamin C actually *reduces* the incidence of several types of urinary stones. And, provided you get sufficient magnesium and vitamin B6 in your diet, even the faint possibility of producing kidney stones is eliminated. Another concern which is commonly voiced about taking large amounts of ascorbic acid regularly is that you will develop a tolerance to it so that it is no longer effective. Seldom has this been reported. Russian scientists eliminate even this possibility by giving high-dose C supplements for three or four weeks and then stopping them for the same period.

Morbidity Index

When ascorbic acid goes to work in your body to detoxify wastes and protect against oxidation and free radical damage, much of it is metabolized into *dehydroascorbic acid*, which is in effect 'oxidized' vitamin C. One of the most useful and interesting ways of using ascorbic acid as a diagnostic and prognostic tool, a way of estimating the biological state of your vitality and resistance to illness and degeneration, is by measuring the ratio of ascorbic acid to dehydroascorbic acid in your blood. Stone calls this ratio the 'morbidity index' (although it could as easily be looked at from the opposite point of view as a 'vitality index'). Normal healthy people have a morbidity index of about 15 – that is, 15 parts ascorbic acid to 1 part dehydroascorbic acid. Critically ill people have a morbidity index of about 1. When they convalesce after serious illness the morbidity index improves dramatically. This measurement is a diagnostic tool which is enormously helpful in indicating the overall state of the body and in estimating just how much oxidation-stress you have been exposed to. It is now just beginning to be used as a biometer for ageing as well.

How and How Much?

Doses of vitamin C are important, both when you are using it for its health-promoting, age-retarding anti-oxidant purposes and when it is being used to treat illnesses. Because it is a water-soluble vitamin, ascorbic acid is not stored in the tissues. Once your tissues have been saturated, any excess is excreted in the urine. Many of the opponents of high-dose therapy complain that the only benefit this leads to is the rather questionable one of having very expensive urine. But scientists with experience in megascorbic therapy for the prevention of illness and ageing say that this flushing and the elimination of excess is an important part of the benefit that the vitamin can bring the body. It neutralizes toxins, free radicals and activated oxygen molecules and constantly keeps undesirable wastes moving through the body, helping to get rid of them.

Ascorbic acid in quantities greater than the body can use beneficially tends to cause loose bowels. Robert Cathcart, an American physician who is known throughout the world for his therapeutic uses of the vitamin, believes this can offer a good indication of just how much at any particular time – ill or not – you need. He uses doses of the vitamin ranging from 10g a day up to 200g taken orally to treat serious illness. To determine the proper dose he 'titrates to bowel tolerance' to determine just what dose is appropriate. It should be just below the point at which this loose-bowel phenomenon occurs, says Cathcart. At least 80 per cent of normal adults, he says, will tolerate 10–15g of ascorbic-acid fine crystals in one half cup of water in four divided doses per twenty-four hour period before this happens.

Vitamin C comes in many water-soluble forms – ascorbic acid, calcium ascorbate, sodium ascorbate, and so forth – both in powder form and in tablet form. Most experts in vitamin C use claim that the best form of the vitamin (and the cheapest) is quite simply the crystalline powder of ascorbic acid itself. This you can stir into fruit juice or spring water and drink three or four times a day (but brush your teeth afterwards as the acid can eat away tooth enamel). High doses of vitamin C tablets sometimes cause distress to sensitive stomachs. Some tablets also contain fillers which, if you are taking megadoses of them over a period of time, you are probably better off without. The advantage of the ascorbate forms of the vitamin is that, unlike ascorbic acid which has a low pH, they are more alkaline. But many people actually come to like the rather acid flavour. Some people take vitamin C by dissolving three 5ml teaspoons of ascorbic acid powder in a litre of sparkling mineral water which they drink throughout the day to supply a steady supply of about 9g of the vitamin per day. It makes a refreshing and stimulating drink and, at the same time, keeps ascorbate levels in the tissues nicely elevated so you can make good use of its natural protection as an anti-ageing nutrient. There is also one oil-soluble form of vitamin C. Called ascorbyl palmitate, it too is a powerful anti-oxidant and it is non-toxic. In the food industry it is used to prevent cut apples from turning brown and to cure meats. Because it is fat-soluble, it may offer far more protection against lipid-peroxidation damage to the cells than the water-soluble forms do. It can be sprinkled on foods or added to salad dressings. It is an excellent complement to water-soluble vitamin C, which is why most longevists take both.

The Amazing Bioflavonoids
In nature vitamin C occurs together with certain pigments of flowers, fruits and vegetables called bioflavonoids. They are a remarkable group of brightly coloured plant-derived substances that were also discovered by Szent-Györgyi and which together with vitamin C make up what is commonly called the 'C complex'. These substances, which are called by various names, include hesperidin, rutin, vitamin P, flavones, flavonals, nobiletin, tangeretin, eriodictyol and so on. They potentiate the effects of ascorbic acid in the body as well as strengthening cell membranes and capillaries. Scientists working with refined techniques which

enable various bioflavonoids to be isolated and tested have shown that some help prevent blood platelets from abnormal clotting by exerting anti-adhesive actions on red blood cells. In the plants from which bioflavonoids come they act as primitive defence systems protecting them from disease. They appear to have similar actions on man. Many studies indicate that various bioflavonoids, either on their own or in combination, actively combat infectious bacteria, viruses and fungi. If you are going to follow a mega nutrient approach to retarding ageing it is probably a good idea to include these substances in the list of supplements you intend to take.

18
Radical Fighters

IT WAS DENMAN Harman at the University of Nebraska in 1957 who first developed the free radical theory of ageing. For more than twenty years it was virtually ignored by the scientific community. Then evidence began to mount that the lives of experimental animals could be extended up to 40 per cent by the use of supplementary anti-oxidants and that the prevention and even reversal of heart disease and some kinds of cancer could be brought about by anti-oxidants. That is when scientists began to sit up and take notice.

In the 1970s Robert Tengerdy and his colleagues at Colorado State University found that when animal diets were supplemented by large quantities of vitamin E the animals were protected against many diseases and poisons which were deliberately introduced into their bodies.

Another American scientist, J. E. Spallhaltz, had similar results when he used the anti-oxidant selenium. In fact immune strength increased fourfold. These studies were then confirmed many times over in other laboratories so that now we know pretty certainly that anti-oxidants supplemented beyond quantities needed for so-called *normal* health enhance immunity significantly.

Anti-oxidant nutrients are helpful in slowing down the rate at which you age, and not only because they deactivate free radicals and unstable oxygen species in the body. As we've seen, the same nutrients enhance the immune system and improve your resistance to disease infections, food and chemical allergies or sensitivities and chronic degenerative illnesses. They also offer protection against many of the life-eroding hazards of twentieth-century life in industrialized societies. These include the vast array of environmental threats to which we are subjected, from the pesticides which are sprayed on our fruits and vegetables to the more than 200,000 chemicals to which we are exposed almost every day of our lives, chemicals which fifty years ago were little present in our environment; water-borne carcinogens formed when the chlorine used to purify our drinking water chemically interacts with industrial effluents; solvents; the halogenated hydrocarbons in air and water; formaldehyde; chlorine gas; heavy metals such as lead and cadmium; asbestos and even radiation. They have become a serious threat to health.

The airborne pollutants are particularly worrying since air is the single thing without which we cannot live for more than a few minutes. The air we breathe contains a long list of nasty-sounding substances which not only erode the marble and granite of buildings but can cause serious harm to lungs and skin and encourage premature ageing on a wide scale. Two of the most destructive oxidant air pollutants are ozone and nitrogen dioxide. The first comes mostly from the burning of petrol in cars, buses and lorries, although gas fires and stoves are another source. The second is created in photochemical smog by reactions involving nitrogen oxides, oxygen and unburnt petrol vapours. Both cause oxidation damage to the lungs by oxidizing the polyunsaturated fatty acids of lung cell membranes. Because they are so useful in protecting from environmentally caused damage, anti-oxidants are on their way to becoming almost necessities in twentieth-century urban life. Where the Hunzas, Vilcabamba Indians and Georgians were able in their unpolluted environment to live long and healthy lives based entirely on natural law anti-ageing practices, for us this appears virtually impossible. We appear to need the high-tech help from extra anti-oxidants for us to manage it. As always they are synergistic – they work best in combination. But three are particularly important in counteracting the destructive effects of environmental pollutants in our air, water and food – vitamin E, selenium and vitamin A.

Tocopherol Power

When vitamin E was isolated from wheatgerm oil in 1936, researchers discovered it was a mixture of several similar substances which are grouped under the name of *tocopherols* – alpha, beta, gamma, delta, epsilon, and so forth. There are seven of them and all of them have biological activity and anti-oxidant power, but each to a slightly different degree. The tocopherols occur in highest concentration in nature in wheatgerm, cold-pressed vegetable oils, whole raw nuts and soy beans. Most vitamin E capsules contain alpha-tocopherol acetate, the most biologically active *isomer* of the series, for which 1mg is equal to one international unit (or IU). Some, however, are made up of a mixture of tocopherols or their *esters* since there is evidence that such a mixture increases alpha-tocopherol's activity in a living system. Vitamin E is a potent anti-oxidant and free radical scavenger, with a particular bent towards looking after the body's lipid-based structures. So far, it's the only anti-oxidant known to prevent lipid peroxidation within the microsomes and mitochondria, so it is terribly important in maintaining cell integrity and ensuring a safe and complete use of oxygen by the cells. It has also been used successfully to treat menopause problems such as hot flushes and chronic muscle cramping as well as to prevent and treat some kinds of anaemia and cancer.

Early research with vitamin E got it rather a bad reputation because it became associated in people's minds as the 'sex vitamin'. This is because tocopherols exist in high concentration in the anterior pituitary gland, where they oversee the production of male hormones, and because animal experiments showed that they are necessary in the female for normal reproduction to take place. Indeed vitamin E does protect sex hormones and other vital hormones from oxidation, but perhaps its most important role in the body is that it encourages a more efficient use of oxygen by the cells. It plays a vital role in cellular respiration and this is why it is so important in protecting the heart from damage. In addition it causes dilation of the blood vessels so that more blood gets through, and it is an effective inhibitor of clots.

Vitamin E also gives your muscles and nerves the ability to function on less oxygen and in this way increases endurance and stamina. It is concentrated in the parts of cells most involved with oxidation and with respiration reactions, such as in the mitochondrial and microsomal membranes. These sites of energy transfer are where nutrients enter to be metabolized and wastes are eliminated. Researchers have found that a vitamin E deficiency dramatically lowers cellular oxygen use at these sites, while it increases peroxidation and the formation of free radicals. This is particularly important in muscle tissue where a shortage of the vitamin can result in a 40 per cent decrease in endurance capacity. That is why vitamin E has long been used by top athletes. The vitamin's ability to minimize oxygen starvation on a cellular level appears to play an important role in protecting the arteries and veins from the build-up of cholesterol which has a tendency to collect in areas where oxygen is particularly sparse.

Pollution and Age-Protector

Experiments with animals have shown that vitamin E even in relatively low doses can protect against the damage which nitrogen oxide and ozone in our air do to lungs and tissues.

American biochemist Roger Williams pointed out that a vitamin E deficiency is often observed to cause physiological and biochemical changes which parallel those of old age. And Russian scientists report that as a supplement for ageing people vitamin E has brought about a disappearance of wrinkles on the face, increased strength and stamina, improved sleep patterns and even turned greying hair back to normal. The tocopherols also offer protection from ageing by enhancing immune responses. This way they also help protect your body from illnesses. When mice infected with pneumonia were given extra doses of vitamin E, over 60 per cent of them were able to resist the disease compared to the control group fed on the ordinary laboratory diet – all of whom caught the illness. But for top immune protection – the kind needed for ageless ageing – it appears that we, like these lab animals, need considerably more of the vitamin than is available in the average diet. One of the world's experts on the vitamin, Robert Tengerdy, says that we appear to require six times more than what is usually thought to be nutritionally adequate.

Vitamin E's anti-oxidant properties are strongly synergistic with other nutrients. For instance, this vitamin reduces the amount of vitamin A you need by preventing it from breaking down and forming other substances that can be harmful to your body. Vitamin E has a similar effect on saturated and unsaturated fatty acids. It also protects the B complex vitamins and vitamin C from oxidation in the digestive tract and enhances the antioxidant activity of both selenium and the amino acid cysteine (see Chapter 19), both of which are central to any nutritional programme for ageless ageing. The more fat there is in your diet the more vitamin E you will need.

How Much Is Enough?

All the experts on vitamin E insist that, thanks to widespread use of refined flour which eliminates the vitamin from it, and to the high-fat diet we eat which quite simply burns it up, few of us get adequate vitamin E to maintain good health, let alone be able to make substantial use of its anti-oxidant properties for age-retardation. Most nutritionists suggest that supplements of 400 IU a day are needed to maintain good immune functions although this need increases with the amount of fat and oils you consume. Many longevists take as much as 1,600 IU a day or more. Although there are no known side-effects of taking such a high dose of vitamin E, there have been some recent reports in the popular media that on prolonged high doses of the vitamin some people develop exhaustion and fatty livers – that is, on doses as high as 1,600–2,000 IU a day for months on end. Laboratory animals have produced abnormalities of the adrenal, thyroid and sex glands on prolonged, extremely high doses. People who have high blood pressure, heart damage from rheumatic fever, or an overactive thyroid usually are advised not to take vitamin E in large doses. In some people, when supplements of very high doses of vitamin E are begun suddenly this can temporarily elevate blood pressure. That is why many physicians begin with a smaller dose of the vitamin, say 100 IU a day, and gradually work up to their optimum amount over a period of several weeks. What is the optimal amount for ageless ageing? Again it depends on the person. Most ageing experts recommend building up to between 600 and 1,200 IU a day together with the other anti-oxidant nutrients. Vitamin E should always be taken with meals, as it is absorbed best where there is some oil or fat in the digestive system, and it is a good idea to take it along with vitamin A and selenium with which it works closely. Because it has a slightly calming and relaxing effect on the nervous system, many people prefer to take it with their evening meal.

Superlative Selenium

In many ways the most exciting of all the anti-oxidant nutrients is selenium – an essential micro-nutrient found in minute quantities in your body. It can preserve elasticity of the skin by preventing oxidation of polyunsaturated fatty acids which can result in cross-linking of proteins. It also helps protect from cancer and premature ageing, and it works closely with vitamin E. How much selenium you get in your diet depends entirely on how much is found in the soils in which the foods you eat are grown, although seafoods, particularly tuna which has been packed in water not oil, are good sources of the nutrient. In areas of high-selenium soils, cancer incidence is significantly lower than in areas of low selenium. For many years nutritionists largely ignored selenium because, like vitamins C and E, in high doses it is toxic: it can inhibit the actions of important enzymes and replace sulphur in biological compounds. These symptoms however have only been reported in areas of exceptionally rich selenium soils, of which there are very few.

A powerful anti-oxidant and free radical scavenger, selenium is part of the glutathione peroxidase molecule which is one of three enzymes that are part of the body's first line of anti-oxidant defence. This protective enzyme is responsible for turning lipid peroxides, which damage cells and collagen, into harmless hydroxy acids. And it cannot function properly in the absence of selenium. This anti-oxidant enzyme is absolutely essential to protect your body from the many forms of environmental pollutants that are linked both to age-degeneration and to the development of cancer. It is also a vital force in protecting you from airborne allergies and environmental sensitivities, and selenium itself appears to be the most important of all the anti-oxidant nutrients for people who are sensitive to the chemical environment. In fact a number of clinical ecologists report that supplements of 400mcg (micrograms) of selenium a day can clear up symptoms in approximately 60 per cent of people suffering from chemical allergies.

The Anti-Cancer Nutrient

Selenium also detoxifies the body of heavy metals such as mercury and appears to be a potent anti-cancer agent. Researchers have only recently discovered this fact. The discovery has a certain irony about it because in the early days of nutritional research selenium was believed by some scientists to be a cancer-causing element.

Its power *against* certain forms of cancer is of particular relevance to anyone concerned about retarding the ageing process, since so many of the changes on a cellular level associated with the development of cancer are paralleled in cellular ageing. It has been demonstrated from several different research approaches. Epidemiological studies have shown that where the dietary intake of selenium is highest, the rate of breast cancer is lowest. For instance, in the United States the average daily intake of selenium is 68mcg and the incidence of breast cancer is 22.2 per 100,000. Thanks to their high consumption of fish, people in Japan have an intake of 287mcg and only a 4.0 in 100,000 incidence of breast cancer. In the Philippines, where the average daily intake is 189mcg, the breast cancer rate is 5.4 per 100,000. Other studies have confirmed these findings and indicate that selenium not only helps protect from cancers of the colon, stomach, lungs, breast, liver and prostate, but from other chronic illnesses as well. These include heart disease, high blood pressure and arteriosclerosis. All of them are less prevalent in areas of high-selenium intake.

Other studies have shown that people with low selenium have an increased risk of skin cancer and still others that selenium supplementation can reduce the incidence of breast tumours in mice from 80 per cent to 18 per cent. In Germany researchers took fifty animals and fed them extra selenium while fifty remained untreated. They were then all irradiated to cause cancer. It developed in thirty-one of the untreated group. Only fourteen of the selenium group succumbed to the disease, however, and the tumours in these animals were less than half the size of tumours in the untreated group. Researchers stated, 'We must infer that selenium must be one of the few chemical elements to which a tumour-preventative effect can be attributed . . . the results of our own investigations enhance and amplify present knowledge of this anticarcinogenic action of selenium.'

Heightened Immune Defences

Selenium's role in glutathione-peroxidase activity and its ability to detoxify the body of carcinogens are no doubt important in its ability to protect from cancer and to retard the ageing process. But so too is the direct action it has on the immune system – improving immune functions as no other single nutrient appears able to do. Selenium is a necessary ingredient in raising your body's defences against foreign invasion from bacteria, viruses and toxic chemicals. Supplements of selenium have been shown to increase the numbers of B-cells – the white blood cells which form an important part of immune defence. Animals treated with selenium show that lymphocytes are also increased in the blood when this micronutrient is given over a period of time. Meanwhile rabbits injected with selenium show increased numbers of white blood cells, heightened phagocyte activity and an increased ability to kill bacteria.

Where From and How Much ?

Seafood is the best source of selenium. Fruits and vegetables are usually poor sources unless they happen to have been grown in selenium-rich soils. Whole grains, onions, garlic, cabbage, mushrooms, asparagus, broccoli and soy beans can all be good sources provided they come from adequate soils. People who live on the average western diet, high in refined and processed foods, are often very selenium-poor. Brown rice contains fifteen times as much selenium as its white counterpart. How much is enough is still a matter of great debate in scientific circles. Most nutritionists err on the side of caution and recommend 200mcg per day despite the fact that the Japanese take in much more than twice that in their daily diet and appear to get nothing but benefits from it.

Selenium *is* a poison in excessively high doses and only a small amount is required. Selenium supplements are always measured in micrograms (millionths of a gram) instead of milligrams. Official reports state that 'chronic selenium toxicity would be expected in human beings after long-term consumption of 2,400 to 3,000mcg daily'.

Most longevists take a minimum of 400mcg a day and a few go as high as 600mcg. When you take this micro-nutrient together with vitamin E and vitamin C both its activity and its safety in the body are enhanced. The most easily absorbed form of selenium is selenomethionine. Nutritional supplements of selenium sometimes include the amino acids it works with in the body to form glutathione peroxidase as well as the other nutrients, such as vitamins A, E and C, with which it is particularly synergistic.

Retinol and the Carotenoids

Vitamin A or retinol is an oil-soluble nutrient named after the retina of the eye which has a special need for it in order to remain healthy. It is also an effective anti-oxidant and free radical protector from damage with a particular role to play in guarding the lungs from damage caused by the airborne pollutants to which we are exposed. Closely related to vitamin A are the carotenoids (named after carrots in which the most well-known carotenoid, the yellow pigment beta-carotene, is found in abundance). Beta-carotene is sometimes called pro-vitamin A because it is converted to the vitamin itself by your body when you eat foods containing it. Much research has correlated a high level of beta-carotene with protection from cancer. Recently many of the other carotenoids have been studied and begun to be used as nutritional supplements. It now appears that each has something unique to offer in terms of anti-oxidant protection and immune enhancement. They can contribute greatly to an ageless-ageing lifestyle.

Vitamin A itself – often with the help of these carotenoids – helps maintain soft, smooth, young-looking skin, protects the mucous membranes of your mouth, nose, throat and lungs, and reduces your susceptibility to infection. Recent studies show that if you are deficient in vitamin A you increase your risk of lung cancer. There is also a definite relationship between your cells' ability to synthesize new RNA and adequate intake of vitamin A or the carotenoids in your diet. As far back as the Forties researchers at Columbia University showed that they were able to extend the lifespan of rats between 10 and 20 per cent by supplementing their diets with vitamin A.

Vitamin A, which occurs in good quantity in liver and fish, is one of the oil-soluble nutrients which can build up in the body. In adults more than 85,000 IU of it a day quickly becomes toxic and can be responsible for symptoms of nausea, vomiting, headache and dizziness. This is why vitamin A is never used in megadoses. Most longevists recommend between 20,000 and 35,000 IU a day – no more.

Beta-carotene is different, however. It is absorbed from your foods through the intestinal wall. And it is non-toxic. Eat too many carrots and all you are likely to end up with is a slight colouring of the skin that looks like a mild tan. Indeed this colouring property of some of the carotenoids is often taken advantage of by people wanting to tan naturally without the sun. How much beta-carotene you absorb depends partly on the kind and quantity of fats that you have also eaten. Some of it is converted into vitamin A in the intestine and then stored in the liver, the rest circulates in the blood. The fact that, unlike retinol itself, beta-carotene *does* circulate in the blood appears to be important in the kind of anti-oxidant protection against age-degeneration which it offers the cells and tissues of your body – particularly the skin and the lungs. To put it simply, it goes easily where it is needed. And the fact that it is non-toxic makes it an important adjunct to vitamin A in the collection of natural anti-oxidants for ageless ageing. Most age researchers and doctors using anti-oxidant nutrients as age-retarders use 15,000–35,000 IU of retinol together with about 25 to 50mg of beta-carotene or mixed carotenoids. This much beta-carotene provides about 40,000 IU of potential vitamin activity.

Natural Support System

All the enzymes involved in free radical protection from damage demand trace elements or B vitamins as co-enzymes. For instance the trace elements copper, zinc and manganese are essential to the superoxide dismutases, selenium is needed for glutathione peroxidase; and iron is essential for catalase and some forms of peroxidase. That is why a truly adequate intake of these trace nutrients is essential for protection against free radical-produced diseases and ageing. They should be included in any effective anti-ageing supplement. In fact several of the B complex vitamins, including vitamin B1, pantothenic acid, B6, PABA, B3, choline, inositol, and B12, and some of the minerals such as zinc, either appear to have their own anti-oxidant properties, are immune-stimulants, or play other specific anti-ageing support roles in the body. For instance the vitamin niacin, B3, is not itself an anti-oxidant but it is used in NADPH – one of your body's major electron-carriers; B2 is also not an anti-oxidant but it is necessary for the natural anti-oxidant-recycling enzyme glutathione reductase. Lecithin is an anti-oxidant. A phospholipid manufactured by your body, it also acts as an emulsifier and has an affinity for water. It breaks down fat into minute particles so it can be dissolved, and appears to bind with cholesterol and to help prevent the buildup of cholesterol in the arteries.

Synergy Has the Last Word

The single most important principle on which any sound nutritional programme must be based is *synergy*. Just as there is never a deficiency of only one vitamin or mineral, there is never any vitamin or mineral action which takes place by itself. It is always the multiple interactions of essential nutrients which constitute the basis of their biological functions. This is never more true than when you are relying on natural anti-oxidants and immune-supporters for age-less ageing. How successful they are in slowing the clock for you depends on their being supplied together with a good balance of all the other nutrients necessary for what you might call 'biochemical housekeeping' – the day-to-day running of things in your body. This means that your way of eating has to be right – not too much, and based on the natural wholesome foods that supply a full range of essential nutrients, plus whatever as yet undiscovered factors are part of the structural information necessary for high-level health. Many high-potency-supplement regimes for slowing down ageing are doomed to failure simply because they forget this principle – so that complementary nutrients are not sufficiently available in the system to make proper use of the high-powered anti-agers. Such an approach is not only a waste of money (anti-oxidant nutrients don't come cheap), it could also seriously unbalance your system. The best way to undertake anti-oxidant supplementation if you decide to do so is to consult a health practitioner or doctor who is well trained in nutrition and biochemistry (see Resources, page 334) and ask them to have your body tested for nutrient levels and heavy metals. They can then outline a supplement programme tailored to your specific needs.

19
The Amazing Aminos

AMINO ACIDS ARE the building blocks from which proteins are made. They are important to know about, for some of them can lend a lot of support to ageless ageing. There are twenty-two of them so far identified which commonly occur in proteins. Eight are called *essential* because your body can't manufacture them itself. They therefore have to be taken in through foods you eat. The rest can be made in the body out of other amino acids. For man the essential amino acids are isoleucine, leucine, lysine, methionine, phenylalanine, threonine, tryptophan and valine. Cysteine and tyrosine are synthesized in the body from methionine and phenylalanine respectively. All these ten amino acids occur in proteins in your cells. Another ten amino acids – alanine, arginine, asparuc acid, asparagine, glutamic acid, glutamine, glycine, histidine, proline and serine – are present in most proteins. Two more, hydroglycerine and hydroproline, are present in collagen. The body has the ability to synthesize these from simple precursors. That is why they are called *non-essential*. Recently however, experts in amino acids have begun to insist that the concept of 'essential' and 'non-essential' amino acids is fallacious and that for high-level well-being and ageless ageing all of the amino acids should be available through the foods you eat. This is because, although your body can itself manufacture the so-called non-essential aminos, some, like arginine, cannot be manufactured in sufficient quantity to supply the need. Further, these can put strain on enzyme systems and use up supplies of co-enzyme nutrients – like zinc, for instance, or vitamin B6 – which are better left free for other duties in the organism.

These twenty-two amino acids can be linked together to form more than 50,000 different proteins. In fact your body is continuously breaking down the proteins you eat into amino-acid complexes and free amino acids, then recombining them to form whatever new proteins it needs to maintain itself. Amino acids supply the raw materials for maintaining the genetic code – DNA – as well as for repairing damaged muscle tissue, for cell division, for making enzymes (together with vitamins as co-factors and minerals as activators), for building new connective tissue and – particularly important – for making hormones which regulate bodily processes and neurotransmitters which are responsible for brain activities.

From Protein to Amino Acid

The common belief amongst doctors and most nutritionists is that deficiencies of amino acids simply don't exist – at least not in the western world where we all eat plenty of protein. But what this belief ignores is the fact that the proteins we eat have to be broken down into their respective amino acids before our bodies can make use of them. This process of break-down is a complicated one, and one which involves the actions of enzymes, which are themselves made from amino acids. The proteins you take in through your foods are first attacked by pepsin, an enzyme secreted in the gastric juices. This is followed by other *proteolytic* (protein-digesting) enzymes from the pancreas and the mucosa of the small intestine. All of these enzymes are themselves made from amino acids. If your system is deficient in the free amino acids which you need in order to make digestive enzymes, your body will be unable to make proper use of the proteins you eat. So despite the fact that you may be taking in plenty of good-quality protein (indeed in Britain and the United States most of us eat far too much) you could be suffering an amino-acid deficiency which, like a vicious circle, only gets worse as the years pass. It goes something like this: if you have insufficient pancreatic proteolytic enzymes, you digest proteins poorly and don't get the amino acids from them that you need. This amino-acid deficiency in turn creates a kind of chain reaction throughout your body. Since proteolytic enzymes are built from amino acids, when these are deficient then digestive enzymes become deficient as well. Also if amino acids are deficient then they fail to evoke proteolytic enzyme secretions from the pancreas. So a deficiency of amino acids at one level leads to a further deficiency at another level, which leads to a further deficiency at yet another level, and so on.

Poor Digestion Leads to Degeneration

This is no hypothetical theory either. Experts say it is a common occurrence as we age. Deficiencies in hydrochloric acid in the stomach, in pepsin and particularly in the pancreatic proteolytic enzymes is widespread in people over thirty who have lived on a typical western diet. They can suffer from digestive degeneration and malabsorption so that they do not break down their food proteins adequately and do not get the amino acids they need to carry out all of the essential biological functions which are dependent on them. Also, when as a result of insufficient enzymes, proteins are incompletely broken down, they putrefy in the small intestine, producing by-products which are toxic and can result in food allergies and mental and emotional disturbances, and which appear to contribute significantly to a number of other problems – from rheumatoid arthritis and gout to poor skin and premature ageing. So important is proper protein digestion in protecting your body from age-degeneration and deterioration that many nutritionally oriented physicians recommend that over the age of thirty-five or forty their patients take supplements of digestive enzymes (usually together with hydrochloric acid) to ensure better protein breakdown in the gut. Many also recommend that a balanced free amino acid supplement also be taken in any serious programme for ageless ageing. This is for two reasons. First because the person can be sure of getting adequate free aminos for enzyme production and second because some free aminos such as methionine and cysteine are themselves superb free radical scavengers. They help protect against the cross-linking and peroxidation damage of the ageing process.

In relation to ageing, probably the most important of all aminos are the sulphur-based amino acids which are themselves powerful anti-oxidant nutrients – useful tools for protecting your system from free radical damage and cross-linking. These sulphur-based aminos are central to any serious programme for ageless ageing.

Stay Young with Sulphur

Seldom do nutritionists concern themselves with sulphur – and yet dietary sulphur is not only an essential mineral and a potent protector against radiation and chemical pollution, it has even been shown to prolong the lifespan of animals. The molecules of most amino acids are made up of carbon, hydrogen, nitrogen and oxygen atoms only. Those which also contain sulphur in their molecules, such as methionine, cysteine and taurine, besides being helpful in building enzymes, hormones and new protein tissue in the body, are also important anti-oxidants, free radical scavengers, neutralizers of toxic wastes and aids for protein synthesis. Their ability to offer protection from radiation of many different sorts – from x-rays to low-level nuclear radiation – makes them particularly important in the late twentieth century when radiation has become such a widespread threat to high-level health. Much of the damage from radiation comes because of radioactivity's ability to steal electrons from water molecules in the body, turning them into hydroxyl radicals which in turn get together to form peroxides. These peroxides emasculate anti-oxidant enzymes such as catalase by damaging their *sulphydryl groups*. When sufficient sulphur amino acids are present in the body then sufficient sulphydryl groups are available to be sacrificed by combining with free radicals and peroxides so that anti-oxidant enzymes remain protected to carry out their jobs. After this occurs the amino acids themselves are simply turned into other harmless substances.

The Methionine Connection
Methionine is a constituent of haemoglobin, tissues and serum and it has an essential part to play in the activity of the spleen, lymph system and pancreas. It is one of the important agents in preventing excessive build-up of fat in the liver and it is often used to eliminate toxic metal loads from the body. Methionine also helps convert a toxic substance, guanidine, to a relatively non-toxic chemical, methyl-guanidine. This is particularly important in countering the kind of fatigue which often accompanies getting older, since guanidine is a major cause of chronic fatigue in the body. Methionine, like many of the natural anti-oxidants, works in a synergistic way with other important nutrients for ageless ageing. For instance, it helps your body make good use of selenium.

Taurine, another sulphur-based amino, as well as being an anti-oxidant and free radical deactivator, plays an important role in cellular health by helping to stabilize membrane excitability in the heart, skeletal muscles and the central nervous system, all of which contain taurine in high concentrations. Taurine has been used therapeutically to lower blood pressure in people with essential hypertension and also as an effective treatment for epilepsy. It also helps the passage of minerals such as calcium and magnesium, sodium and potassium through cell walls. Taurine is found in very high concentration in human breast milk. Many scientists now believe that it is an important substance in the healthy development of the brain and in the prevention of strokes. Taurine is often not included in anti-oxidant formulas for ageless ageing simply because it can be synthesized in the brain from other amino acids, but many experts in the field of amino-acid biochemistry insist it should be.

Cysteine – the Youth Connection

Cysteine is probably the most important sulphur-based amino acid of all. It has a pleasant garlic-like taste and you can sprinkle it on your foods instead of using salt. But you have to be sure to keep it in a tight container since it is also an amino which tends to draw water from the atmosphere. In fact many serious longevists include it in good quantity in their list of supplements by taking between 500 and 2,000mg of L-cysteine hydrochloride a day, which is really a stable form of the sulphur-rich amino acid cysteine. One gram of cysteine hydrochloride contains about 180mg of sulphur. Your body can convert one into the other as it needs it. Cysteine occurs in good concentration in the hair and nails and is one of the most useful supplements in improving the health and good looks of both. It is equally important in keeping your skin smooth and young-looking and in helping skin recover from damage. Like selenium, cysteine is particularly useful in protecting the body from chemical pollutants. It can also help protect the body from the destructive effects of radiation.

Cysteine is a central component of the body's important anti-oxidant enzyme glutathione peroxidase. It is also able to chelate or tie up metals such as copper, cadmium and mercury and help eliminate them from the body. And it is an important agent to counteract the effects of acetaldehyde and other chemicals which build up in the body as a result of smoking and drinking. When researchers dosed rats with enough acetaldehyde to kill 90 per cent of a control group, an amazing 80 per cent of those treated with cysteine half an hour before testing survived the challenge. Cysteine is particularly bound up with the use of vitamin B6 in the body. That is why it is important if you take the one that it is complemented with the other. Cysteine is not given as a supplement to diabetics except under medical supervision since it is capable of inactivating insulin. And most ageing experts agree that if you are going to take a very large dose of cysteine as an anti-ageing supplement you should also take three times the dose of ascorbic acid. This, they say, will protect your body from any possibility of its developing kidney or bladder stones from very high doses of this amino acid.

Don't Forget the Eggs and Garlic

Your body contains about 140g of sulphur, almost a gram of which is lost every day and which needs to be replaced through the foods you eat. Foods which are a good source of sulphur amino acids include eggs, cabbage, garlic and onions. Eggs can be particularly important as part of any nutritional programme for ageless ageing. Each egg contains about 65mg of sulphur. Unfortunately, over the years, as a result of the notion that eggs contribute to the accumulation of cholesterol, many people have been shortchanging themselves of the support that these sulphur-rich foods can bring. Recent research has shown that this belief is completely unfounded. For although eggs do indeed contain cholesterol they also are a good source of iron, lecithin, zinc and sulphur as well as other trace minerals which are active elements in converting cholesterol into useful steroid hormones and other substances in the body. As twice Nobel laureate Linus Pauling says, 'We must educate people away from the dangerous idea that you can control heart disease by not eating foods such as eggs, butter and milk. This oversimplified idea is totally wrong.' Don't neglect your eggs. Years from now you will be glad you didn't.

Tri-Peptide Anti-Oxidants and Immune-Supports

Some of the amino acids do appear to have a strengthening effect on the immune system. They have been shown to improve immune response to bacteria, viruses and tumour cells in animal experiments. They have also been used to increase the weight of the thymus gland – the master gland of immunity – and to increase important T-cell production. These immune-supporting functions, coupled with the anti-oxidant capabilities of some amino acids we have already mentioned and the characteristics that many of them have of being able to detoxify the body, and of encouraging full functioning of the body's anti-oxidant enzymes and digestive enzymes, make free amino acids potent nutritional tools for ageless ageing.

One particular *tri-peptide* known as glutathione which is composed of three amino acids – L-cysteine, L-glutamic acid, and glycine – offers particular support to the body's anti-oxidant defence system. You may remember we spoke of the body's first and second lines of defence against free radical attack and cross-linking. The second line of defence is composed of all of the anti-oxidant nutrients from ascorbic acid to methionine which act as free radical scavengers in the system. Glutathione plays an important part in our first line of defence. It works something like this. The primary enzyme defending against activated species of molecules is composed of superoxide dismutase (SOD), glutathione peroxidase and catalase. SOD takes care of converting activated oxygen molecules to hydrogen peroxide. But hydrogen peroxide itself is still mildly toxic. It has to be further metabolized either by catalase or by glutathione peroxidase. Glutathione has been used for many years in injectable form to stimulate glutathione peroxidase activity in the body with excellent results. Recently it was discovered that, unlike SOD, whose effect when taken orally is highly controversial, glutathione taken orally as a nutritional supplement appears helpful in guarding against fat peroxidation as well as in detoxifying the body of wastes. It has been used with particular success to clear away debris and harmful bacteria from the lungs in the case of infection or when a person has been exposed to a high level of air pollution. Like all of the free radical scavengers it works best in combination with others. Selenium is particularly important since it is essential for the formation of glutathione peroxidase in the body.

Make Friends with Aminos

If you want to make use of some of the benefits which have been reported from using free amino acids as part of a programme of ageless ageing, how do you go about it? And what kind of cautions do you need to exercise? Let's look at cautions first. Arginine and ornithine are not usually given to schizophrenics; tryptophan is not given to pregnant or lactating women; cysteine is not given to diabetics and is always taken with three times the amount of vitamin C; phenylalanine is given with caution in cases of high blood pressure; histidine is taken with an equal quantity of vitamin C and not by people who already have high histamine levels or by manic depressives; tyrosine is not given to people who are taking the MAO inhibitor anti-depressant drugs; neither is phenylalanine or tryptophan.

Robert Erdmann, who has spent twenty-five years researching the clinical and preventative use of free amino acids as nutritional supplements, advises anyone taking them long term to ensure they have a 'complete' formula in addition to any specific free amino they may be using for a certain effect – say cysteine as a means of improving hair condition – as well as a well-balanced formula of vitamin and mineral supplementation. For like all anti-oxidant nutrients it is important to ensure that you get sufficient co-factors for their use, vitamins such as B6, B12 and C, selenium, zinc and so forth – to be able adequately to draw from them all of the support for high-level energy and well-being which they potentially offer. This way one can be absolutely sure of supplying the body with all of the nutrients – amino acids as well as vitamins and minerals – it needs to function at a high level of vitality. This way too, you can be sure of not causing any imbalances in the system. An example of a good balanced formula would be one which has been based either on the amino acid balance naturally found in an egg or in spirulina – a freshwater alga. Again I believe it is important to work closely with a nutritionally informed doctor or health practitioner (see Resources, page 334) in designing an individual supplement programme which incorporates free amino acids.

Most free amino acids are best taken on an empty stomach at least forty-five minutes before a meal. They are available from health-food stores and by post from suppliers. By far the best way to take any of them is in pure white crystalline form simply by stirring a teaspoon or more of the powder into a glass of mineral water or in simple gelatin capsules, since this means you avoid any of the incipients (i.e. the binding ingredients) which are used to put them into tablet form. Be sure when buying amino acids that you buy absolutely the best and don't be misled by manufacturers who are trying to get on to the amino acid bandwagon by putting inferior products on the market.

PART THREE

THE AGELESS BODY

20
Move Back Through Time

NOT ONLY WILL regular exercise firm your muscles, keep your body young-looking and improve your self-image, it can also rejuvenate your body by altering what are ordinarily considered age-related parameters towards more youthful levels. Research has shown that it can:

- Prevent and reduce overweight
- Help keep hormones at optimum levels
- Improve the heart's output and efficiency
- Make skin look younger and function in a younger way
- Protect the cardiovascular system from arteriosclerosis
- Improve glucose-tolerance against degenerative changes leading to diabetes
- Lower triglycerides
- Increase the level of high-density lipoproteins (HDL) associated with protecting the heart
- Strengthen bones and prevent their shrinkage
- Increase lean muscle mass
- Improve the oxygen-carrying capacity of the blood
- Lower high blood pressure
- Banish anxiety and depression
- Improve mental functions
- Heighten vitality
- Help you live longer

Go for Muscle
Animal bodies, like ours, are made up of two basic components - *lean body mass* (LBM) which encompasses our muscle tissue, and *fat*. Lean body mass – that part which is not fat – is the part of

you which is most alive. It consists of your organs such as the heart, the liver, the pancreas, bones and skin, as well as your muscle tissue. Your LBM demands oxygen, uses nutrients from your food, thinks and feels, moves, grows and repairs itself. Wild animals have a high percentage of LBM. That is what gives them their power, their ease of movement, their stamina and their sleek bodies. The rest of you is fat. The hardest thing for most of us who have been brainwashed by low-calorie slimming nonsense to understand is that it is your body's *fat* stores that are the enemy, not your weight as measured by the scales.

Fat tissue is very different from your muscle. It does not need oxygen, does not create movement or activity, and cannot repair itself. In fact body fat is just about as close as you can get to dead flesh within a living system. Dr Vince Quas, American expert on body change and fat loss and author of an excellent book on the subject *The Lean Body Promise*, says it better than anyone else I have ever met: 'Your lean body mass *is* you,' he says. 'Your fat is *on* you.'

It is the muscle portion of your LBM you will need to work with, through both dietary change and exercise for ageless ageing. Doing so will not only help keep energy levels high but also keep hormones responsible for young skin and strong sex drives flowing. Building more lean muscle through exercise is a fascinating metamorphosis to experience. It does not change you in any intrinsic way, nor does it turn you into someone else's idea of the perfect body. It only makes you more what in essence you really are. What happens is your lean body mass slowly but inexorably begins to metamorphose a body distorted over the years through stress, poor eating and lack of movement, into the true form that is hidden within it.

Body Sculpture

Many years ago I read that Michelangelo claimed never to have sculpted any statues. 'I only took my chisel and removed the extraneous marble in order to reveal the form that was hidden within the stone,' he said. Beginning to be conscious of your own LBM and to work through exercise with that part of it which is muscle sculpts your own body from within. In the process it releases quite astounding levels of energy, creativity and joy. More about the power of LBM in a moment. First let's look more specifically at why exercise is such an important element in ageless ageing.

Exercise and Live Longer

The word is out: exercise helps prevent degenerative diseases such as cancer and heart disease. An eight-year study, which followed more than 10,000 men and 3,000 women and was reported in the *Journal of the American Medical Association* not long ago, looked at the long-term effects of physical fitness. It found that sedentary women – women who are not fit and therefore have a low LBM to fat ratio – were 460 per cent more likely to die than those who took exercise more regularly. Men in the low fitness category were 340 per cent more likely to die. Being a lounge-lizard is a major risk factor for degeneration and disease. Many data-research projects exploring links between exercise and longevity now show strong evidence that exercise is a powerful tool for age-retardation and life extension – even rejuvenation – for it alters many parameters such as blood-pressure and cholesterol levels, bone mineralization, vitality, and the oxygen-carrying capacity of the blood – all towards more youthful levels.

Exercise can not only make you look and feel younger, it can actually help you live longer. A study by Harvard and Stanford University of nearly 17,000 graduates carried out over five decades showed that regular exercise delays ageing. It is also an important factor in preventing coronary heart disease (CHD). Researchers found there was 'a strong inverse relationship between exercise and death from *all* causes, total cardiovascular diseases (including both CHD and stroke) and total respiratory diseases'. They discovered that the adjusted death rate for the most sedentary of the men studied was almost twice that of individuals who regularly burned 2,000 calories a week in exercise. But to reap benefit from the life-lengthening effects of exercise it has to be carried out steadily – not in spurts and spells. For even university athletes have a high risk of death if they later become sedentary, while sedentary ex-athletes are able to lower their risk if later on they return to regular exercise. Bruce B. Dan, editor of the *Journal of the American Medical Association*, which reported the study, commented, 'We can now prove that large numbers of Americans are *dying from sitting on their behinds*' [my italics]. Researchers noted, 'If everyone studied had been physically active there would have been a 23 per cent lower incidence of coronary disease.' They also found that how much physical exercise you get can influence your other lifestyle habits for the better. Physical activity reduces your desire to smoke, lowers the chance of your becoming obese, helps control blood pressure and leads both to a better diet and better stress control.

Exercise for Fun and Live Longer

In 1977 Charles Rose and Michel Cohen at the Veterans' Administration Hospital in Boston examined the death records of 500 men by interviewing living relatives about their lifestyle. They discovered that while exercise on the job appeared to have little effect on longevity those men who exercised regularly in their leisure-time lived 7.1 years longer than those who let their exercise decline steadily after their twenties. They also showed that regular exercise carried out throughout life extends lifespan. Meanwhile in Canada Terence Kavanagh and Roy Shepherd examined 128 men and 7 women participants – some top athletes, others simply enthusiastic amateurs, some as old as ninety – who exercised regularly and who were playing in the 1975 World Masters' Golf Championships in Toronto. These exercisers showed significantly fewer signs of ageing than the average person does. For instance, where most of us lose height at a rate of about half an inch per decade after the age of 45, they had lost less than half that much. Those between forty and ninety years of age also showed less body fat, had larger muscle mass in their body and better heart and lung function. Their bodies looked younger and stronger, their physiology functioned better and they were able to maintain their bodies even under conditions of 'haphazard' nutrition, thanks to the powerful anti-ageing effects of exercise.

Use It or Lose It

This old adage is never better applied than in the realm of age-prevention. A large part of what generally passes for age-related degeneration in the human body is instead a result of simple *disuse*. In fact, some of the latest research indicates that disuse may be even more important than disease or the passage of time in determining the rate at which you age. Your body was built for movement, just as your digestive system was designed to deal with natural foods rich in fibre and structural information. When – thanks to our sedentary occupations and the hours we spend driving around in cars instead of walking or running from place to place – your body does not get the rhythmic vigorous exercise for which it was designed, it begins in a hundred ways to degenerate. This degeneration is easily measured in terms of loss of calcium and a thinning of the bones, increases in blood pressure and certain blood fats, poor muscle tone and sagging skin. But what has only recently been recognized (indeed even many age-researchers have not tumbled to this fact yet) is that changes in the body due to low levels of physical activity are very close to those commonly attributed to ageing. These changes can come on fast. In only twenty-four hours of inactivity your muscle tissue begins to deteriorate. Let a year go by without exercise and 50 per cent of the health and age-control benefits you may have gained from a lifetime of sports will be lost. For lounge lizards this is the bad news: regular rhythmic exercise as well as weight-bearing exercise are essential to holding back the ravages of time. But there is good news too: it is never too late to begin.

Space-Age Research

Much of the awareness of how disuse (far more than the passage of time) is central to the processes of ageing and degeneration has come out of the scientific work involved in putting man into space, in particular plunging him into that novel physiological state known as *weightlessness*. Weightlessness in physiological terms is a kind of intensified disuse in which the human body does not even have to make the effort to resist the force of gravity. When researchers started to investigate weightlessness they naturally studied the two conditions which most closely approximate to it – being in water and being at rest in bed. In either of these states you rapidly lose precious minerals from the bones, making them weaker and more susceptible to breakage, you slow down the elimination of wastes from the tissues, and you get muscle shrinkage and a wasting of the skin and muscles that most people associate with old age.

Disuse or Dynamism

Break your arm and it will shed half its muscle and a third of its bone mass within a few weeks simply because you stop using it. When the cast is taken off it will have shrunk to as little as half its size. If you are forced for any reason to stay in bed for a few months the loss of minerals from your bones and the ageing of your muscle tissue can speed up by ten years. That is the bad news. Here is the good news: your body responds amazingly to exercise – even to a little of it. Start now to make demands upon your muscles by doing both aerobic and weight-bearing exercise – go nice and easy, especially if you are not used to it. Not only will your muscles grow stronger and smoother, your bone tissue will become denser. Stop exercising again and your body turns to flab, your energy levels drop, your muscle mass shrinks (as does your ability to burn calories) and with it goes your overall sense of wellbeing. Exercise for ageless ageing needs to do two things – enhance your body's ability to use oxygen (this calls for aerobic exercise) and help build lean body mass (weight-bearing exercise).

The Oxygen Connection

Your body's single most important function is its use of oxygen. Unlike food or water, you cannot go without oxygen for even a few minutes without suffering damage. And when an organ such as the brain or heart is deprived of oxygen, even for a short time, it brings about catastrophic results – a stroke or a heart attack, for instance. Studying the effects of weightlessness and immobility on the body, researchers such as Walter M. Bortz II at the Stanford University School of Medicine have found that by far the most serious effects of disuse lie in the way it decreases the body's ability to extract oxygen from the atmosphere and to transmit it via the bloodstream to the tissues which use it for energy. They claim that it is not a pill, magic potion or some glamorous and expensive youth treatment which can best reverse the long and rather depressing list of changes that have come to be associated with ageing, but exercise – simply because it dramatically improves your body's ability to extract oxygen.

The measurement of how well you do this is expressed in scientific terms as *VO2 max*. Bortz began studying the relationship between age-related changes and inactivity as a result of having his own leg in a cast for six weeks. He noticed when the cast was removed that the 'withered, stiff and painful leg' looked as if it belonged on a body which was forty years older than he was. Researching the subject in depth, he discovered that by almost every measurement that could be taken, a lack of exercise produced bodily changes which paralleled those associated with ageing. Put yourself into a programme of regular, sustained physical activity and you can not only prevent them but even help reverse them when they have already occurred.

VO2 Max – Key to Youth

In most people VO2 max steadily declines after thirty – at a rate of about 1 per cent per year. The decline takes place simply because, unlike our primitive ancestors who remained physically active all through their lives, we lead a largely sedentary existence. As a result we appear to age quite rapidly: our bodies decline in cardiovascular and lung fitness, we lose muscle and bone tissue, our skin wrinkles and thins and we experience a progressive stiffening of the joints. Curiously, these age-related changes occur at just the rate at which your V02 max declines. But what some of the exciting new studies show is that a decline in V02 max is not inevitable. When an ageing person of thirty-five, fifty-five or even seventy-five works out regularly he or she can restore their V02 max levels to that of someone much younger. And as V02 max increases, energy levels rise, measurements of the state of the cardiovascular system such as heart rate, cholesterol levels and blood lipids return to more youthful parameters, skin looks younger, high blood pressure decreases, joints regain their flexibility, the loss of minerals from the bones is halted, muscle mass increases and fat is lost. Even intelligence levels improve.

Turn Back the Clock

Physiologist J.L. Hodgson at Pennsylvania State University has carried out studies which show that when an inactive seventy-year-old starts a programme of moderate activity he can expect to improve his oxygen-transporting ability by some fifteen years. If he then goes on to achieve an athlete's level of conditioning, says Hodgson, he could potentially regain forty years of V02 max and experience many of the physical and physiological effects of rejuvenation in the process. So exceptional is the ability of regular exercise to reverse age changes that, as Bortz has written in the *Journal of the American Medical Association,* 'It seems extremely unlikely that any further drug or physician-oriented technique will approach such a benefit.'

Regular sustained physical activity can go a long way towards preventing age-related changes of all sorts from cardiovascular ones to the look of the skin. It also dramatically increases a person's energy levels. Herbert de Vries, age expert at the Andrus Gerontology Centre at the University of Southern California has shown in a study involving more than 200 people that men and women of sixty or seventy can become as fit and energetic as people thirty years younger. 'Regular exercise turned back the clock for our volunteers,' says de Vries. When questioned about what they considered the greatest benefit of their regular exercise programmes his subjects most often answered 'greater energy'. The fitter you are the more energy you have. It is the 'body so unused to activity that tires at the slightest effort', he says.

Muscle and Transformation

Now let's go back to lean body mass, for there lies the secret of permanent weight control. Your LBM is always changing – increasing or decreasing. When it changes, this is not because of alterations in your organs or bones but rather because of alterations in your muscle. Under-muscled people have low levels of energy. Studies show they are at as great a risk from degeneration and early ageing as people who are over-fat. When your muscles are strong and dense and alive, aches and pains vanish. When muscles are in tone your posture is good too, for posture depends upon muscle alone. So does the proper elimination of waste from your cells. The lymphatic system, which carries waste products away, is not powered by the heart but by muscle movement. The more muscle movement you get the better it works. This is particularly important for women – even slim women. For unless your lymphatic system is working properly you can end up with deposits of water, wastes and fat on localised areas of your body, better known as cellulite. To shed fat and keep it off you need to increase your LBM. For energy, beauty, health and weight control, most physiologists would say that 90 per cent LBM to only 10 per cent fat is ideal for men. For women 80–85 per cent LBM is just about perfect, which means carrying no more than 15-20 per cent of your weight in fat.

How your body performs both biochemically as well as physiologically is determined by the ratio of LBM to fat on it. When for any reason, such as being inactive or going off and on slimming diets, you shed lean muscle tissue, your energy and the way your body performs is undermined. In most of us this is a slow decrease, often so slow that you don't notice it. You awaken in mid-life only to find that your body is flabby even if you have remained thin and that you suffer from chronic fatigue. There are other things too that can decrease muscle mass, such as illness, or too much exercise, or the wrong kind of exercise. Then, even if you appear to have stayed the same weight on the scales, the fat on your body will have increased and your body will have lost a great deal of its tone. The important thing to remember about weight control is to stop worrying about how to whittle away just a bit more flab from your hips, thighs or tummy and concentrate instead on improving your muscle mass.

Check it Out

There are a number of methods for measuring body composition. They are most often used by physiologists concerned with improving the performance of athletes. It is sometimes done in sports clinics by hydrostatic weighing – that is immersing your body in a large tub of water and then weighing you when you are entirely under water. For your LBM is heavy and the fat on your body is lighter than water, which is why fat people tend to float very easily when they swim. Sometimes physiologists use what is called an impedance unit, where a very small current is sent through pads placed on your wrist or ankle to determine LBM to fat ratios, or sound or light waves are sent through the body. These methods, too, can give quite an accurate reading of the fat/lean body mass measurement because your muscle tissue is heavier in water – which is a better conductor of electricity than is fat – so the current travels faster when you have a lot of muscle tissue.

The most common way of measuring – although not by any means the most accurate – is done with skin calipers where you pinch your skin at various parts of the body, then measure the thickness of the pinch and do some complex calculations to determine LBM to fat ratio. This method is a lot less accurate than the others, but is a lot easier to carry out. Easiest of all is to reach down and pinch your own flesh with your fingers at the area at the bottom of the ribs, on your thighs, upper arms, belly, bottom and hips. If your pinch is thicker than half an inch to one inch your LBM to fat ratio is not as good as it could be.

Forget Your Age
There is widespread belief that as you get older your body metabolism naturally slows down and therefore you are less and less able to prevent yourself from becoming fat. Actually, age has absolutely nothing to do with it. It doesn't matter how old you are or how much you weigh now. What limits your ability to burn fat and stay lean is how long you have been inactive. It is long-term inactivity that wastes lean body mass and results in the mitochondria being unable to burn the calories you take in from wholesome food as energy. Start now to improve your LBM by increasing the amount of muscle on your body and you can forget the days of calorie-counting for ever. Once your LBM becomes prominent enough you will become one of those people you have always envied, who can eat whatever they like without ever gaining an ounce. But you have got to exercise to keep it that way.

That is where exercise designed specifically for building muscle comes in. Don't worry, this does not mean that you will end up with a killer body. Quite the contrary. Exercise to build muscle, such as weight training using very light weights but many repetitions, is the most effective way of building LBM and uncovering your true body form. It chisels and defines arms, legs, torso, hips and bottom, even if they have been neglected for many years and have lost their natural tone and shape. So good is this kind of body building at improving LBM that until recently no-one considered that it might be an excellent form of protecting against degenerative diseases such as coronary heart disease as well. There was a time when aerobic exercise was considered king for health, fitness and longevity. Now, thanks to new research into the effects of weight training at prestigious centres such as McMasters University in Ontario, we know that aerobic exercise combined with weight training is the very best you can get for health, fitness and longevity as well as good looks, stamina and energy. As a result the much respected American College of Sports Medicine has recently revised its long-standing assertion that aerobic exercise held the key. Its new programme advises a minimum of two sessions of weight training a week using ten different exercises to enhance the large muscles of the chest, back and legs as well as three sessions of aerobic exercise.

Many sports centres throughout the world now offer excellent weight training equipment and instructors to teach you how to use it at very little cost. Even if you have never tried any form of weight training before you might enrol at one and have a go. If, for any reason you are house-bound, get yourself a couple of dumbbells and a simple book on weight training and get to work.

Work Out Your Stresses

De Vries has also explored in depth how exercise might be used to relieve anxiety and depression – two conditions from which so-called middle-aged and older people are believed to suffer greatly. It has long been established that there is a direct correlation via the autonomic nervous system between anxiety and the level of electrical activity in our skeletal muscles. Electromyographic instruments are designed to measure even minute electrical changes in muscles and this in turn indicates the degree of muscular tensions present. De Vries has taken these kind of measurements and correlated the relationship between resting muscle action potential and the body's oxygen consumption as a whole – something which also reflects both neuromuscular tension and emotional status. He has discovered that even a few minutes of moderate exercise, where you are breathing deeply and your heart is beating well, significantly reduces emotional anxiety. And when you exercise regularly and aerobically by brisk walking, swimming, jogging, cycling and so forth, you dramatically decrease your anxiety levels. The right kind of exercise for the right length of time can bring about a better tranquillizing effect than drugs, with none of the side effects. According to de Vries, to make the most of exercise's tranquillizing effects you need to practise it from five to thirty minutes each session at between 30 and 60 per cent of maximum heart rate.

Defeat Depression

No one is absolutely sure why exercise has such a tranquillizing effect on body and mood. At least in part it probably comes from the decrease in the muscle irritability and the increase in deep muscle heat which it brings about. Partly too it must be a result of how exercise alters brain chemistry. For moderate aerobic exercise has at least two important effects on the brain. First it encourages the production of *noradrenaline* or *norepinephrine*, the neurotransmitter which makes you feel 'up'. Athletes tend to have high levels of this hormone in their blood while endogenously depressed people usually show very low levels. Putting sedentary people into a regular exercise programme quite soon leads to an increase in noradrenaline and therefore to an improvement in mood, making them more optimistic and giving them feelings of having power over their life. Second, exercise greatly increases the body's production of *beta-endorphins* – natural opiates produced in the pituitary gland and in various structures of the brain which, through their action on the central nervous system, have a calming effect on the whole body as well as uplifting mind and mood. Study after study has shown that when chronically depressed people get into exercise programmes even as simple as taking long brisk walks a few times a week, their depression lifts.

Rejuvenate Your Skin

Regular physical exercise four or five times a week also makes you look younger. It suffuses your skin with blood and increases the ability of your body to carry oxygen and nutrients to the skin's cells and to remove waste products from them. Exercise physiologist James White at the University of California at San Diego carried out an interesting study to discover just how effective exercise can be at retarding and reversing the effects of ageing on skin. He paired older women on a programme of rebounding using mini-trampolines with sedentary women and discovered that the exercisers looked younger, had better skin and colouring and fewer wrinkles than non-exercisers. White was surprised to find that exercise reduces bags under the eyes as well. So, while forty minutes a day of an aerobic activity may not sound as mysterious and romantic as a visit to one of Europe's glamorous rejuvenation centres, in the long run it may do you a lot more good. Not to mention the amount of money it can save. You don't have to be an enthusiastic jogger or visit the gym four times a week to reap the benefits of exercise. Activities as gentle as yoga and as pleasant as long brisk walks can do it for you. One of the most important factors in exercising for ageless ageing is the way when it is done with ease and enjoyment it can be a tool for the integration of mind and body. So important is this factor that it merits closer scrutiny.

21
Free the Body – Charge the Mind

WE ARE SUPPOSED to live in an age of aerobic fitness. Joggers pound the pavements summer and winter, dance studios brim with all sizes and shapes of sweaty women in pink leg warmers, and every month or so a 'new' system of physical exercise appears on the scene. You'd expect to find the world full of strong, supple bodies brimming with grace and energy. The reality is somewhat different. The fine muscle tone, buoyant energy and rich mobility of a coordinated, supple and responsive physical body is a rare occurrence in the western world, even amongst those who consider themselves most fit. Instead we are faced with contracted shoulders and sunken chests, distorted thighs and faces which have aged before their time thanks to poor muscle tone and flagging energy. Meanwhile too many of us – fitness freaks and lounge lizards alike – experience our body not as a joy or a finely tuned instrument of expression for our inner being, but rather as a prison incarcerating the Self which cries out for physical expression but is rendered mute by walls of chronic tension, fatigue or postural distortions. Most of us live at only a fraction of our capacity for vitality and we have not the least notion of our body's potential for beauty and for pleasure. For exercise to be of real benefit in ageless ageing, it needs to be an *integrating* activity which draws together mind and body.

The Body as Energy
For, just as it's important to recognize that the ageing process as a whole is not only a biochemical phenomenon but is also dependent upon energy changes – structural information that comes to us through our food and our environment, and our mental attitudes and expectations – so a new approach to exercise is needed to make

the most of its potential for ageless ageing. Thinkers such as von Bertalanffy and researchers such as Szent-Györgyi and the American orthopaedic specialist and expert in electrobiology Robert Becker are helping to create a new awareness of the physical body and the mind as a single complex. They demonstrate that it is no longer enough to consider the body as a physiological and biochemical phenomenon alone.

Beneath our physiology and biochemistry lies a unifying system of *energetics* which is subtle and complex as well as enormously potent in its effect on body, mind and overall vitality. Becker has even uncovered a second 'nervous system' previously unrecognized by science – which he insists controls growth, healing and regeneration of broken bones. This energetic system appears to be influenced by both our environment and by our thoughts. It is currently being used to explain such diverse phenomena as why acupuncture can be used for pain relief and how hypnosis works. So far very little of the new scientific findings about the body as a unified energetic system has filtered down into the awareness of exercise physiologists and teachers. As a result there are still a great many people for whom even a dedicated and dynamic exercise programme followed regularly but mechanically does little good. To an unfortunate few it can even be harmful. To make the most of aerobic exercise for ageless ageing, you need not gear yourself up for some superhuman effort. You only need to leave behind the mechanical approach to exercise which tends to treat your body as a machine to be put through its paces – and to get back to basics.

Try Walking for a Start
A number of studies show that, for a variety of reasons, walking is the best form of aerobic exercise available for most people – provided it is done regularly, briskly and with true enjoyment. There is another important proviso too: vigorous exercise in any form will serve you best, and you will only avoid strain and injury if you have worked out enough of your chronic residual tensions to enable you to give your body over to the rhythmic movements it involves (more about that later). Outdoor sports such as tennis, golf, riding and sailing can be fun and helpful although, unlike walking and the other specifically aerobic activities, they do not create a steady demand on your body because of their stop-and-start nature, so it is best to include some aerobic exercise in your lifestyle even if you are an avid games player. If you like more challenging activities

than walking, try jogging or running, rowing or swimming, cycling or cross-country skiing – all excellent aerobic activities. Like regular brisk walking, they too get heart and lungs working well and help keep you looking and feeling young. They are great if you want to achieve a high level of fitness and, most important of all, if you really like doing them. This sense of enjoyment is a central consideration in whatever exercise programme you choose for ageless ageing. Any physical activity which you carry out with your teeth gritted virtuously thinking that you are, after all, doing your duty – though you hate every minute of it – can only be counterproductive. For mind and body are inextricably linked and for you to get all the benefits of exercise you need to make that link a positive one.

Charge the Body – Free the Mind

That's why, for most people, walking is so good. There is something quite extraordinary about the way that walking briskly in low-heeled shoes – particularly if you can walk in the country or in a park amidst trees and flowers – seems to revitalize the body while it sets the mind free for thought. Thoreau used to say, 'The moment my legs begin to move, my thoughts begin to flow.' And Dr George Sheehan, the highly respected cardiologist and sports-medicine expert, himself a passionate marathon runner – wrote recently of walking, 'You will read of this phenomenon again and again in the journals of the great thinkers, writers and artists. They were all great walkers. They found that not only can one train the body while one is using the mind, the mind actually works better when the body is in motion.'

Some interesting scientific studies confirm the notion that walking helps clarify mental processes. At Purdue University, after giving subjects psychological tests to determine their decision-making abilities, researchers put people into a fitness programme in which regular walking was a central feature. They found that after six months on the programme they had improved their decision-making skills 60 per cent more than subjects in the control group who did not exercise. George Macaulay Trevelyan, Britain's highly respected historian, who had a real passion for long walks, used to say, 'I have two doctors, my left leg and my right.' Latest research into the effects of regular brisk walking more than bears out his belief that this kind of moderate exercise can play a central role in keeping the body healthy, young and fit. Besides, walking is the form of exercise least likely to cause injury, it is inexpensive to practise, natural, and efficacious for ageless ageing. It will lift your spirits and keep down your weight, tone your muscles and reduce your risk of cardiovascular disease.

Walk Your Way to Wellness

So good is brisk walking as a means of strengthening heart and lungs and improving cardiac resistance that in some studies of different forms of exercise it comes out better than cycling or running. At the University of Wisconsin, for instance, when researchers examined the effects of brisk walking (at a rate of 4 miles an hour or more) on men they found that it pushed some heart rates up to 87 per cent of capacity, which was the same as the cyclists achieved and only 3 per cent lower than the runners. This measure of maximum heart rate is a useful one, whatever kind of exercise you choose to follow. It is determined by subtracting your age from 220 beats a minute. And it will tell you just what kind of workout you are giving yourself.

In an interesting study by David Mymin and Dan Streja at the University of Manitoba in Canada researchers discovered that the rejuvenating effects of strenuous exercise such as running – including a significant increase in high-density lipoprotein (HDL) and decreases in circulating insulin levels – also take place when people are put on exercise programmes based on walking, even at a pace lower than 4 miles an hour. HDL is a lipoprotein in your blood. Statistics indicate that when it is high the chances you will suffer a heart attack are low. Before the Mymin study it was assumed that only long-distance runners and other active exercisers would have high levels of HDL in their blood. But the study showed that such beneficial changes can take place just from walking. Walking's ability to lower circulating insulin levels is also important for high-level wellness and age-retardation. Many people past the age of forty have disturbed insulin levels which can lead to adult-onset diabetes and heart disease. The walkers in Mymin's programme experienced a definite decrease in circulating insulin. Other research confirms the Manitoba findings and shows as well that walking is an excellent way of increasing the amount of oxygen that reaches the cells all over the body. Like any form of rhythmic aerobic exercise it improves lymphatic drainage, stimulates arterial and venous circulation, and promotes the elimination of wastes and morbid materials which can cause free radical damage and cross-linking on a cellular level. It also brings increased blood supply to all the body's organs. Brisk walking is particularly good for people whose work tends to be mentally or physically passive because it counteracts the tendency of their circulation and their eliminative processes to become sluggish. Max Bircher-Benner always insisted his patients rise early. Then he sent them out into the hills and forests around Zürich for an hour's brisk walk before breakfast. Walking was an important part of his 'order therapy' and still is in every naturopathic clinic in Europe.

Free and Often
To get the most out of walking do it every day. Choose some place you want to walk to, and wearing low-heeled shoes and loose comfortable clothes, set out with your arms swinging free from the shoulders. Breathe deeply and carry your body high. Every few minutes draw in a breath and then after a few seconds, without exhaling, draw in another and after a further interval of a few seconds still another. After the third inhalation vigorously expel all your air. This helps inflate your chest to its full capacity. Most of us don't breathe fully and deeply. We therefore miss out on the full benefits of oxygen for brain and body. After a walk of, say, 2 or 3 or 4 miles, if possible take off your clothes and rub down your skin with a flannel which has been dipped in cold water, or take a brief cool shower followed by a brisk rub with a Turkish towel. It will leave you refreshed and renewed with energy to spare in the hours ahead.

And how intense should an aerobic activity – walking or other – be, for best results? Most experts insist you should exercise somewhere between 40 and 60 per cent of maximum capacity. This you can figure out by following a few simple steps:

1. Find out what your resting heart rate is by taking your pulse for six seconds and multiplying by ten while you are seated comfortably. You do this by putting two fingers on the artery just inside your wrist.
2. Subtract your age from 220 to determine your maximum heart rate. For instance if you are fifty then your maximum heart rate would be 170.
3. Now find out your *heart rate range* by subtracting your resting heart rate from your maximum heart rate. Say, for example, you are fifty and your maximum heart rate is 170 with a resting rate of 70. Then your heart rate range would be 100.

4. With this information you can now calculate your best exercise level to achieve a good anti-stress, anti-ageing effect. Calculate 40 per cent of your heart rate range (which is 100 in our example, so that's 40). Now add this to the resting rate of 70 and you get the figure of 110 beats per minute – your target heart rate for exercise.
5. For middle-aged and older people who are not athletes, walking moderately or briskly will raise their heart rate to that target rate, which is 40 per cent of ultimate capacity. Younger people and highly trained people will need to run or exercise more vigorously to reach it.

One of the best things about taking a daily walk is that it is such a natural and easy thing to do. You need no special equipment – apart from a good pair of shoes – and because the easy flowing movement of putting one foot in front of another can be so wholehearted it often brings a sense of freedom to the body which so many more mechanical approaches to exercise miss out on.

Exercise and Self-Transformation

Not only is such wholeheartedness important if one is to realize the full potential for exercise used as a tool for ageless ageing, the enormous power for self-expression and physical transformation which can come through movement only takes place when muscles and exercise are also linked through mind-body awareness. We are not machines, no matter how much flashy books on exercise would have us believe otherwise. When we have treated ourselves as such, either by neglecting to care for our physical needs or by forcing our bodies through exercise routines like automatons, we both create distortions of posture and body shape and dissipate precious adaptive energy instead of renewing it. In fact most of us have quite literally grown up with postural distortions which over the years become so much a part of us they are almost like physical symbols for our personality. When you begin to approach exercise from a more unified perspective, it's important to find ways of unlocking some of the residual tensions which underlie these distortions and to set the body free to move naturally so we can make the most of whatever form of exercise we choose to do. A good yoga teacher can help you do this gradually over a period of time. So can some very simple exercises which I learned from a quite extraordinary movement teacher called Lilla Bek.

Herself a longtime teacher of yoga as well as an acclaimed healer and writer, Lilla Bek's approach to movement is an ancient one, based on the principles of sacred dance where the body is put through its physical paces not only to tighten muscles and firm contours but to balance the body's energies through what in mystic tradition are known as the *chakra centres*. There are believed to be seven of these, starting at the base of the spine and rising through the solar plexus to finish at the crown of the head. Each chakra is said to be connected with specific endocrine glands and to influence the functions of organs related to it as well as energy in the part of the body it governs. Each is also believed to have specific psychic qualities – the one in the belly, for instance, is said to be connected with the actions of the will, while the chakra at the throat is a centre for creative energies, particularly artistic ones and for self-expression. The purpose of sacred dance is to revitalize the energetic circuits of the body and mind and to unify the system so that one connects up both with the earth as well as one's own energies and is fed by them. Whether or not the chakra system is ever validated by scientific research, working with exercise and movement in this way can be a superb means of integrating mind and body as well as working out long-standing bodily tensions and postural distortions that make you look and feel older than you are. After a while your body really does become a vehicle for the expression of the inner being. Its movements become naturally graceful and authentic. Over a period of time even the most distorted frame seems to untwist itself as the muscles are freed from chronic postural habits and tensions which deplete energies and undermine natural beauty. But for me the most rewarding thing of all in beginning to work in an energetically aware way with movement is the extraordinary levels of energy it brings. It is as if you create for yourself a link with the earth which supports you at a high level of calm vitality long after the other, more disconnected exercisers have fallen by the wayside.

Postures for Transformation

To begin working energetically rather than mechanically with your body it is necessary to do two things. First, you need to identify areas of chronic tension which are distorting body shape and posture, and eliminate them by an active process of *letting go*. Second, you need to begin drawing conscious awareness to the ways in which even the smallest movement, whether it takes place while running, dancing, speaking or whatever, affects muscle groups and energy-focus in other areas of the body not directly related to the muscles doing the work. Lilla Bek has worked out some gentle but useful postures which do both.

'Most people,' she says, 'even very active people, have many areas of residual tension which restrict full movement and interfere with the free flow of energy so that they become unnecessarily fatigued. These areas are really the result of how we live and how we use our bodies. Our waking hours are largely spent using only a small amount of space right in front of us – for instance as when we are driving a car or eating, working at a desk or watching television. Every group of muscles in the body has another which works in opposition to it. When we restrict our movement to such a small space we tend to contract the muscles of one group without ever doing any kind of contra-stretch to bring its opposing muscles into play. This is how chronically tense muscles lead to body distortions such as dowager's hump, slumped shoulders, excessively curved backs and the rest.'

Undoing the Kinks
The postures Lilla Bek uses to undo long-standing kinks in the body are designed specifically to create a contra-stretch for each group of chronically tightened muscles. At the same time, because they are done slowly and deliberately in a deeply relaxed state, they make it possible for the person practising them to begin experiencing just how connected up his or her body is energetically. Take the movements implied in Leonardo's famous spread-eagled man, for example. Hold yourself in this position and slowly move your arms from your sides to above your head – palms turned outwards. At each level of movement you will find that a different group of muscles come into action which are quite separate from those of the arms and shoulders involved in the movement. First the lower abdomen is tightened and the energy there is stimulated, then the solar plexus, the chest and the area of the heart chakra come into play. Then the jaw line, the lower face and ears, the roof of the mouth, the eyes, cheeks and forehead each in their turn are activated as you move your arms higher and higher. To someone who has never had any consciousness of the energetic phenomenon of exercise and the unification of body movement, such an experience is like a revelation.

Practise a few of the postures which heighten your body

awareness and you will find very soon not only that your posture changes as your body becomes more fluid and more supple and a more articulate expression of your being, but when you turn to your aerobics or your yoga or your running or your sacred dance there is a lightness and a freedom which you have never experienced before. Here are five of Lilla Bek's simple postures. Spend two to five minutes on each once a day and you are likely to experience new energy levels as well as a sense of authentic natural grace which no amount of mechanical jogging around the park or sweating it out in pink leg warmers can match.

'The Opening'
This position has a remarkable ability to open out the body, expanding the chest, releasing chronic tension from the neck and shoulders, gradually smoothing out hollow backs, and greatly expanding contracted hip joints.

Here's How
Lying flat on the floor, relax and close your eyes. Ask a friend to take a look at the position of your chin. If it is higher than the illustration, place a book under your head to bring it back into alignment. As the natural alignment of your spine improves you will need a thinner and thinner book until you can do without one altogether. Does your back lie flat against the floor or is there a hollow? An arched spine indicates that you normally hold your chin wrongly which stretches the skin of the neck and creates a double-chin look. How far are your shoulders off the floor? Do they differ in this? As chronic tension is released by doing the exercise regularly your shoulders will come closer and closer to the floor, your back will lengthen and your chin will naturally align.

Draw your right foot up while placing your palms downwards on the floor and rest it near your buttocks. Do the same with the other foot, placing your heels together, soles flat on the floor. Now, starting with your palms against the sides of your hips, begin to explore space with your arms and notice the parts of your body which slowly moving your arms outwards and upwards activates. Moving your arms up and out you begin to activate energy first in the pelvic area, then the solar plexus, heart, thymus, forehead and top of the head. When you get to the level where you are lying with your arms in line with your shoulders, let your hands open slightly and you will have reached the level of the throat energies. Explore

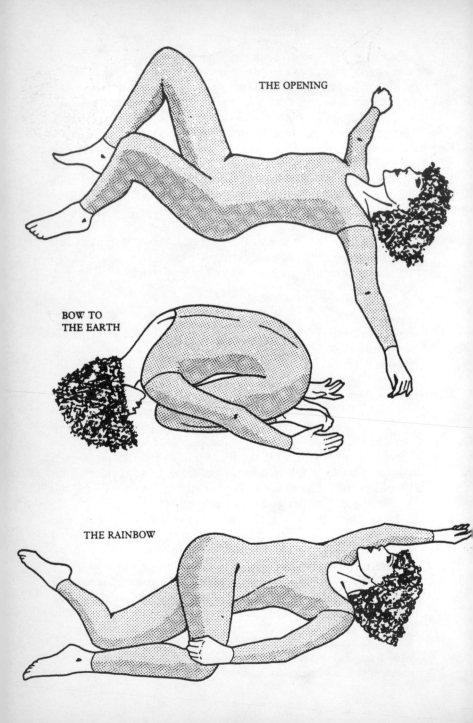

THE OPENING

BOW TO
THE EARTH

THE RAINBOW

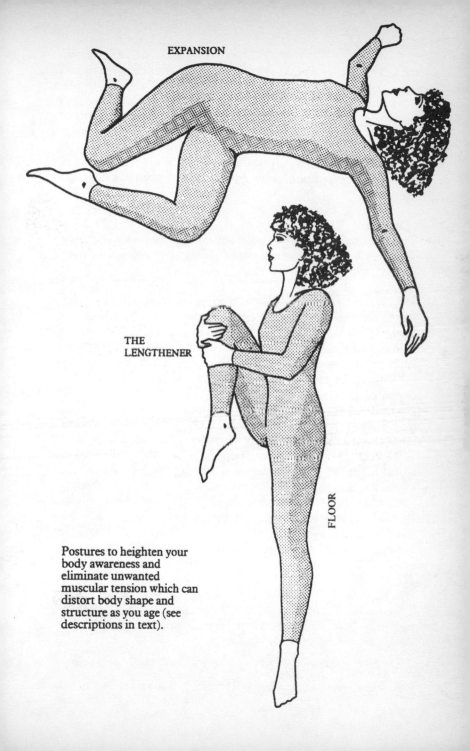

EXPANSION

**THE
LENGTHENER**

FLOOR

Postures to heighten your
body awareness and
eliminate unwanted
muscular tension which can
distort body shape and
structure as you age (see
descriptions in text).

the feel of each level of the arms in turn by moving them slowly and then leaving them at each level to sink quietly to the floor. If while doing this you gradually open out or close your fingers you will produce many interesting changes in energy at different levels of your body. With your arms extended like this at the sides, shoulder blades will separate, and then by letting your knees open outwards to the natural pull of gravity you will discover your breathing opens up. Explore this position for two or three minutes before going on to the next.

'Expansion'
This position opens out a collapsed midriff, lengthens the body, energizes the solar plexus and even tightens the muscles of the face.

Here's How
Moving from the first position, now place your feet about 18 inches apart with soles flat against the floor. Leave your arms at shoulder level and very slowly roll your hips to the right side, simultaneously rolling your head to the left. Return to the centre, keeping your lower spine in contact with the floor, and repeat the movement to the other side. Your knees should gradually fit into the arches of the opposite legs. Don't worry if they don't touch the floor. They will eventually. Most people have a shortened midriff and the solar-plexus chakra which provides the body with dynamic physical energy cannot function properly when this is the case. This position has a remarkable effect on the look of the face when it is practised regularly and can make you look considerably younger. But for this to work you must 'connect up' your face with your body – particularly in the spaces through which the knees move in your awareness as you carry out the movement. Take a full breath before you begin and exhale as your hips roll to the side then inhale again slowly as they return to centre, exhale in starting position and repeat to the other side.

'The Rainbow'
This is a position of natural grace. It brings a superb stretch to the waistline, lengthens the whole body, flattens and firms the abdomen, and integrates body energies.

Here's How
Lying flat on your back take a full breath, exhale and roll to the left

side, bringing your arms together in the same direction. Now bring your right knee across and exhale. Keep your knee down by holding it with your left hand to make sure it will not go back up. Now very gently try to take your right hand up and around your body. If it does not come in contact easily with the floor above your head then the energies from your heart and throat areas are not freed for use. Have a friend calculate in this position how much your arm is off the floor. If it is more than 6 inches then problems of distortion will be exaggerated in your body and it will take a bit of time to correct. If it is exaggerated it is a good idea not to exercise vigorously until the exaggeration disappears.

'Bow to the Earth'

Not only is this position profoundly relaxing – an excellent way to relieve stress after the end of a long day – it is also wonderful for alleviating lower-back problems and period aches and it encourages energy to rise up the spine flooding the whole body with new vitality and clearing a fuzzy mind.

Here's How

From a kneeling position, bend your body forward, pushing your hands out in front, and stretch forward like a cat. On the in-breath, bring your hands to lie at the sides of your feet and lower your buttocks. If you have difficulty in doing this be gentle but persevere, since chronic contraction here can lead to lower-back problems later. On the out-breath, bring the top of your head down in front of your knees. Rest a moment and then bring your hands forwards and place them one palm on top of the other. Rest your forehead on top. Close your eyes and relax for two minutes or more. The de-tensing effects of this position work slowly. It can be held for longer than most. It too is excellent for the solar plexus but it is also good for releasing energy that has been blocked at the base of the spine.

'The Lengthener'

This position and the gentle movement which accompanies it activate the base of the spine, improve blood flow to the brain, take pressure off tired legs, alleviate lower-back tensions, improve circulation in the pelvis and are a superb antidote to stress.

Here's How

Lying flat on your back relax as fully as you can. Now start to raise one leg slowly up as high as you can go. Be aware as your leg moves through the arc that, with each 6 or 8 inches it passes through, different parts of your body become energized, starting with the base chakra and moving up through the belly, heart and throat when it reaches a right angle. If you can go beyond this upright position you can also activate head energies. Now with your hand on one knee, don't pull by force but hold your knee with your hands and see how far you can bring it into your body. On the in-breath raise your forehead to the knee. Breathe out as you bring them together, relax and lie back. Repeat with the other leg, going through the whole sequence for two or three minutes. If you are unable to bring your knee all the way to your body do persist with the exercise. It will help protect you from lower-back troubles later. You will get a splendid feeling of lengthening over your whole body after working through this position.

Combine these simple 'untwisters' with a habit of regular aerobic activity – walking, swimming, rebounding on a mini-trampoline, cycling, running, jogging or rowing – and you will not only strengthen your lifestyle for ageless ageing significantly, you will also find a new sense of integration takes place. And your energy levels will soar.

22
Water Works

AT THE CORE of a lifestyle for ageless ageing is *pure* water – lots of it – internally and externally too. Remember that old adage your grandmother used to chant about drinking 6 to 8 glasses of water a day? Well, she was right. Except that you may even need *more* than that.

Water is the most important nutrient of all. It is the stuff from which your blood, your cells, your muscles – even your bones – are mostly made. A healthy person who weighs 65 kilos carries about 40 litres of water around – 25 litres inside the cells, 15 litres outside, including 5 litres in the blood. Let yourself become dehydrated and the chemical reactions in the cells involved in fat-burning become sluggish. Also your cells cannot build new tissue efficiently, toxic products build up in your blood stream and your blood volume decreases so that you have less oxygen and nutrients transported to your cells – all of which are essential to fat-burning. Dehydration also results in your feeling weak and tired and can lead to overeating as it disturbs appetite mechanisms so you think you are hungry even when you are not. The role of water in weight control and health in general is almost completely ignored. The brain, too, is 75 per cent water. This is why the quantity and quality of water you drink also affects how you think and feel. Thoughts and feelings become distorted when your body gets even mildly dehydrated. For mental clarity and emotional balance you need plenty of water. But if the water you drink is polluted by heavy metals or chemicals then the biochemical reactions on which clear thought and emotional balance depend will become polluted as well.

Liquid Energy
Drinking water liberally brings dynamic energy. When Sir Edmund

Hillary set out to conquer Everest he had a shrewd doctor named George Hunt on his ascent team. Hunt knew this precept well. He had studied the records of the recent failed attempt by the Swiss team and discovered that their climbers had drunk less than two glasses of water per day per man. So he ordered special battery-operated snow-melting equipment for the kit and urged the British climbers to take a minimum of twelve glasses of water each day of the climb to reduce their fatigue as they scaled the peaks.

Since then, research with athletes at Harvard University and Loma Linda University in the United States carried out to explore the relationship between water drinking and energy has demonstrated that drinking extra water reduces fatigue and stress and increases stamina and energy to a remarkable degree. During one of the Harvard studies, researcher G.C. Pitts set athletes walking at 3½ miles an hour, allowing them to rest regularly, but not allowing them to drink extra water. They reached exhaustion after 3½ hours with temperatures of 102 degrees Fahrenheit. Under the same conditions, he allowed them to drink as much as they wanted. The same athletes lasted 6 hours before collapsing. The third time around athletes were forced to drink more water than thirst dictated – in quantities calculated by researchers to replace what was being lost in perspiration. This time the athletes were able to continue indefinitely without fatigue or fever until finally, after running out of time, researchers were forced to bring the experiment to a close. Few of us drink as much water as we need to remain in top form. Even if you pay attention to your thirst and quench it regularly you are likely to replace only about a half to two-thirds of the water your body needs for optimal health.

Water Power
Water plays a major part in digesting your foods and absorbing nutrients, thanks to enzymes which are themselves mostly water. If you fail to drink enough water between meals, your mouth becomes low in saliva and digestion suffers. Water is also the medium through which wastes are eliminated from your body. Each time you exhale you release highly humidified air – about two big glasses' worth a day. Your kidneys and intestines eliminate another 6 or so glasses every 24 hours while another 2 glasses' worth are released through the pores of your skin. That makes 8 glasses a day – and this is on a *cool* day. When it gets hot, when you are exercising, or when you are working hard the usual 10 glasses lost in this way can triple.

On average, in a temperate climate – not sweating from exertion or heat – we need about 6 pints a day for optimal health. Few of us consume as much as 2. The important thing to remember is that how thirsty you are is *not* a reliable indication of how much water you need to drink. If you want to grow lean and stay that way you need to do as French women have done for decades. Keep a large bottle or 2 of pure, fresh mineral water on your desk and make sure you consume your quota of this clear, delicious, health-giving drink. Here's how to figure it:

> Divide your *current* weight in kilos by 8. If you weigh 58 kilos then 58 divided by 8 equals 7.25 big glasses. Round the figure upwards to the next glass and there you have it: 8 glasses a day. But remember, that is only a base calculation for a cool day. *You will need a lot more during exercise or on a hot day.*

Provided you do not suffer from a kidney or liver disease, drinking 8 big glasses or more of water a day not only helps you lose weight and keep it off permanently, it improves the functioning of your whole body. This kind of water-drinking forms an important part of the total regeneration and weight-loss programmes carried out at the best clinics for natural healing and health education such as Weimar in northern California or the Centre for Health Promotion at Loma Linda University. It has long been advocated by Adventist health experts whose assertions have only recently been validated by sports physiologists and others.

Appetite Control

The control centre for both thirst and hunger is in the same place in your body: the hypothalamus. Often when you think you are hungry what you body is trying to tell you is that you need to take in more water. Perhaps the best kept secret in the world about weight control is this: reach for a glass of water every time you feel hungry between meals and you will find your hunger diminishing within a few minutes. Try it and see.

There is another way in which drinking optimal quantities of water plays a central role in weight control and ageless ageing. It has to do with your kidneys. The kidneys are responsible for recycling all the water in your body – some 800 glasses of it a day – and for filtering out any wastes present before they can lower immunity, create fatigue, make you feel hungry even though you have had enough to eat, and cause the kind of water retention which plagues so many who have gone on and off slimming diets for years. The filtering mechanism responsible for all this in the kidneys is made up of millions of microscopic bodies known as *glomeruli*. They identify waste products such as urea which need to be removed, as well as screening out other chemicals and unwanted metals and minerals, while at the same time other bodies known as tubules pour back into the bloodstream the minerals you *do* need and regulate your body's acid-alkaline balance.

When some part of you needs more water, your kidneys make sure it arrives. For instance, when you are hot and sweating a message is sent to the pituitary gland in the head telling it to release the anti-diuretic hormone which in turn tells your kidneys to let more water be reabsorbed into the blood. Your urine at such times can become highly concentrated and a dark colour. But provided you replenish the water you are losing in sweat by drinking more, your kidneys remain happy and well-functioning and the appetite/ thirst messages from your brain do not become confused. When your body's water level gets too low, however, from not drinking enough, your kidneys cannot carry out their cleansing efficiently. Then your liver has to come to the rescue – trying not to let the side down. The trouble is the liver's main function in weight loss is to mobilize body fat and help transform it into usable energy. The liver is also an organ for detoxifying the body. When it has to take on some of the kidneys' work the liver is unable to do either of these things effectively. Drinking lots of water – far more than you think you need – helps your kidneys to help your liver to do what *it* does best.

Only Water Works

Water is also better than any diuretic. If your body tends to retain water this is often because you don't drink *enough* so it tries its best to hold on to the water there is. Once you do begin to drink enough this tendency to waterlogging decreases and usually disappears completely. And by the way, if you are worried about puckered thighs, the best way to help eliminate them easily is simply to *drink more water*.

What about other drinks – coffee and tea, soft drinks, fruit juices and herb teas? Won't they do just as well? No, they won't. Quite apart from the other negative effects of caffeine – an ingredient in coffee, tea and many soft drinks – drinking coffee messes up blood sugar. Caffeine, technically known as trimethyl xanthine, is a habit-forming drug. It has frequently been shown to be responsible for headache, insomnia, nervousness, anxiety, and that familiar wired mental state which keeps you buzzing for a time intellectually but tends to disconnect you from your instincts and in some people even from having a good grip on reality. Caffeine gives you a quick lift and the illusion of energy, only to let you crash down a couple of hours later when you are inclined to reach for more – or for a sticky bun or chocolate – just to keep going.

Caffeine has a *mutagenic* effect too – that is, it is capable of crossing the placenta to cause permanent damage to an unborn child as well as breaking apart the chromosomes in your own cells and interfering with the repair of DNA. Drinking coffee also stimulates the secretion of acid in your stomach, disturbing natural appetite control mechanisms and making you far more likely to end up with an ulcer than your non-coffee-drinking cousin. In fact, caffeine acts as a stimulant to the central nervous system in a rather curious way. It makes you *feel* more mentally alert. But tests show that in reality it creates more confusion and nervousness. In animal experiments very high doses of caffeine have been shown to create psychotic behaviour. Coffee also tends to raise blood pressure and to increase the risk of coronary thrombosis. Drink five cups each day and your heart attack risk goes up by 60 per cent.

What about tea? It too contains caffeine – 100mg to coffee's 120mg in a regular sized cup. Tea also contains tannic acid – an irritant to the digestive system. In high enough concentrations tannic acid is carcinogenic. There is also evidence that drinking tea in quantity interferes with iron absorption from foods. And it's surprisingly easy to over-consume fluoride as tea, if you drink a lot of it. Even if you have always been a committed 6 to 8 cups a day tea or coffee drinker, after a couple of weeks on good water you will find you don't miss it. Then when you have an occasional cup it becomes a simple pleasure rather than an addiction.

Herb teas such as peppermint, camomile, vervain, lemon grass are also OK. By all means drink them and enjoy them. But stay away from the fancy packaged ones unless you read the labels carefully and make sure they are entirely natural. Many contain artificial flavours which you don't need. But don't count them into your daily water quota. Think of them as extras. The bottom line is simple: water is best by far. The only problem these days is how do you find water that is fit to drink?

Is Pure Water an Illusion?

The quality of water you drink affects every biochemical reaction on which leanness depends. Hundreds of millions of people in the western world now drink water contaminated with levels of toxic chemicals far in excess of official standards of safety. Even in sparsely populated countries like Australia, Canada, and New Zealand, water is becoming more contaminated each year with toxic heavy metals such as lead, cadmium and aluminium, as well as herbicide and pesticide residues and industrial chemicals – pollutants which are expensive, difficult and sometimes impossible to remove using present water purification methods. In the United States the Environmental Protection Agency, responsible for monitoring the purity of water, have issued official figures that show as much as 85 per cent of tap water is contaminated to a degree where there is virtually nothing that can be done to improve it significantly. In Britain – by the most conservative estimates – 1.6 million people are now drinking water that breaks the European limits for nitrates alone, quite apart from the 2,000 other possible contaminants. Another 2 million are at risk from high lead and aluminium. As Tom Birch from the environmental pressure group Greenpeace observed as far back as five years ago, 'The water authorities and industry are involved in a giant chemistry experiment, using the environment as a test tube.'

Impossible Task

What is going on? In theory, our governments are obliged to provide pure water. In practice, however, carrying out this obligation is now so costly that no taxpayer would tolerate the burden. As a result of the ubiquitous environmental pollution world wide, it would be nearly impossible to implement. Nitrates from our farms, acid rain, weed-killers, fertilizers and pesticides, nuclear wastes and the chemical by-products of runaway industrialization have polluted our rivers, dumps, and land-fill sites. From there they seep back into the water table to show up as far as 100 miles away. Even in the most remote regions of Antarctica man-made chemicals such as the polychlorinated bi-phenyls (PCBs) now pollute fish and wildlife despite their living thousands of miles from the so-called civilized world. Yet the public remains largely unaware of how bad it has become.

The technology we still use for cleaning our water is obsolete. We add chlorine, aluminium and other chemicals as part of the attempt to purify water for drinking. Yet many of the chemicals we still use are themselves pollutants that can make matters worse. Chlorine, which we use to kill bacteria, has been linked to the development of anaemia, high blood pressure and diabetes. It reacts with industrial effluent, polluting our ground water to form cancer-causing compounds. In the United States, where the awareness of these water problems and water treatment itself is believed to be the most advanced in the world, only fifty of the 60,000 public water systems use up-to-date water purification methods. The whole issue of water pollution and the effect it is having on health – yours and mine – is a huge one. But what is important is this: if you want a strong, beautiful and healthy body you need to find a source of water that is clean.

The Clean-Up

This is not an easy task. Most water filters only do part of the job, and for any filtering system to work it has to be cleaned and serviced frequently. Boiling your water will kill most bacteria and boil off some of the chlorine, but won't move heavy metals and chemical pollutants. Filtering your water through carbon filters will remove pesticides, chlorine and suspended particles, but bacteria from contaminated water poured through them tends to colonize and grow between the carbon particles so they need to be cleaned and changed often. Some manufacturers have added silver to these units to inhibit bacterial growth yet silver itself is a contaminant when taken in quantity. This kind of filter won't touch heavy metals like lead and aluminium which have become *dissolved* in the water.

The effective removal of all impurities from water demands large, multi-staged and highly complex filter systems operated under carefully controlled conditions. Few home filtering systems are capable of removing anywhere near the cross-section of contaminants. Friends of the Earth will let you have information about how to check out the condition of your own tap water and what your statutory rights are. Put pressure on government and read everything you can on the state of your local and natural water. This is a huge issue for the health of yourself and your family and without massive public pressure it is unlikely to change. In the meantime take a good look at what inexpensive jug filters are available and start using one – for cooking too. Be sure to change the filter it contains often and regularly. If you can afford it, use the best bottled water for drinking.

Drink Your Health

Bottled waters differ tremendously from one to another. Some which come in plastic containers or glass bottles in the supermarket are nothing more than tap water which has been run through conditioning filters to remove the taste while doing nothing to improve the quality. And just because they say 'spring' on the label that doesn't mean a thing. The word may be nothing more than the brand name used to sell the product. Other bottled waters are excellent in taste and quality. Few countries do much to regulate standards for bottled water, and what regulation there is is generally even poorer than that applied to tap water. Except in France.

There are some 1,200 springs in France. Several dozen of them supply bottled waters, the quality of which has been long monitored and controlled by official government bodies. A few have been granted the title *eau minérale naturelle*. This means that they maintain a constant mineral content. It also means that they have a reputation for specific therapeutic properties. These waters should be safe from bacterial or chemical contamination and you can be sure they have not been mixed with any foreign substance when they are bottled.

Two of the best mineral waters are Volvic, an exceptionally pure still water from the Auvergne mountains in central France, and the sparkling Perrier which arrives in a carbonated form from a spring in Vergèze in Southern France. The Volvic spring is surrounded by seventeen square miles of countryside free from industry, intensive farming and other nearby sources of pollution. Volvic is lightly mineralized with a lot of character and a vibrant quality. The well-known Perrier has long been recommended by French doctors after strenuous exercise. It is a refreshing drink, popular with athletes. I like the taste of it. I also approve of the responsible way in which the Perrier company chose to withdraw hundreds of millions of bottles from the market a few years ago when they discovered that some had been contaminated with benzene from a faulty filter. It shows a sense of responsibility I would like to see copied by other companies. Finally, from the Western region of the Vosges mountains in France comes one of the finest of them all: Vittel Bonne Source. Pure and delicate in flavour, Vittel water wends its way through rock tunnels, then pours forth clean and fresh from a source surrounded by 12,000 acres of conservation land in North Eastern France. Vittel is low in sodium and rich in calcium – an ideal everyday drinking water.

Provided you have no kidney disease or other condition which would mean your doctor would disapprove, whatever water you choose to drink, start now to drink a lot of it. So long as your kidneys are normal you need not worry about taking too much. Professor of Paediatrics at Harvard Medical School, Dr Jack Crawford, discovered that healthy adults can tolerate up to 80 glasses of fluid in a day. But drink your water *between* meals, not with them. Water drunk with meals dilutes the potency of digestive juices needed to properly break down and assimilate nutrients from your food. It also makes you more likely to overeat.

Two Each Morning

It takes a bit of practice at first to make sure you get your water quota each day but soon it will become second nature. Start by drinking two glasses of water first thing in the morning when you get up, either neat or with a twist of lemon or lime. You can heat the water if you like. This helps with elimination. Then drink two or three glasses between breakfast and lunch and another two or three between lunch and dinner. When you exercise or when it is hot remember to drink more. Getting the water habit will quench your appetite, improve your body's ability to eliminate wastes, heighten your energy levels, improve the look of your skin and help your metabolic processes function at peak.

Kneipp Water

Water is not only good for drinking. It is also one of the most potent of nature's tools for the ageless-ageing body from the outside. That is why hydrotherapy forms an important part of treatment at most of the world's clinics and spas which are dedicated to using natural law methods of age-retardation and rejuvenation. Yet it has been little used in Britain and the United States. Would you consider pouring a stream of cold water over your face to banish fatigue or prevent your skin from wrinkling and sagging? Would you apply a hot compress of hay flowers to get rid of an aching back or knee, or tennis elbow? Walk in ice-cold water up to your knees every morning to increase your vitality and ward off premature ageing? Or even have jets of cold water directed against your back and legs to help you lose weight? Extraordinary as these things may sound, they are natural methods of treatment with over 100 years of clinical validation behind them. In fact they are part of one of the most elaborate, effective and well-researched methods of healing, health enhancement and age-retardation in the world: Kneipp therapy.

An Officially Supported Treatment

Virtually unknown in English-speaking countries, Kneipp therapy is practised in some seventy spas and 6,000 hospitals in continental Europe. There, treatments are supervised by physicians who have been highly trained in the various methods it involves, the most important of which is a complex set of water applications which have profound regenerative and protective effects on the body. Far from being some kind of far-out alternative therapy used only by nature freaks and old women, Kneipp hydrotherapy is supported by government health-insurance schemes in Europe and subsidized by the state both as a preventative and a prophylactic treatment against ageing as well as a means of curing and rehabilitating the seriously ill. The anti-ageing prophylactic use of Kneipp's water treatments is steadily gaining ground simply because it has proved to be less costly to prevent the degenerative conditions of ageing than to cure them. Now Kneipp therapy is used in its various applications – from *affusions*, where water in a steady stream is poured over specific parts of your body, to *hot and cold compresses* – as a treatment for a wide variety of these conditions, from arthritis, abscesses and heart disease to asthma, diabetes and allergic eczema. Kneipp methods use water in all its many forms and can greatly increase your vitality, enhance athletic prowess, help you handle stress better, banish insomnia and counteract a myriad of negative effects usually connected with the ageing process.

The Kneipp system is a means of improving health and raising vitality without resorting to drugs, drastic methods or great expense. As such, in Europe it has become increasingly valued in a world of soaring medical costs and increasing *iatrogenic* (doctor-caused) diseases. As far back as 1900 Kneipp's water therapy was already being practised all over continental Europe. Since then his methods have been researched, applied, refined and adapted to contemporary needs by a large number of medical scientists – most of them German – who form the basis of the Kneipp movement worldwide. There are prizes of thousands of German marks given each year to scientists now investigating how the simple application of water can have such a profound effect on the health of the human body.

A Bid to Save His Life

Sebastian Kneipp, after whom European hydrotherapy is named, was born in Bavaria in 1821, the poor son of a humble weaver with an ambition to become a priest. In youth he experienced brutally hard work coupled with extreme poverty.

While studying for the priesthood he contracted tuberculosis. His physicians pronounced him incurable and advised him, in effect, to prepare for death. But Kneipp was unwilling to accept their judgement. He came across an old book written by a German physician on the curative powers of water. He began to experiment on himself by applying water in various ways. This, together with a growing awareness of the body's own ability to heal itself in accordance with certain laws of nature, brought him back to full health. This was much to the consternation of some physicians who did not believe (as most still don't) that water applications could have potent healing power, and much to the delight of many of his fellow students who themselves were cured of various minor and serious illnesses by his suggestions. He then went on to develop hydrotherapy into the remarkable therapeutic and preventative system which bears his name.

In 1855 he was sent to the tiny Bavarian village of Worishofen to supervise a Dominican nunnery. Many of his friends insisted that the church had only sent him there to get him away from his fascination with water-healing, in the belief that it was interfering with his clerical life. There he acted as father-confessor to the nuns, revived the village's stagnant economy and advised farmers how to improve their agriculture. But his fascination with health and healing continued even when later he was made parson of the village. Despite the fact that his days were filled with ecclesiastical duties, he found his time increasingly taken up by a growing number of ailing people who had heard of his 'miracle cures', and either did not have enough money to pay for medical care or had been given up as 'hopeless' by their physicians. Kneipp treated them with his water techniques and he taught them to treat themselves, gradually developing a complete system for prevention, cure and rehabilitation, based on the theory that a human being is a unity of body and soul and that whenever this unity is threatened, or whenever the harmony of nature is disturbed, illness ensues.

Total Therapy

His methods – which include water applications, herbal treatments (many passed on to him by local peasants), nutritional therapy using fresh natural foods simply prepared, movement therapy and the development of a positive attitude to life, formed a course of treatment designed to restore physical and mental unity of the human being with a particular emphasis on the use of the forces of nature (sun, water, food, movement etc). His therapy was intuitive, empirical and directed towards the specific needs of the individual patient.

Kneipp collected his own herbs, taught people how to use them and how to be moderate in the way they lived. He rapidly developed a reputation unequalled amongst nineteenth-century healers – physicians or no. He treated emperors and popes, the peasants and the clergy, all of whom flocked to Worishofen for his care and advice. Kneipp was farsighted enough to insist that his methods be put into the hands of doctors to be further developed and improved. He taught many physicians and bequeathed his herbal formulas to a pharmacist with whom he had worked for several years before he died. The pharmacist began to manufacture them late in the nineteenth century. The same company, Kneipp-Werke, still does. And Worishofen, the village where Kneipp settled, became Bad Worishofen – the largest spa centre in Europe and a centre completely devoted to Kneipp treatment. The town, which now has been carefully developed by the German government, boasts 7,000 beds in its many hotels, sanatoria and clinics where people can go to take a 'Kneippkur' and to walk the miles of beautiful pathways through the woods.

100 Ways with Water

What makes Kneipp hydrotherapy unique as a part of a lifestyle for ageless ageing is its exceptional versatility. It uses water in more than a hundred ways of widely varying intensity. They begin with such gentle stimuli as a compress or an ankle or foot bath, measures which involve almost no strain on the body – and range on to highly strenuous treatments such as the *Blitzguss*, where a powerful stream of cold water is directed at specific areas of the body to stimulate immunity, strengthen vitality and encourage the complete elimination of harmful waste products from the system. Depending on the general condition of the person, and the kind of ailment being treated, the water can be hot or cold: some treatments involve the use of steam.

Warm water is generally used in Kneipp baths, to which herbal extracts such as melissa, rosemary and pine (either alone or in combination) have been added. Some baths involve the immersion of the whole body, others only a portion. Many Kneipp treatments are based on the use of compresses – to quell fever, to detoxify the body, to bring relaxation to a stressed person. These are applied to various parts of the body for measured lengths of time. Kneipp also developed all kinds of other local applications, from treading cold water – Bad Worishofen is full of beautiful pools in the woods and in the hotels for people to walk in – to walking through dewy grass, on wet cobblestones and even in snow. These treatments, at least one of which is meant to be part of your daily routine, all aim at enhancing immunity and increasing vitality. The system is highly complex and versatile, so physicians prescribing it can carefully gear the treatment to the state of the circulation and the reactive powers – Selye would have called them adaptive abilities – of each individual patient. Each patient is advised to carry out a controlled, gradually intensifying training programme.

Water as a Source of Information for Health

The way each treatment, from the most sophisticated to the simplest form of water treading, is to be carried out for good results is carefully regulated by a number of absolute principles. For hydrotherapy is not something 'innocuous'. These seemingly simple water techniques can be detrimental if used wrongly. There is a real science to it all. It is the temperature of the water when applied to the surface of the body in specific ways which brings about beneficial results. It causes a stimulation to the skin which is transferred by way of the nerves and blood vessels to the organs. The greater the difference between the temperature of the water applied and the body itself, the stronger an effect its application will have.

In terms of information theory applied to biology, specific applications of water could be said to bring to an organism what Brekhman and others call *absolute*, *connected* or *structural* information which acts beneficially to bring the body the kind of stimulation it needs to thrive. Augustin de la Peña, author of *The Psychobiology of Cancer: Automatization and Boredom in Health and Disease* describes the kind of beneficial total-body reaction that such stimulation can bring when he says:

Presentation of a novel or unexpected stimulus produces a

generalized orienting reaction. This orienting response is accompanied by an increase in the level of CNS [central nervous system] activation relative to the pre-novel stimulus baseline. The purpose of the physiological changes, in general terms, is to make the individual more sensitive to incoming sensory stimuli so that he is better equipped to discern what is happening and to mobilize the body for whatever action may be necessary.

Water applied to your body, like spring-cleaning 'cures', exercise, and a number of the other natural law tools of ageless ageing, can 'stress' your system in very positive ways – ways which make you stronger and more resistant to illness and which can increase overall vitality and improve biological functioning as well as even providing a healthy mental stimulation which takes one away from the habitualized ways of thinking and being that result in boredom and degeneration of a living organism.

Do-It-Yourself Kneipp

Not every Kneipp treatment has to be administered by a professional in a clinic or a spa. One of Kneipp's most important principles was that hydrotherapy should be simple enough that any otherwise healthy person should be able to benefit from it – both as a prophylactic treatment against ageing as well as to improve the condition of the skin, to eliminate stress and to treat minor ailments from a headache to a cold without professional help. Simple at-home water treatments can fortify your body against sickness in general, improve circulation and calm frayed nerves. If you decide to make use of water applications as part of a programme for ageless ageing, you need to know a few principles, for good results depend on each application being carried out in the correct way. Whatever water application you make, these are Kneipp's general rules to follow:

- Apply cold water only to a warm body, never to a chilled one. It's best to warm up with exercise or be wrapped up snugly in bed just before you begin. If your body doesn't get warm quickly afterwards, then it is best to use alternate warm and cold applications instead of cold ones only, until your system becomes stronger and more resilient.

- Your body should always regain its warmth within fifteen or twenty minutes after a water application. It is a good idea to move about afterwards or rest in a warm bed.

- After any form of warm Kneipp bath, either a full bath or a half bath (if not followed by a cold affusion), you should rest for half an hour to get the full benefit of the treatment.

- Wait until at least an hour after a meal to carry out any water application.

- Don't dry your skin with a Turkish towel after a water application as this can lessen its benefits. Instead pat dry the wet parts of your body with your hands then cover yourself quickly with warm clothing in natural fibres which are porous.

- For women, during a menstrual period, only make use of applications on the upper part of your body.

Here are a few of the simplest and most useful Kneipp treatments which have good applications for ageless ageing.

Face Affusions for Perfect Skin

An *affusion* is literally a pouring of running water over a particular area of the body. The fact is, affusion stimulates blood supply to the skin and restores lost tautness and freshness to sagging or faded skin. It is a popular natural treatment in Europe amongst men and women who want to retain their youthful good looks. It helps prevent premature ageing of the skin, eliminates feelings of fatigue and can even cure a migraine.

Here's How

Make sure your body is in a well-warmed state to begin with. Then, using a hose with an opening of about ½ inch (it can be a bathroom hand shower with the head removed) turn on the cold water so that a sheet of water is delivered to the skin when the hose is held 2–4 inches from it. (There should be no great pressure of water.) When an affusion is done right the water flows smoothly and evenly and there is no 'splashback'. Now, resting your neck on a towel and bending over a sink or the bath, begin by circling your face with the water from just below the temple. Then go back and forth from one side of the face to the other. Now guide the stream several times from up to down starting at the left side and working towards the right. End by circling the whole face again. The entire process is done with cold water and should take only a couple of minutes. Now pat your face gently to remove excess water and then let it dry completely in the air.

To Boost Vitality and Strengthen the Immune Functions

There are several techniques designed to increase vitality and bring protection against illness and age-degeneration. Which you choose depends on your current state of stamina and health. They range from the body wash, which is gentle enough for almost anyone, to the cold *Blitzguss* which top athletes and other very fit people favour.

The Body Wash

This is quite different from the usual cleansing wash you carry out in the bath or shower using a flannel. It involves the uniform spreading of water over your skin with a rough linen cloth. Afterwards you should not dry yourself. Instead get into a warm bed for a few minutes. It helps relax the body while bracing and strengthening it, and activates natural warmth to eliminate and to prevent the build-up of toxic substances in the blood and tissues which can cause the cellular damage and cross-linking that come with ageing.

Here's How

Having dipped the linen cloth into cold water, begin on the back of the right hand and sweep upwards over the shoulder then down again on the inside to the thumb. Now turn the cloth over and wash the inside of the hand and arm to the armpit and finally the back of the palm. Now dip the cloth in water again quickly and carry out the same movements on the other arm. Then quickly dipping the cloth in water again, with half a dozen vertical movements wash over the chest, abdomen and the fronts of legs. Another dip and do the back (or have a friend help here since it is easier). Finish the body wash by quickly rubbing the soles of the feet. The whole procedure, which must be carried out in a warm room, needs to be very quick (only thirty to forty seconds); then take off excess water from your body's surface, dress warmly and move about, or pop into a warm bed for a few minutes. (It can be a superb way of refreshing yourself after a long day before going out for the evening.)

Water Treading

This takes a couple of minutes. In Bad Worishofen there are beautiful pools in the clinics and hotels and even the woods, where you can take off your shoes and socks and walk barefoot in water every morning – summer and winter – even when there is snow on the ground. If you are lucky enough to live near the sea or by a brook both are ideal. But you can get the same results at home using a bath filled with cold water.

Here's How

Dressed warmly, but with your legs and feet naked from the knee down, step into the water and 'walk on the spot', lifting first one foot and then another up out of the water. The sharp reaction will be either a pleasant warm feeling flooding the feet or a sharp cold ache, followed by warmth. Begin by treading water for only thirty seconds or so, then work up to a couple of minutes as your system gets stronger and more resilient. Immediately afterwards put on dry warm socks and shoes and move about. (This is also an excellent treatment for insomniacs – done just before going to bed.)

Blitzguss

A real *Blitzguss* has to be done by a professional in a special shower using a powerful water-force. But you can get many of its beneficial effects in the shower, particularly if you happen to have a hand-held shower which you can direct on to different parts of your body.

Here's How

Take a warm shower until your skin is really glowing with the warmth. Turn off the hot water and use only cold – directing it over your face, down your arms and legs, over your trunk and abdomen and down your back. The whole process should take no more than thirty seconds. Get out of the shower, pat off the excess water and dress warmly. This will leave your skin glowing with warmth thanks to the reaction against the cold water. Practised every day or so, it will also strengthen your immune system not only against age-degeneration but also against colds, flu and other illnesses. And it will greatly increase your vitality. This is a favourite of top athletes in Germany. It is also my favourite of all the prophylactic treatments with water – and I am a long way from being a top athlete. But I had to work up to it in the beginning by starting with the body wash and with water treading (which I still do when I feel tired but unable to sleep). You shouldn't use the *Blitzguss* until you are already quite strong.

De-stressors for Better Sleep
The next two techniques are particularly good if you feel stressed or you tend to wrestle with insomnia at the end of the day.

Wet Socks
A favourite of Kneipp himself, this is an easy way to apply a foot compress. It is quite extraordinarily relaxing.

Here's How
Wet a pair of cotton socks in cold water and wring them out so that they are no longer dripping. Put them on and then cover them with a pair of dry woollen socks, then pop into bed. Leave the socks on for at least half an hour although it doesn't matter if they stay on all night should you fall asleep.

Cold Sitz Baths
These last only ten to thirty seconds, according to how quickly and how well you react. They are carried out with the upper part of your body well clothed, always in a warm room. This is also an excellent way of boosting immunity and protecting against minor illnesses – particularly throat and chest conditions – eliminating flatulence, constipation and stress.

Here's How
Fill the bath with enough cold water to reach to your waist. Climb into the bath and stay there for a few seconds, then get out, gently pat the excess water from your skin and immediately climb into a warm bed.

Hot Compress for Digestive Upset
This is enormously helpful when you have eaten a meal the size or content of which you regret. It rapidly restores normal digestive processes to a stomach overloaded with rich or too much food. It can be a godsend after holiday revelry.

Here's How

Take a linen or pure cotton cloth large enough to be folded twice and still cover your abdomen from waist to upper thighs. Dip it folded into hot water and wring it out well, then lay it over your abdomen. Now place a hot-water bottle filled with very hot water over that and cover the whole abdomen with a warm blanket which is wrapped all around your body. (An electric heating pad won't work.) Now relax for half an hour or more.

Once you begin to experience some of the extraordinary benefits from these simple treatments you may find you want to explore some of the other natural therapies which are also carriers of vital information for health and ageless ageing. They include air baths, saunas and Turkish baths, herbal treatments using the adaptogens and dry skin-brushing. Not only can each one of them leave you feeling vibrantly well and looking good, together with good nutrition, exercise and relaxation they are some of the means by which your body/mind/spirit can in Schrödinger's words 'drink order' from the environment – just the quality and kind of information needed to keep you well, youthful and vital long after those around you have succumbed to the ravages of time.

23
Shed the Skin of Age

MEN ARE MORE fortunate than women when it comes to ageing skin. Wrinkles on the male skin give 'character' lines. Thanks to the higher production of male hormones in men their skin boasts larger quantities of sebum. Men also have additional supporting fibres in their skin to make it thicker, stronger and less susceptible to sagging and wrinkling. For most women, wrinkles strike horror into their hearts. No single aspect of ageing seems to worry people as much as the look of their skin. Nobody likes to see their face look old. To slow down the rate at which wrinkles appear you need to treat your skin not as a superficial covering to your body but as the living, breathing organism it is, and you need to provide optimal conditions for its health and functioning on a cellular level. This involves both internal and external care. It means making sure you are well supplied internally with free radical scavengers and antioxidant nutrients, detoxifying your body periodically, protecting yourself from ultraviolet light damage and from water loss, and using specific substances on the surface of the skin either to guard against age-related damage or to encourage cellular repair when it occurs. The time to begin is long before those worrying lines start to show. But if that time has already passed, don't despair. It is never too late to get significant improvement in the smoothness of your skin's surface and its overall appearance, provided you are willing to work for it.

The Mystery of the Wrinkle

For generations dermatologists and cosmetic scientists have been trying to find out why skin wrinkles. They have chemically analysed old skin and compared it to young. They have examined the differences in cell structure between young and old skin and in the ground substance, all of which help give skin its cushiony feel and smooth contours. They have even taken skin samples from wrinkled areas of a body and compared it with skin taken from smooth areas of the same body. What they have discovered is that there are no fundamental differences between skin taken from wrinkled and from unwrinkled areas. A wrinkle is simply a crease in the skin where the collagen beneath it has been imprinted by continual muscle actions such as smiling or squinting. Wrinkling is but one phenomenon within the whole matrix of complex changes associated with age-degeneration. To prevent it we must prevent them. The more we can protect from them systemically – by treating and caring for the whole organism – the more slowly they will occur.

As skin ages, distinct fine lines appear, skin grows dryer and rougher and can become discoloured. There is a loss of elasticity and of tone. The rate at which skin ageing takes place depends on your genetic inheritance and your exposure to ultraviolet light, as well as your diet and general state of health. It involves the kind of alterations to the mesenchyme as well as to the cells' genetic material and to cell walls which we've been looking at in previous chapters. These changes tend to lower cell metabolism and to interfere with proper cellular use of nutrients. They also tend to slow down the elimination of wastes.

Atrophy of the sebaceous glands, resulting in lower secretions of sebum, also takes place with age. This makes your skin's surface dry. A decrease in the volume of circulating blood and a loss of subcutaneous fat which gives youthful skin its smooth cushiony look are also part of the process which results in wrinkling. So is a slowing down of cell reproduction at the base of the epidermis, and a decrease in the water content of the dermis. Most of these age-related changes occur from free radical and peroxidation damage and to cross-linking of collagen in the body. One of the major factors in bringing these things about in your facial skin is being exposed to ultraviolet (UV) light day in, day out, throughout your entire life.

UV light in its many wavelengths acts on skin in a number of ways – all of which can make it look and feel older. It disorganizes and hardens the collagen fibres and it damages the skin's elastic fibres, destroying its 'stretchability'. Both of these effects encourage the formation of wrinkles and sagging. Free radical damage and cross-linking also disrupt the natural balance of your skin's *muco-*

polysaccharides which form the gel-like medium in which the cells live which helps your skin retain water. Finally, they damage the cell membranes and even the ability of a cell to reproduce accurately so that, gradually, as cells divide, they come in time to be quite different in structure and functioning from the young cells from which they are descended.

Protecting DNA and RNA

As in every other cell of your body, within the nucleus of every skin cell lies the genetic material which makes it possible for that cell to reproduce by dividing – ideally making perfect replicas of the original cell. What ensure this continuity, what make sure that each cell is therefore able to carry out perfectly and efficiently its functions without the skin tissue, are the minute 'blueprints' clustered by hundreds of thousands in every chromosome. These blueprints come in the form of a long spiral molecule which looks like a twisted ladder. This is deoxyribonucleic acid – DNA. And although there is nothing very special about the components of this molecule, its superb architecture makes it unique among chemicals. Without DNA no life would exist on earth. DNA is simply made up of phosphates and sugars (which form the spirals of the twisted ladder) and bases, which are the nitrogen-containing adenine, thymine, guanine and cytosine. The 'rungs' of the spiral ladder are made out of any combination of two of these bases. The ingenious way in which the DNA molecule is structured in these two intertwined spirals connected by thousands of these rungs enables it to 'spell out' an incredibly complex coded message. Even more important, DNA has an ability which is totally unique in biology: it can reproduce itself.

Your skin's health and good looks depend heavily on this unique skill. It makes it possible for cells to replicate themselves perfectly, thanks to the carefully coded message. That is, it should. But, as we have seen, DNA can become damaged by free radicals and highly reactive oxygen molecules that are present in the body as a result of exposure to chemicals in the atmosphere, cigarettes, alcohol, caffeine from coffee, drugs and metabolic wastes. When such damage takes place, the cell can usually repair itself and continue to reproduce itself (that is unless the damage is so great that it dies) but its genetic coding will no longer be perfect. And unless the damage to the genetic material can be repaired, future generations of cells which come from it will be flawed. An accumulation of such errors in the genetic message can lead to a decline in cellular functioning and promote skin ageing. Of course the human body, like all biological systems, is programmed for success and for survival. So there are trigger mechanisms which come into play when damage to the DNA occurs. One of the most important is a process called *excision repair* or 'dark repair'. It stimulates the production of specific enzymes which excise or cut out the damage. Then a new section is made to replace the damaged one which has been removed, so that the DNA strand is restored to normal; the offspring cells which are produced by this one will remain perfect.

The only problem is that when skin is exposed to UV light and to other sources of oxy-stress and free radical damage, as it is every day, year after year, the DNA can accrue more errors than the normal repair mechanisms can handle before the cells reproduce themselves. Also as you get older the natural repair mechanisms appear to work less efficiently.

Skin cells become less active and the skin's metabolism slows down. The exchange of blood and lymph can become sluggish and the basal layer beneath the epidermis which in young skin is wavy tends to flatten and thin, further decreasing the amount of nourishment that reaches the cells. At the same time there is a decrease in the levels of natural moisturizing factors, including not only the lipid protective film but also hyaluronic acid – a powerful moisturising agent in the skin's ground substance. Skin also becomes more sensitive and reactive to external threats as it ages.

Together these degenerative changes result in a significant lowering of vitality in the skin and in the build-up of wastes in the tissues. The lower the vitality and the higher the levels of wastes, the more cellular degeneration takes place and the more rapidly your skin is inclined to show signs of ageing. To counter the ageing of skin one needs to increase cell activity, decrease free radical damage and increase the skin's moisture-retaining ability.

Cosmetics and Nutrients to the Aid
In recent years a number of products have appeared which contain active ingredients, including free radical scavengers like vitamin C, E, A, zinc and selenium, that are designed not only to mop up free radicals but also to accelerate the skin's natural repair process, thereby increasing the number of repaired cells for reproduction by somewhere between 40 and 50 per cent. Such a complex is Estée Lauder's Advanced Night Repair. Even more potent help however

can come from providing your system with an *optimal* supply of the nutrients known to promote DNA repair. They include ascorbic acid, biotin, choline, chromium, the amino acid cysteine, folic acid, manganese, methionine, molybdenum, nucleic acids, orotic acid, pantothenic acid, pyridoxine, thiamine, vitamin E and zinc.

Surreptitious Cosmetics

Cosmetic counters are also full of products – from night creams, eye creams and neck creams to ampoules and masks for both men and women – which contain special ingredients claiming to help prevent and counteract wrinkling and other age-related changes in various ways. The best anti-ageing skin care products are based either on vitamin A, fatty acids and minerals such as vitamin E and biotin, analogues of natural metabolites found in the skin such as ATP (adenosine triphosphate which controls energy supply), hyaluronic acid and ceramides, or natural substances and compounds such as fruit acids and extracts of *Ginkgo bilopa* or other plants.

The 'anti-wrinkle' substances used in most products usually work in one of two ways. Either they aim to increase the skin's water content – something which in itself has been shown measurably (although only temporarily) to decrease the depth of facial lines by 'plumping' up the epidermis – or, more important, they attempt – often surreptitiously – to stimulate skin tissue biologically. A good example of such biological stimulation (and an approach which a number of cosmetic manufacturers take in formulating their products) is the use of specific factors known to increase cell reproduction at the base of the epidermis. Another is to heighten circulation in the dermis, thereby bringing increased blood-flow and nutrients to the skin's cells, or to improve the cells' use of oxygen and thereby stimulate skin metabolism.

The reason I say that such stimulation is often 'surreptitious' is because by law cosmetic products are only allowed to treat the epidermis – the skin's outer layer. Anything which is absorbed into the dermis and which has a biological effect on skin's deeper layers is supposed to be classified as a drug. However, many of the most effective anti-ageing ingredients in skin-treatment products undoubtedly improve the look and feel of skin and help work against age-related changes, not only because of the way they act on the epidermis but because they are in fact absorbed much deeper, where they bring about a stimulation to skin tissue which can improve cell metabolism, strengthen cell walls and even encourage the natural repair process to genetic material, thus helping to slow down the ageing process at a cellular level. Most of the best cosmetics have more than 'cosmetic' – that is superficial – actions. One of the ironies of maintaining such strict controls on cosmetic advertising is that cosmetic ads tend to sound all alike since manufacturers of genuinely active products can say little more about them than those who produce jars full of empty promises. The old idea that cosmetics are only superficial, because they sit on the surface of the skin, is an evasive half-truth. Many biologically active ingredients are drawn deeply into the skin where they act for good or ill.

Slough it Off

Gentle exfoliation of skin – the removal of the very top layers of the epidermis, either by chemical or physical means – can help refine ageing skin and smooth it out. It can also make your skin more receptive to whatever treatment products you use afterwards – moisturizers, anti-oxidant creams and lotions. But it needs to be only a *gentle* sloughing, otherwise you risk irritation and damage.

Alpha hydroxy acids (AHAs) or 'fruit' acids are currently being used for this purpose although they offer bonuses in other ways too. The four most common are glycolic acid, derived from sugar cane; malic acid from apples; lactic acid from milk; and pyruvic acid from papaya. They come in different strengths and help dissolve the intercellular 'glue' that makes old skin cells on the surface stick together. When they are cleared away the skin looks finer and brighter since it refracts light better. AHAs are also believed to increase the level of hyaluronic acid and enhance the making of collagen which makes up the skin's supporting connective tissue. Good AHA products include Chanel's Formule Intensive, Fruition by Estée Lauder, All You Need by Prescriptives, Elizabeth Arden's Ceramide Time Complex Moisture Cream, and Vichy's Novactia Skin Re-Activator.

The Vital Positive Response

In order for any of these biologically active substances to be of use, your skin's potential for good cellular function has to be good. A fairly high level of potential vitality is necessary for skin to benefit from whatever treatment-product stimulation is being offered it. This is something that the low-calorie-high-potency diet helps provide. The adaptogens can help too (see Chapter 27). So can many specific nutrients with special actions on skin. But without a high degree of potential energy in your skin's cells themselves, using any treatment product, no matter how well formulated, is rather like beating a dead horse. The single most important action to take to improve the responsiveness of your skin to whatever treatment products you are going to use on it is simply to detoxify it by detoxifying your whole body (see Chapter 16). Most skin needs detoxification badly, for people living the sedentary life common to western man and eating the average western fare, a diet high in fat, protein and refined carbohydrates, not to mention too much food and alcohol, cannot help but store up waste products in their system. (This is also a major cause of cellulite in women and hair loss in men.) Once there they tend to build up, and impede microcirculation so that the supply of nutrients carried to the cells via the blood is decreased and the elimination of cellular wastes is also slowed down. This results in a kind of tissue sludge which dulls the responses of the skin's cells, not to mention those of the cells in the rest of the body, so that no matter how good the biological stimulation you are offering it you will get little positive response and therefore little improvement in its health and beauty.

Going on a seasonal 'cure' – a detoxifying diet for from ten days to two weeks – or a well-monitored juice fast, or a regime which is ultra-high in fresh raw vegetables and fruits, can help with elimination and stimulate skin's responsiveness. Even on its own this will lessen the depth of wrinkles and leave your skin looking smoother, softer, better moisturized and firmer within a fortnight. A dynamic exercise programme followed regularly over a few months can do the same thing. So can many of the European treatments for overall body 'rejuvenation' – such as cell therapy or organ-specific RNA treatment. They can also work wonders for some skins because of the way they can improve microcirculation and cell metabolism all over the body.

The Water Margin

Youthful skin holds an amazing 14 pints of water on which its good looks largely depend. Most of its water is found in the deeper layers – the dermis and hypodermis – where, bound within the cells and in the interstitial network, the water forms a semi-fluid gel with glucosamino glycans (GAG) or mucopolysaccharides and poly-saccharides which together with healthy collagen give your skin its healthy and youthful look and feel. So long as the water balance of your body is good, the water content of these deeper layers will be right too. If, however, you take diuretics, you will lose too much water and in time your skin can become flaccid and desiccated looking. If you eat too many refined carbohydrates – which no ageless-ager would ever dream of doing – or if you suffer from hormone imbalances such as an excess of oestrogen, the opposite can happen. Your skin can grow puffy with too much fluid.

The outer layers of your skin are different. A mere 8 per cent of the skin's water is found in the epidermis – the superficial horny layer of cells on the outside of the body which cosmetics set out to treat. Yet the softness and the smoothness depend greatly on it. Unlike the deeper layers, the moisture level here is strongly influenced by outside factors such as temperature and relative humidity as well as by chemicals you come in contact with – from airborne pollutants to cosmetics. In the modern world, full of artificially heated and cooled buildings and chemical assaults of various kinds, every type of skin is fighting a battle against water loss.

Your skin is always giving up moisture into the air. We lose up to 3½ pints of water a day through the skin. When this water loss is excessive, the skin tends to become fragile and cracked. If the cracks are deep, as in those on hands which have been repeatedly exposed to harsh detergents, then chapping develops. When they are more superficial, the skin flakes. Sometimes these flakes are large enough to be seen with the naked eye. Sometimes they simply give skin a dull, flat look.

Protection from Water Loss

The epidermis itself does its best to control water loss in two ways. First, in the most superficial layer of the epidermis, the horny scales of the cells separate, leaving spaces which are then filled in with the skin's own natural protective emulsion made up from sebum, water and salts. This has an acid pH and thus helps retain some of the available water on the skin's surface. It creates a film which holds water in, rather as petroleum jelly might, although not as success-fully. One of the ways that moisturizers work is by creating such a film artificially on the skin's surface.

Naturally oily skin has an advantage in that its sebum is richer in lipids, which give better natural protection against water loss. The second way the epidermis works to retain its moisture is internal.

The cells of the skin themselves act as a selective filter, regulating both the passage of substances through the skin from outside and also the loss of water from within. They contain hygroscopic (moisture-attracting) substances carefully protected by membranes which are rich in lipids. Another cosmetic approach to moisturization has been to supply the skin with some of these natural moisturizing factors – such as urea, lactates, sugars, electrolytes and other humectants, phospholipids, sodium-pyrrolydocarboxylic acid (Na-PCA), lactic acid, propylene glycol, and hyaluronic acid.

There are a number of good moisturizers on the market which incorporate both approaches to moisturization in their products. And there is a third approach too. It uses oils that are particularly rich in essential fatty acids such as gamma-linolenic acid which occurs in evening primrose oil. A few moisturizers now offer all three. Sometimes I prefer home treatments both to encourage moisture retention and to retard skin ageing with anti-oxidants applied as you would expensive ampoules on the surface of your skin. Let's look at do-it-yourself moisturization first.

Moisture-Gatherer
Some of the best (and most expensive) moisturizers, face creams and treatment ampoules rely heavily for their effectiveness on a concentrated solution of Na-PCA. This ingredient is perhaps the skin's most important natural moisturizing factor. So powerfully hygroscopic is Na-PCA that it quite literally pulls water from the air to moisturize the skin. It is found in human skin and is synthesized in the body from glutamic acid, a 'non-essential' amino acid. As we age, both the ability of the skin to retain moisture and the concentration of Na-PCA decline. For a long time, unless you happened to be a chemist yourself, you could only take advantage of Na-PCA's ability to improve moisturization of skin – and therefore both its texture and look – by buying products which were very expensive. Now however it is available on its own in a spray bottle. You can spray it all over the body after a bath, on the face before make-up and even on hair which has become dried out. It is non-oily and an excellent and inexpensive way of moisturizing skin and it is available in chemists and health-food stores and by post from manufacturers.

Simply the Best
Among the best moisturizers on the market is Shiseido's Bio

Performance cream, based on GLA and anti-oxidants – it is one of the best creams for dry skin ever invented. Also based on GLA are the Scandinavian cosmeceutical Super Glandin Intensive Day and Night creams which are very good value.

RoC do some first-rate moisturizing treatment for the face called Hydra+ Integral, and Hydra+ Optimum Moisturizing Body Lotions and Hydro Nourishing Cream for the body. Christian Dior offer highly sophisticated multi-action skin care for every type of skin in their Hydra Star range; and Estée Lauder's Skin Perfecting Lotion is excellent. Vichy, leading-edge skin care at an affordable price, has a top-quality smoothing anti-wrinkle and restructuring serum, Renovital Skin Energizing Concentrate.

Internal Skin Care

The latest discovery in internal cosmetics is the use of nutritional supplements of fish cartilage and marine extracts. It is the *only* naturopathic formula ever double-blind tested in hospitals and reported in international medical journals. It supports the bio-chemical processes in your skin that produce new elastin and new collagen, enabling them to work in an optimal way. The result is smoother, firmer, younger-looking skin. This is just the beginning of a whole new revolution in internal cosmetics.

Nail, Hair and Skin Help

Essential fatty acids or EFAs – the most recently discovered tools for improving skin quality and moisturization (see Chapter 13) – are useful both taken internally through foods or supplements and spread directly on the skin, either from their capsules or in products which contain them. They can dramatically improve the texture, functioning and look of your skin. Rapidly absorbed through its surface, they reinforce the hydrolipidic film and the intercellular cement, strengthen cell walls so you get better cellular exchange of nutrients and elimination of wastes, and increase your skin's moisture-holding capacity. There are now skin care products on the market which are beginning to make use of various forms of EFAs. And what has come to light recently, as a result of experiments with various EFAs used to treat such conditions as premenstrual tension and in the prevention of heart disease, is the fact that used as nutritional supplements for many people they offer a number of highly desirable 'side-effects'. For instance many people using these supplements have found that broken and brittle nails become strong and grow long and healthy, while hair texture and quality also improve. I use both Na-PCA and evening primrose oil daily, spraying my skin with the former after cleansing it or after a bath and then, as soon as it has dried, applying the contents of a capsule of evening primrose oil, which I have pierced with a pin, to my skin and massaging it in morning and evening.

Vitamins for External Use

The notion that you can use vitamins to advantage on the surface of your skin was long dismissed by the uninformed who insisted that these relatively large molecules cannot be absorbed into the body through the skin and that they have no therapeutic effect. In fact just the opposite is true. Since just after the last world war scientists have known that the fat-soluble vitamins – A and E and essential fatty acids – were rapidly and easily absorbed through the skin's surface. They found that this was the only way in which they could treat many of the vitamin deficiencies of the concentration-camp victims, because their digestive systems had degenerated so greatly that they could not get adequate nutrients through their foods. The effect of topical applications is anything but superficial. It can affect the body systemically. At the Unilever Research Laboratory in Bedford, scientists reported that daily skin applications of sunflower-seed oil rapidly corrected essential-fatty-acid deficiencies which had been brought about by massive small intestine reactions. Recently much work has been done with the water-soluble vitamins and some of the minerals as well, using them in topical applications with remarkable results, and most of the top skin care manufacturers have got on the band wagon, producing anti-ageing products such as RoC's Special Wrinkle Treatment and Christian Dior's Capture Lift. The advantage of using vitamins and nutrients this way is that they can reach the area you are trying to treat, in this case the skin, without being used up or converted into some other metabolite in the body. So even relatively small doses of them applied topically can be helpful.

Topical C for Collagen

Vitamin C, zinc and the bioflavonoids are essential for the production of new collagen in the body. The condition of your skin is to a great degree dependent on how efficiently you can use them to manufacture it. Vitamin C is therefore an important factor in wound healing. Anthony N. Silvetti, director of the Wound Healing

Intensive Care Unit at West Lake Community Hospital in Melrose Park, Illinois, has found that, used in a wound-healing nutrient solution, vitamin C can successfully heal even chronic bedsores – lesions which in some cases are thirty years old. Vitamin C stimulates the skin's fibroblast cells to produce new collagen. Another American physician, Lawrence Schachner, director of paediatric dermatology at the University of Miami School of Medicine, uses zinc applied topically in a similar way to heal skin rashes and eruptions. Meanwhile doctors at Hadasah University in Jerusalem have discovered that topical zinc almost halves the healing time of herpes simplex sores, and Swedish studies have shown that the continued use of zinc after sores have been healed helps prevent their recurrence.

Vitamin E has a long history of being used topically. Because of its anti-oxidant properties, applied to the surface of the skin it can help protect cells from the damage caused by exposure to UV light or chemotherapy. It can also reduce inflammation and heat on sunburnt skin and, thanks to its potentizing effect on vitamin A, it can make this vitamin more available for healing and good skin-cell functioning. But there are some more interesting things which have recently been discovered about vitamin E. Peter T. Pugliese of the Xienta Institute for Skin Research in Bernville, Pennsylvania, has found that this nutrient also helps restore damaged capillaries that are leaking excessively into surrounding tissue – something which is common with age and in people who have been living on a typical western diet. Japanese researchers as well have found that vitamin E topically applied constricts capillaries and reduces the kind of excessive permeability which also comes with inflammation. Vitamin A has also been used with good results on the surface of the skin. One form of it – retinoic acid – which is strictly on prescription, even accelerates cell turnover, which is something that slows considerably as the skin grows older. It enhances wound healing, increases blood flow to the skin and stimulates fibroblasts to produce new collagen, but it must be used with extreme care – something even some doctors prescribing it don't exercise. It makes skin highly sensitive to light and can burn. It is best to begin at very low concentration (0.025 per cent) and increase only gradually. It must not be used by pregnant women and can cause adverse reactions in many people. The 'fruit' acids are gentler and, most experts say, better too.

Skin Cocktails for Ageless Ageing

But most important of all perhaps, when it comes to making use of nutrients applied to the skin for ageless ageing, is the fact that vitamin E, as well as zinc, vitamins C and A and gamma-linolenic acid from evening primrose oil, have anti-oxidant properties. They can mop up free radicals and highly reactive oxygen species before they have a chance to damage cell materials and cause cross-linking of collagen to occur. And when you apply them to clean skin instead of only relying on nutritional supplements taken orally, you get them right where you need them to do their work – you don't have to worry about what has been metabolized into other forms which don't have such a powerful effect on skin.

Having spent several years in search of a simple, relatively inexpensive yet highly effective external anti-ageing treatment, more than ten years ago I made my own mixture which I used for years. It was no glamorous cosmetic product, however. Indeed it left my skin smelling more like a kitchen or a chemist's shop than a beauty salon. But it was truly a powerhouse for protecting skin, built from the latest research into free radical biochemistry and anti-oxidant therapies. Now, however, skin care manufacturers have awakened to the power of anti-oxidants and most of the best products contain one or more. They are far easier and more pleasant than my old Anti-Ox recipe which contained an oil-soluble form of vitamin C, vitamin E, evening primrose oil, and a few other 'goodies'.

Some of the very best skin care products – such as Christian Dior's Capture Lift, Lancôme's Niosôme Plus, Estée Lauder's Resilience, Lancaster's Skin Therapy and L'Oréal's Plenitude Eye Contour Cream Gel – rely on sophisticated delivery systems such as microspheres or liposomes to target specific fatty acids or other ingredients to the exact place in the skin's cells where they can be of most use. In fact, some skin care products may still be horribly expensive because of the costs of advertising, promotion and packaging, but these days you can find some of the best of leading-edge formulas at low prices. Take a look at L'Oréal's Plenitude range and at Vichy's products. They are a lot nicer to use and just as effective as my old Anti-Ox mixture.

24
To Tan or Not to Tan?

EVERYBODY KNOWS THAT sun damages your skin. UV radiation is the single most powerful accelerator of skin ageing to which you are likely to be exposed on a day-to-day basis. Radiation triggers free radical and oxidation damage. It also causes collagen to break down so that skin wrinkles, weakens elastin so that it sags, and brings about unsightly pigmentation blotches which are sure signs of getting old. Happily, fashions are changing away from the half-baked look to paler skin. Trouble is, though, many people still love a tan. Until recently you had only two choices – tan and age or stay pale and preserve your skin. Now that is changing, thanks to new advances in cosmetic chemistry and new formulations which make use of them, as well as special natural substances which can help you fake a tan while actually providing you with some protection against the sun's ageing effects when you are exposed to it. And while no one in their right mind should toast themselves in the sun, with a little bit of careful manoeuvring and a clear understanding of what is involved in the tanning process you just might be able to have your cake and eat it too.

Solar Radiation and the Skin Challenge
You hear a lot about UVA, UVB and the kind of filters in sun preparations designed to protect from them. In fact 'UVA' and 'UVB' are only rather arbitrary designations for wavelengths of radiation. Until relatively recently manufacturers of sun tanning preparations concerned themselves mostly with using filters which block out all or part of the shorter-wavelength UVB radiation which is most responsible for sunburning. But 95 per cent of short wave UVB radiation is absorbed by the uppermost layer of the skin. It gets no further. They paid little attention to the longer UVA waves

which are more implicated in the tanning process. The thinking was that if you cut out the burning rays and let the tanning ones through then you would be getting the best from a sun-protection product. It is also on this theory that most of the new so-called 'safe' sunbeds – those which cut out all or most of the UVB rays while letting the UVA rays through – have been sold as well. What they didn't know (or what they chose to ignore for commercial reasons) was the fact that it is the longer UVA rays which are most implicated in premature ageing, simply because they penetrate the skin far more deeply than UVB radiation. 80 per cent of UVA radiation passes right through the outer layers penetrating right into the dermis – or deep skin. There it goes to work disorganizing bands of collagen and producing wrinkles and sagging. Short of tying people to sunbeds in laboratories for ten years, there is really no way absolutely to validate this, but leading dermatologists such as Albert Kligman at the University of Pennsylvania have referred to these sunbeds as 'automatic ageing machines'. Both UVA and UVB rays in excess are detrimental and both need to be reckoned with. For they react with the constituents of both epidermis and dermis, causing changes in the skin's vital systems which rapidly accelerate skin ageing.

The Harmful Changes
First exposure to UV radiation releases chemical messengers in the skin which produce vasodilation. Your skin rapidly becomes reddened and puffy as plasma proteins pass through cell walls and cause the accumulation of water in tissues. Such exposure also reduces the population of the cells which form your skin's true protective shield, making it more vulnerable to damage on a molecular level. And it is at the molecular level that UV radiation does its most fundamental damage, by acting on four kinds of *macromolecules* – DNA, RNA, the protein of connective tissue and the lysosome membranes. It causes breakages in the molecular chain of the DNA – the cell's genetic material – due to free radical reactions, and in the RNA, the chemical messenger for the transfer of genetic information in the birth of new cells, so that a breakdown in protein synthesis and cell mutation occur. DNA damage sends distorted signals to the epidermal cells. This alters the structure of the collagen and the elastin, which are responsible for skin firmness and elasticity. It damages the membranes of some important parts within the skin's cells, called lysosomes, which you may remember

contain enzymes, so that even more damage is done to the cells. Cell reproduction speeds up, replicating damaged cells rapidly. Cells *keratinize* or mature too early and produce fewer lipids so skin becomes dry and rough. The skin's protective lipids break down and its moisture-binding elements such as hyaluronic acid are lost so skin becomes even dryer and vulnerable to further damage.

The biochemical consequences of such UV-induced responses are many, including a decrease in your skin's ability to hold moisture in its outer layer, a decrease in elasticity and an increase in the number and depth of wrinkles. And skin ageing as a result of UV exposure is both cumulative and irreversible.

The Natural Protectors
You have two. First, the urocanic acid contained in sweat, has a weak filtering action on UV light reaching the skin's surface. Second, the natural process of tanning itself – provided it is *carefully controlled*. The new approach to sun tanning reflected in some excellent new formulations does just that. They not only provide *both* UVA and UVB protection, they also do a lot of other, sometimes highly sophisticated, things either to accelerate the tanning process or to provide skin with specific help in resisting and repairing UV damage at a deeper level, or both. In fact we are seeing a real breakthrough in skin protection and sun tanning. To understand how the new ranges work their wonders, you need to know a little about how the process of tanning itself occurs.

Exposure to UV light brings about two quite separate effects – the immediate pigment-darkening you get after even a few minutes in the sun and real tanning, which is called *melanogenesis*. The first effect is only the result of a photo-oxidation and changes in colour of the melanins or tanning pigments already synthesized in the skin. But real tanning takes place only when new melanins are synthesized. It involves two kinds of cells. *Melanocytes* at the skin's reproductive layer produce the melanin pigments which are based on an amino acid, tyrosine. Under the action of an enzyme called tyrosinase, tyrosine is converted into pigment in specialized organelles within these melanocytes. Then the second kind of cells, the *keratinocytes*, come into play. For while the melanocytes are stationary cells, they only manufacture the tanning pigment; it is the job of the keratinocytes to carry these pigments to the skin's surface where they form a coloured screen. Provided no degenerative damage is done in the process, this gives your skin a natural protection from further UV damage as well as creating a beautiful tan.

Recently animal studies have shown that although normal sunscreens can protect against sunburn they don't necessarily protect against ageing or cancer. It is relatively easy to make an efficient and stable UVB filter against sunburn but cosmetic scientists have long struggled to create the same quality UVA screens for protection against premature ageing and cancer. UVA filters have tended not to be photostable – that is, they have tended to break down in light and become ineffective. Forward-looking cosmetic companies such as L'Oréal, Estée Lauder, and Shiseido, set out to create new molecules and discover new substances that would overcome these problems. What they have come up with are excellent UV screens so good they can be rightly called 'Sun-Ageing Protection'. The new L'Oréal sunscreen, Mexoryl SX, is so good it has won much scientific acclaim. Vichy have incorporated it into their Capital Soleil range. Estée Lauder have developed an excellent *physical* sunscreen which is used in all their advanced skin care products.

Most sun-tanning products are aimed at optimizing the natural protective process while guarding against damage within the skin. They incorporate highly selective UVA and UVB filters which transmit only a controlled amount of UV radiation – just enough to stimulate the formation of melanin. Many are also formulated to increase melanin synthesis in the melanocytes. This they can do not by using the *psoralenes* as has been done in the past (since these substances may be harmful), but by providing skin with a melanocyte-stimulating substance to accelerate the activity of tyrosinase as well as other factors such as beta-carotene, glyco-proteins and glycopeptides which can also influence the activities of melanocytes. Many of the new products are also formulated to influence the formation of keratinocytes which carry the pigments to the skin's surface so that they have a good capacity for renewal, perfect integrity, perfect elasticity and so that your skin is in the best possible state of hydration, elasticity, smoothness and firmness. Some of these new ranges also incorporate anti-wrinkle and hydrating agents and both can be shown by objective laboratory measurements to leave skin in better condition (firmer, smoother, more moist, fewer lines) *after* tanning with them than *before*. But just in case you think these new advances in sun-protection make it possible to throw caution to the wind, think again. The sun's rays are still powerful forces for ageing. Go easy with them.

Safe Alternative with a Bonus

Tanning, then, is nature's way of putting limits on the amount of damage the sun can do your skin. There are other ways of providing such protection as well, for instance by ensuring you get optimum quantities of the anti-oxidant nutrients needed. Some nutrients, such as PABA, one of the B complex vitamins, are particularly helpful. It can be used either as a nutritional supplement or spread on the skin. In fact it is the main ingredient in many sun-protected products. But the protectors which fascinate me most are the carotenoids – colorants which occur naturally in our foods, such as carotene, which turns carrots orange and which, as a precursor to vitamin A, has potent free radical-scavenging abilities.

All of these things can help protect from UV damage on an internal level. But by far the best protection is no tan at all, or simply the palest golden glow, augmented if you like with one of the excellent new generation of self-tanning products. These rely on the presence of a chemical called dihydroxacetone that reacts with skin proteins to darken them. Apply them once a day and after four or five days you will have built up to maximum colour possible. Some of the best are Clinique's Self-Tanning Formula, Vichy's Moisturizing Self-Tanning Care, and Lancôme's Self-Tanning Milk. Remember, though, that these products offer no protection from exposure to UV light. For that you need to apply a broad-spectrum sunscreen product every day, summer and winter. This is important, as UVA radiation to which we are exposed remains pretty constant in its intensity. A sunscreen in a moisturizer will do day to day, with an SPF of 4 or more on cloudy days. This should go up to on SPF of 15 when the sun shines, and far higher – up to 25 – on very sunny days.

25
Cellular Therapy

THE MOST CONTROVERSIAL of all the natural treatments for revitalizing the body is cellular therapy – the injection of fresh animal embryo cells into living organisms. It is a treatment which is outlawed in Britain and the United States, where it has been the focus of orthodox medical hostility for more than thirty years. Meanwhile in Germany, Switzerland and Austria (and now in Mexico and further afield) some 8,000 physicians and surgeons have been regularly using it not only to treat chronic skin diseases, and those connected with ageing and degeneration such as arteriosclerosis and arthritis, but also as a technique for improving Down's Syndrome in children, a treatment for resistant obesity, and as a way of eliminating sexual dysfunctions.

Secrets of Royalty
Live cell therapy is often called the therapy of kings, no misnomer for a treatment which numbers popes and emperors, the wealthy, the powerful and the privileged of the art and entertainment world among its devotees. Those who take it regularly every two or three years claim it not only slows down degeneration in the body but also stimulates the immune system and even reverses signs of premature ageing.

For half a century cell therapy has been decried by the orthodox medical profession in the English-speaking world, who claim that it is little more than an expensive hoax used to pamper the spoilt and gullible in overpriced European clinics. Meanwhile, and within the halls of the same orthodoxy, a new variation on the cell therapy theme called *foetal cell transplants* has been written up (although, believe it or not, many of the scientists and doctors working with it don't connect what they are doing with live cell therapy). This new approach entails not the injection of foetal or young animal cell and tissue suspensions into the body but those from an unborn human, with all the ethical implications that implies.

Foetal cell transplants, which researchers currently hope to use as a treatment for a score or more of intractable conditions from stroke and some forms of cancer to diabetes, sickle cell anaemia and Parkinson's disease, first made headlines at the time of Chernobyl when American surgeon Robert Gale from the University of California at Los Angeles went to the then Soviet Union to implant liver cells from aborted human foetuses into some of its victims. Gale's hope was that the cells would multiply and supplant the bone marrow by restoring the victim's ability to produce blood cells which had been destroyed through radiation exposure. Sadly, his patients died from their burns before the results of the therapy could be seen. Australian-born immunologist Kevin Lafferty has cultivated foetal cells taken from the insulin-producing islet in the pancreas to use in the treatment of diabetes. At Shanghai People's Hospital too, Chinese doctors have been treating diabetics with foetal islet cells. But perhaps most interesting of all is the promise that foetal cell transplants, this new form of an old treatment, may bring help in the treatment of Parkinson's disease – the neurological disorder associated with age that affects at least one million people in the United States alone.

Surgeons in Mexico, Scandinavia and the United States have been taking out adrenal glands from Parkinson's victims and injecting adrenal cells 'harvested' from aborted human foetuses into the brain's basal ganglia. The assumption is that these embryonic cells will secrete dopamine, a brain hormone vital to the control of tremors associated with Parkinson's disease, and so allow the body to move normally. Dr Abraham Lieberman of New York University Medical Center has commented that brain transplants using foetal tissue, 'are to medicine what superconductivity is to physics'.

Now biotech companies are starting to offer treatments for diseases by transplanting specific cells from new-borns or foetuses. Under the title of *cytotherapeutics* they are also taking the adrenal cells from cows, wrapping them in polymers and inserting them into the human spine for chronic pain. Soon they hope to put similar implants in the brain as a treatment for Alzheimer's and Parkinson's diseases.

A New Twist

A few years ago in France yet another application for foetal cell transplants was introduced when two prominent physicians in Lyons – Dr Jean-Louis Touraine, an immunologist at Edouard-Herriot Hospital, and Dr Daniel Raudrant, an obstetrician at Hôtel-Dieu Hospital, took 7cc of an isotonic body-compatible solution containing some 16 million immune cells from the liver and thymus of two aborted foetuses and injected them into the umbilical cord of a baby suffering from a fatal hereditary disorder called bare lymphocyte syndrome. The results so far have been excellent. However, organizations such as the National Right to Life Committee in the United States and elsewhere voice concern that such techniques, dependent as they are on a steady supply of aborted human foetuses, may be creating a kind of black market in human life, particularly in third world countries. They speak of a 'brave new world' where men in sterile (or not so sterile) white coats traffic in human life and women, in need of money to buy food for their families become living abortion factories. What is so surprising about all of this is that within the rapidly burgeoning foetal-cell transplant scientific community there appears to be no recognition of something that any cell therapist experienced in using animal tissues knows like the back of his own hand: thanks to the biological closeness of all mammal tissue and the immunologically naive characteristics of all embryo tissue, cells from any mammalian embryo – human, rabbit, sheep, etc. – will do equally well.

Embryonic Wonders

Live cell therapy used for its anti-ageing properties, like its human counterpart foetal cell surgery, is a simple biological technique which relies on fresh live cells taken from specific embryo tissue – the brain, the liver, the thyroid, and so forth – being injected or 'implanted' into the body of an ailing or ageing person. What makes such implants valuable is the fact that cells from the unborn are *immunologically naive*. That is, because they are in a primitive state of development, the body does not yet recognize them as its *antigens* – distinctive proteins which it identifies as foreign and then rejects. That is why, unlike organs transplanted by surgery such as the kidneys or the heart, they cause low or minor immune reactions and therefore no dangerous rejection.

In fact, the non-antigenic quality of embryo cells plays an important role in the development of the life of every mammal. For instance, each of us has a different blood group from our mother and a completely different tissue type and yet, thanks to immunological naivety and to the protection offered by the placenta and its umbilical cord, a child can live at peace in the body of its mother for nine months without either being hurt by her immune reactions or harming her body. So when embryo cells from either animal or human origins are injected into the body, except in very rare cases, it accepts them.

Live cell therapy has ancient antecedents. As far back as 360 BC Aristotle spoke of a group of healing preparations taken from animal or human organs. In the 16th century the Swiss doctor Paracelsus voiced similar basic principles when he said, ''The heart heals the heart, the kidney heals the kidney.' And that is exactly what happens in cell therapy treatment – cells from a foetal liver are used to treat an ailing human liver for instance or cells from an unborn spleen are given as treatment for a troubled human spleen. Then at the beginning of this century a Russian surgeon named Professor Serge Voronoff became famous – even notorious – for implanting cells from apes' testicles in human men as a treatment for premature ageing and impotence.

Early Success

The father of modern cell therapy was another controversial doctor – the Swiss surgeon Dr Paul Niehans. At first Niehans transplanted whole glands from animals into his patients through surgical incisions. Then he found he could simply embed fine slivers of organic tissue into muscle pockets and get the same results. That is, until he discovered a better method: injecting cell suspensions of specific organs, glands and tissues into the buttocks of his patients using large hypodermic needles. His first injection was given in 1931 to a woman suffering from severe convulsions who had been transferred to Niehans' care following an unsuccessful operation on her thyroid gland. Niehans saved her life by giving her a suspension of fresh live cells of animal parathyroid glands. From then on, however, Niehans began to work not only with glands (which were customary in his branch of therapy) but other types of tissues too: heart, liver, brain, etc. Niehans was also the first to use different types of cells from unborn donor animals. For he recognized, long before any understanding of immune reactions was present in the scientific community, that foetal tissues are more easily tolerated by the patient and also have a more powerful therapeutic effect.

Niehans was an eccentric, outspoken and opinionated man who fought hard, and some say not always completely honestly, with anyone fighting him. This, coupled with the unorthodox (i.e. non-drug) character of the treatment he had developed, gave both the doctor himself and cell therapy a highly controversial image. During his lifetime Niehans' patient records were filled with the names of the rich and famous. He numbered among his clients Churchill, de Gaulle, Eisenhower and Adenauer as well as the Duke and Duchess of Windsor, Picasso, Noël Coward and Somerset Maugham. But what first brought cell therapy to the attention of the world at large was his treatment of Pope Pius XII.

Summoned to the Vatican to inject fresh cells into the critically ailing Pope, Niehans drew popular attention, especially when Pius went on to live for another four years and insisted that the Swiss doctor had saved his life. Since then it has been practised throughout Europe and been shown to be successful in the treatment of a wide variety of conditions from Down's Syndrome in children to endocrine disorders and immune-deficiency diseases in adults and (most commonly) as an antidote to premature ageing. In the past fifty years, between four million and five million cell-therapy treatments have been given in former West Germany alone.

Europe Leads the Way
Although cell therapy is often challenged on the grounds that there is no evidence that it has any beneficial effect on the body, in truth since the early Fifties some 2,000 experiments and clinical reports have been published about it – about half of them from university-based scientists – in European medical publications. These reports not only support the contention that cell therapy can be a highly effective treatment for a wide variety of illnesses and degenerative conditions, but they also indicate that European scientists have considerable understanding of how cell injections function in the body – something which doctors working with the new human-based foetal cell transplants admit they are still at a loss to explain. Cell therapy consist of several injections made all at once. The injections are made up of cells and tissues from animal embryos which have been carefully chosen to meet the individual needs of the patient. These are determined by the doctor giving the treatment from results of blood and urine tests on the patient and from taking a complete case history. Usually the doctor chooses

cells from between 20 and 25 different tissues. They can range from cartilage, connective tissue, lung and bronchi to eye, parathyroid, pituitary, spleen, muscle and thymus – there are nearly forty different possibilities in all. When the patient's 'cocktail' has been prepared from freshly sacrificed animal foetal tissue it is immediately injected into his muscle and he is required to spend at least two or three days in bed so that the biological actions which begin almost immediately can continue without excess stress.

Early on cell therapists believed that cells from each specific tissue migrated to the site of that particular tissue in the human body and settled there. Now researchers know that it is nowhere near as simple as this. Yet what does appear to happen in the living body is, if anything, an even greater miracle. On injection, the embryo tissue particles are loosened and their chromosomes become 'despiralized' within the first 20 minutes. At the same time, human microphages – white blood cells – migrate to the site of the injection to link up with particles from the implanted cells and break them down into smaller particles. The whole process of breakdown takes as little as twenty-four hours, by which time the entire embryo cell material has been degraded and absorbed by these microphages which are in turn engulfed by our larger white blood cells – the macrophages.

And as this decomposition is taking place, so is something else important: the biological materials from the breakdown of embryo cells are being rapidly distributed throughout the body in an exponentially declining curve – the main activity being about forty-eight hours after the first injection.

Radioactive Proof
Measurements by radioactive tracers indicate that one hour after the injections have been given, a high concentration of the implanted material has reached the various organs of the body, and, even more astonishingly, the lion's share of each particular embryo tissue can be found in the specific tissue to which it corresponds in the body. Laboratory investigations even indicate that the degree of absorption of substances from a particular organ or tissue in the body is directly related to the need of that organ for regeneration.

Yet, despite the rapid assimilation of embryo cell material, it can be months before the person receiving cell therapy begins to experience the full benefit of the treatment. This is because cell therapy, unlike drug treatments or the artificial stimulation which comes with using specific hormones, works *biologically*, at the speed of nature. But when improvement does come (in seven out of ten people) it is often dramatic. Over half of patients given the treatment report they feel better within the first two weeks. In fact live cells stimulate repair processes in different organs at different speeds depending upon how rapidly specific organs or tissues renew themselves. The conditions for which cell therapy has a good reputation include many of the disorders for which foetal-cell transplants are currently being tried: Down's Syndrome, brain damage in early childhood, constitutional sickness and diseases of the immune system such as antibody deficiency syndromes or blood ailments including sickle-cell anaemia. It also appears to work remarkably well in the treatment of skin diseases, neurological disorders including Parkinson's disease, infertility, endocrine imbalances and circulatory problems. But the fields in which clinical reports on cell therapy are most abundant and most glowing are still those of treating age-dependent weaknesses – restoring lost sexual functions, revitalizing the body, banishing arthritis and the rest.

Like foetal-cell transplants, the benefits of cell therapy are based on the ability which immuno-competent embryonic cells, when injected into a living organism, have to stimulate a regeneration of tissues in the recipient body. The mystery is all about how they do this. What do these live cells contain that makes them such potent vehicles for the restoration of normal biological function?

Mysteries of Bio-Engineering

Most cell therapists and researchers agree with Professor Franz Schmid, renowned throughout the world for this treatment of children with the technique. He insists that foetal tissue contains a high concentration of biochemical substances, such as enzymes and their substrates, which are designed to bring about the high growth rate of foetal structures.

These substances, when injected into the body, appear to be absorbed by it and made use of in the way it needs to stimulate its own living processes at the most fundamental levels. And when you heighten cell 'aliveness' in such a way, say experts in cell therapy, you ultimately improve the condition of the whole body.

We will probably never know the complete answer to the questions these treatments raise. But one of the factors which appears to be particularly important in bringing about enhancement of energy is the presence of specific growth factors in high concentration in embryo tissue. So when embryo tissue is introduced into the body, these growth factors stimulate the body's repair mechanisms, both on a cellular level and in the immune system, resulting in a total revitalization of the organism.

As Dr Claus Martin, director of the Institute for Live Cell Therapy in Rottach-Egern, Germany, says, 'Live cell therapy is so far our only available form of molecular bio-engineering therapy, so that is why it is probably the best way to stay young longer and healthier.' In a recent study Martin and his associates compared the complaints and the state of health of patients before and six months after treatments of more than 370 participants. The results showed more than 80 per cent of patients valued the therapy as an alleviation of their complaints and an improvement of their state of health.

A highly-trained surgeon with an exceptionally orthodox background and medical training that literally spans the globe, Martin came to look at cell therapy only as a result of a family health problem for which he could find no solution. His eldest son Patrick had developed Perthe's disease – a kind of degeneration of the hip bone in which the centre of bone-growth breaks up and the bone doesn't grow.

This resulted in the child living in constant pain. It was so bad that Patrick could no longer walk. Martin consulted all the top specialists in the world. They insisted that his son needed a complex operation in which the hip bone is cut and turned around. This would mean the child remained in a cast for two months. And afterwards, according to other parents who allowed the operation on their children, there was a likelihood that he would suffer great pain and remain crippled for the rest of this life.

Martin had heard about Schmid's work with children using cell therapy in Aschaffenburg. He contacted him only to find that Schmid had treated 10 children with Perthe's disease, with good results, so Martin decided to give it a try. He administered the embryo tissue himself and, to his amazement, in two months Patrick began to walk again. Within a year x-rays showed that the hip joints were completely normal. But that was many years ago. Now, Patrick is in his twenties, six foot three inches tall, handsome, athletic and perfectly normal.

Martin took this experience as an indication that he should pursue cell therapy as a career. This he has done. Several years ago he established a clinic, the Four Seasons, by the beautiful Lake Tegernsee in Bavaria.

Fresh, Frozen or Dried

Until recently cell therapy came in three different forms: fresh cells taken from live embryos and injected almost immediately; deep frozen cells; and *lipolized* or freeze-dried cells purchased from pharmaceutical houses. The potency of the treatment, in terms of its healing and regenerative capacities, depended largely on which kind was given. Live cells were best, with deep frozen next and lipolized last. Six years ago however, as a result of reports of allergic reactions to the injection of lipolized and frozen cells by untrained practitioners, authorities in what was then West Germany forced a halt to the selling of commercially prepared cell therapy preparations. There has been much controversy and speculation around their action. There have even been suggestions that pressures from conventional drug companies may have been behind such changes since in reality reports of allergic reactions to cell therapy have been very few and far between. In any case as of now this rather splendid biological 'therapy of kings' is only available at three or four clinics in the world, and there only in its original (and best, as it happens) form – fresh cells from live embryos. It is sad to think that a biological treatment of such value is now only available to an elite few fortunate enough to know about it and rich enough to afford it. But, thanks to the new research into foetal cell transplants, the growing interest in non-drug biological alternatives, and growing moral concerns over using human foetal material in any kind of treatment, in the next five years there is a good likelihood that this 'treatment of kings' will not only enjoy a renaissance but may even for the first time in its existence be properly honoured by the scientific community for its power.

Hopefully this is a first step. For in a world in which degenerative diseases for which we have no effective treatments in our repertoire of drug therapies have reached epidemic proportions, we cannot afford to ignore the clinical experience of physicians like Franklin Bircher and the methods they use for restoring harmony and balance to the person as a whole. Cellular therapy certainly has a place among them.

Hormone Magic and Nucleic Wonders

AS FAR BACK as the papyrus of Eber, physicians have prescribed raw glandular substances for healing and rejuvenation. Homer tells how Achilles took bone marrow from lions for strength. In 1400 BC the Indian doctor Susrata counselled eating sex glands from tigers to cure impotence. In the past hundred years numerous reports have appeared in scientific journals about the successful use of raw glands such as thyroid, pancreas, pituitary and so forth in the treatment of disease and age-related degeneration. In fact it was the discovery that these raw glands from animals, or extracts derived from them, could dramatically improve glandular insufficiencies in human beings that led pharmaceutical companies at the beginning of the century to make these preparations available for common medical use, and which lent power to the newly developing science of endocrinology. In recent years, however, orthodox medicine has tended to discard the use of whole glands and glandular extracts in favour of specific hormones such as insulin, pancreatin and thyroxine, which have either been isolated from them or chemically made.

Out of this work has come the development of the contraceptive pill, the use of insulin in drug therapy for diabetes and a number of other important treatment modalities using powerful chemicals which have potent actions. The problem is they can also have powerful side-effects. For the entire endocrine system is a delicately balanced interwoven complex of chemical messengers – the hormones – which are interdependent. Giving excessive amounts of one of them on its own can *seriously* imbalance the whole system, leading to harmful side-effects.

Isolated hormones such as testosterone (the male sex hormone), oestrogen, insulin and so forth are not as safe as the whole raw glands from which they have been derived, which is why they are only available on prescription and why they need to be handled very carefully by specialists. Whole-gland extracts are different.

Natural Chemical Messengers

Glands, or more specifically endocrine glands, secrete hormones. They release these chemical messengers directly into the bloodstream. The hormone messengers are then carried through the circulation to specific points in the body where they excite action. It is largely because of the minute quantities of hormones and polypeptides which glands secrete – usually measured in micrograms per millilitre of blood serum – that the body's organs and systems can communicate with each other. In the body there are complex biochemical cycles involving hormones from one gland which trigger actions in organs and other glands, and there are also superbly controlled feedback loops for slowing or stopping the functions of an organ or another gland when a particular task is finished. Ten glands are known to have endocrine functions, including the pineal, the hypothalamus and the pituitary in the brain, the thyroid and the parathyroid in the neck, the thymus in the chest, the adrenals, kidney and pancreas in the abdomen and the gonads or sex glands in the pelvis.

As the body ages, many essential hormones are in increasingly short supply, while at the same time imbalances between various hormones and the glands that secrete them tend to develop. According to experts in cell therapy, one of the reasons why, when properly administered, it can be so useful in restoring vitality to an organism and improving immunity is because the majority of cells used are taken from endocrine glands. And, provided these are well chosen according to a patient's need, they appear able to rebalance the endocrine system and are able to a remarkable degree to restore depleted hormone levels to nearly normal.

While not as potent in its actions as injected cells, oral glandular therapy – the clinical evidence for which was established as long as sixty to eighty years ago – appears to have considerable therapeutic value as an anti-ageing tool. That is provided of course that the glandulars are carefully processed. The major controversy now is not so much *whether* they work but *how* they work.

Oral Glandular Therapy

For many years after the endocrinologists began to isolate

individual hormones and use them for treatment, the idea of giving the extract of a whole raw gland orally instead was dismissed on the belief that, because the biologically active hormones and enzymes in these glands were proteins and polypeptides, taken orally these would only be broken down into their constituent amino acids and peptides in the stomach and therefore could exert no specific action on the body's own endocrine glands or hormonal secretions. Recent investigation has shown however that even very large molecules such as enzymes can penetrate the gut. It has been suggested by researchers such as W.A. Hemmings that about half of the food proteins which pass through the stomach into the small intestine are not broken down into amino acids and small peptides in the gut but pass as intact molecules into the circulatory system. There is also biochemical evidence that a significant percentage of the food proteins which have left the bloodstream and entered the tissues – possibly more than 20 per cent – retain their original characteristics as complex animal proteins. Clinically too, there is evidence that substances in properly prepared glandular tissues – factors such as enzymes, hormones, polypeptides, essential fatty acids and even prostaglandins – have clinically significant effects which may account for the therapeutic value of oral glandular therapy.

There are a number of glands which are available for oral use. They can be purchased from health food stores and by post from manufacturers of nutritional supplements. Because proper endocrine balance and the restoration of good hormone levels are so important to ageless ageing, these natural substances are commonly used by physicians employing non-drug methods for age-retardation – usually after a careful consideration of the endocrine status of the individual patient. The most commonly used gland is the thymus because this gland, which is often called 'the master gland of immunity', governs immune functions, which in turn play such a central role in how rapidly the body ages. It is usually given in amounts of between 200 and 800mg of thymus tissue a day, in two doses.

Other common glands used orally in anti-ageing treatment include the pituitary, the pancreas, the thyroid, the adrenals and the male and female sex glands. Most longevists agree that raw glandulars can also be useful taken as a complex which includes not only the glands themselves but other bodily tissues particularly susceptible to age-degeneration: liver, stomach, heart, brain, kidney, spleen, pancreas, duodenum, thyroid, thymus, adrenal, parotid, parathyroid, pineal, adrenal and pituitary. This can be taken together with an ovarian and uterus glandular extract for women and a prostate and orchic (taken from the testicles) glandular concentrate for men. Raw glandulars are usually taken for a period of about six weeks at a time, three or four times a year, and they are best utilized when the body has good supplies of the nutrients needed to make use of them – vitamins C, A, E, folic acid, B6, zinc, B12, manganese, B1 and B2.

The Key Lies in Processing
Health-food stores abound in glandular products many of which are of very poor quality, either because they have been heat processed, which destroys much of the biological activity of the raw substance, or because they have been extracted from animals which are not healthy or which have been treated with growth hormones such as di-ethyl stilbestrol (DES) to make them fatten quickly for market. Avoid them. Poorly processed glandular material cannot be effective if the biologically active materials it contains have been eliminated or destroyed. These materials tend to be stable at temperatures below freezing but they can be destroyed by heat. There are three ways of processing raw glandulars which are widely used: the azeotropic method of co-distillation, salt precipitation and freeze-drying.

While the azeotropic method produces a final product which is quite high in enzyme activity, it removes the fat-based substances present. And, since many of the active fat-soluble hormones are present either in the fat surrounding the gland or in the interstitial fat these are removed in the process. So are essential fatty acids and prostaglandins. The salt precipitation method involves maceration – steeping the fresh frozen glands in liquid – after which salt and water are added and then the mixture is centrifuged to separate the fat. But even after the processing is finished the salt remains.

The best way of processing glandular extracts is by freeze-drying them. This process, in which they are treated under vacuum, avoids removing the fat within the glands and produces a product which is stable over long periods when exposed to air. You end up with a product which has at least five times the raw coagulable protein and enzymes of glandular tissue prepared by other methods. It is also very important to make sure that the glandular materials themselves come not from animals which have been raised on feed lots but from livestock which has been grazed. Glandulars from New Zealand are particularly good since there are strict regulations there prohibiting the use of insecticides or synthetic hormones, and their livestock is range-grazed. When choosing a supplement for oral glandular therapy it is also important to look for one which is prepared in such a way that each tablet is protected from stomach acid so that as much of the biologically active glandular substances as possible reach the small intestine where they can be absorbed by the lymph system.

Nucleic Acids for Prolonged Youth?

You may remember from Chapter 23 that one of the major problem areas in ageing on a cellular level is the missynthesis of proteins and especially the nucleic acids which carry the cell's genetic information – DNA and RNA. When this occurs, amongst other things cell vitality is lowered and, unless the damage is repaired, a cell can no longer reproduce itself accurately. Nucleic acids – DNA and RNA – have continually to be synthesized in the cells and there has long been a controversy about whether supplying these substances dietetically or in the form of supplements, together with the various vitamins, minerals and amino acids needed to manufacture them, can promote the repair of damaged genetic material and boost the synthesis of healthy protein. There is some evidence that taking between 1,200 and 2,000mg of nucleic acids five days a week for a two-month period at a time can do this.

This theory has mostly been propagated by a Swiss-trained American physician, Benjamin Frank, who has written several books on the subject of nucleic-acid supplementation and who has for more than twenty-five years been using nucleic acids either as dietary supplements or encouraging people to eat foods which are high in them, such as sardines, very often. Frank claims that the body is not always able to synthesize enough DNA and RNA. This results in a breakdown of genetic encoding that eventually leads to degeneration. He asserts that 'by providing supplementary nutrients, exogenous RNA, especially when combined with meta-bolically associated B vitamins, minerals, amino acids and sugars, will enter the cell and aid in normal regeneration of the decayed metabolic organization of the cell, and in so doing will bring about normal enzyme synthesis and activation.'

Frank believes that supplementing your diet with nucleic acids increases the production of ATP – the cell's basic energy currency

– and that this in turn stimulates cell repair and normal functioning. ATP itself can be synthesized from nucleic acids. If one can increase the production of ATP, claims Frank, then your cells are able to use oxygen more efficiently and therefore oxidation damage to them will be reduced. He claims that several weeks on such a regime brings improvements in health, including an increase in stamina and vitality. Facial lines become softened and begin to disappear while the skin becomes moist and glowing as a result of improved cell functions and increased production of one of the skin's most important moisture-retaining factors – hyaluronic acid. The Frank diet stresses foods which are particularly high in nucleic acids such as brewer's yeasts (the richest source), sardines, pinto beans, lentils and so forth. Nucleic acids are also available as supplements from health-food stores.

The Nays
The most common objection to Frank's techniques is twofold. First, dissenters claim that nucleic acids are not needed in the diet because the body can make them out of proteins and carbohydrates. Frank is quick to counter this argument by pointing out that nucleic acids are actually taken in when we eat many foods and that we have both digestive enzymes which are able to break nucleic acids down into nucleotides as well as biochemical pathways for resynthesizing nucleic acids from these nucleotides in the cells. So, he claims, it would appear that nature intended us to get at least some of them in our diet. The second common objection to nucleic-acid therapy lies in the fear that they might increase the level of uric acid in the blood and encourage gout. But provided vitamin B5 and thiamine are present in sufficient quantities this should not happen. Vitamins C, A and E as well as the essential fatty acids also help detoxify the body of excess uric acid.

Unfortunately nobody so far has done much to try to validate Frank's work, so there is little more than his clinical records to go by in evaluating the treatment. However there has been quite a lot of research into how exogenous nucleic acids affect animals. For instance, as long ago as 1928 Australian scientists experimented by feeding yeast-derived nucleic acids to mice from weaning to death. They recorded a 16 per cent increase in lifespan. If this were to be translated into human terms you would have to eat a lot of yeast – about 70g (2½oz). Another researcher, T. S. Gardner, later fed yeast-derived nucleic acids to mice, starting when they were 600 days old, well on the way to old age. He found they lived 9 per cent longer than the control group and also that they kept their vigour and had significantly less tendency to senile changes than their counterparts.

Organ-Specific RNA

In Europe, particularly in Germany, there is a well-established tradition of using RNA and DNA derived specifically from glands and organs for rejuvenation and restoring hormonal balance. The best-known mixture is called Regenerensen or RN-13. It is made up of organ-specific RNA from testes, ovaries, placenta, hypo-thalamus, adrenals, liver, pituitary, thalamus, spleen, blood vessels, brain and kidneys plus some yeast-derived RNA. It is meant to encourage proper protein synthesis in all the corresponding glands, organs and tissues of the body. (This treatment is an offshoot of the original cellular therapy.) Organ-specific RNA is usually given by injection but it is also available in tablet form. Anyone taking either organ-specific RNA or dietary supplements of yeast RNA orally is usually advised to take the tablets five out of seven days a week, to ensure he or she gets all of the vitamin and mineral factors which are particularly important in the synthesis of new nucleic acids, and to drink plenty of water while following the treatment. I personally have never tried either, while I have several times used oral glandulars with good results. People I know, however, claim to have found them very helpful. Most of them insist that Frank is right – dietary supplements of RNA do improve the look and feel of the skin dramatically.

27
Nature's Anti-Agers

AMIDST THE GROWING awareness of what high-tech bio-chemistry boasts in the form of the anti-oxidant nutrients against degeneration and what expensive treatments such as cell therapy can do to improve your appearance, to slow down the rate at which you are ageing and to revitalize your system, we often give little thought to what simple natural substances have to offer. Take herbs and roots and animal tonics, for instance – some with a history going back several thousand years. Amongst them all, the most exciting, the finest and most effective belong to a group called *the adaptogens*. The adaptogens, which include a number of very different natural substances – from *Panax ginseng* and *eleutherococcus* (sometimes called 'Siberian ginseng') to an exotic-sounding preparation made from the horn of a deer – have been widely investigated in recent years by Soviet and Russian scientists and, in centuries past, mostly by the Orientals.

Most of the adaptogens belong to long traditions of folk medicines and most have been held in high esteem for thousands of years in the pharmacopoeia of the world's medicine. What is so special about these natural products and why they are grouped together under the name is that they are all substances which, in carefully conducted laboratory and clinical studies, have been shown to enhance an organism's 'non-specific resistance' to ageing, illness and fatigue. In practical terms, they enhance your body's ability to adapt itself to all forms of stress – from the stress of fatigue, of illness, of exertion and of ageing to emotional hardship – while at the same time helping to normalize biochemical activities. Taken as 'medicines for well people' they can be remarkably helpful in keeping your body young and full of vitality. So remarkable are the positive effects that adaptogens have been shown to have on a living organism that it is a constant source of wonder to me that they have not been more widely investigated and used in Europe and in America. Meanwhile Soviet, Russian and Oriental scientists have spent the last forty years working with certain natural products which, when taken in a form unadulterated by heat or heavy processing, have a remarkable ability to improve health. They appear to be high in *structural information*.

Structural Information for High-Level Health

As Russian scientist I. I. Brekhman and others have shown, not only are the chemicals and nutrients which can be extracted from natural plant or animal substances in the laboratory – vitamins, minerals, protein, organic acids, oils, etc – important for health, so is the complexity of the way they and other as yet unidentified factors are synergistically combined. In Brekhman's terms certain natural products (many of them folk remedies) are rich in structural information, a high-quality, health-supporting energy which cannot be measured in chemical terms alone. He is particularly interested in certain natural pharmacological substances such as ginseng which appear to supply a high degree of structural information to an organism and thereby support a high level of health and energy. There is something quite special in the way the constituents of such natural products seem to work together and have a natural affinity for the body. They have been shown to increase physical stamina and endurance, stimulate protein repair on a cellular level, protect from radiation damage, increase antibody production, detoxify your body and improve your stamina and vitality. In a way the adaptogens could be considered the 'elixirs of life' in the late twentieth century. They are perfect natural tools for ageless ageing.

Stress without Distress

It was Soviet scientists who first developed the notion of an adaptogen, from the work of Hans Selye, Director of the Institute of Experimental Medicine and Surgery at the University of Montreal, whose work on stress has become universally accepted. His *general adaptation syndrome*, the GAS, you may remember from Chapter 6, describes the way in which when your body is stressed by whatever agent – from cold to fatigue to emotional upset to overwork to chemicals in your air or foods – its homeostasis, that is, its natural balance, is threatened. Immediately it draws upon its resources to resist the threat and to maintain well-being. And indeed, provided you are young and strong and well it can go on resisting any damage from stress for a long time. But, alas, eventually it enters the final stage of the GAS in which exhaustion takes over. Then your body's weakest system starts to break down and chronic illness, fatigue and (if the stress is great enough) even death can follow. What in effect has happened is that your body's adaptive energy – its ability to cope – has finally become exhausted.

Selye pointed out that the ageing process itself can be viewed as the GAS on a wider scale. He emphasized that the capacity to adapt virtually disappears in old age and that this loss, equivalent to a loss of vitality, is characteristic of senescence. Selye was always fascinated by the notion that it might be possible to discover or to develop 'medicines for well people' which could enhance the body's own adaptation mechanisms – substances which could prolong your body's ability to resist age-degeneration and exhaustion. They would be different from usual medicines in that, unlike drugs, they would not be aimed at a specific effect such as lowering blood pressure or eliminating pain. Nor would they be intended for the treatment of illness. Instead they would belong to a new category of medicines for health, for they would improve the body's *non-specific resistance* to illness, ageing and fatigue.

That's where the *adaptogens* come in – substances which can increase your general capacity to overcome external stresses through adaptation. Their use has an important part to play in protecting skin from ageing, in maintaining a high level of health and vitality and even in enhancing mental abilities. I. I. Brekhman, at the Far East Scientific Centre of the Academy of Science, Vladivostok, has done more than any other single scientist to explore adaptogens and to test their effects on both animals and humans. In fact it was Brekhman's teacher, the Russian expert in pharmacology N.V. Lazarev, who first coined the word in order to describe these substances with the remarkable ability of strengthening and rebalancing the whole system. One of the first natural substances which Brekhman and his co-workers investigated and which they found had this ability was *Panax ginseng* – the root that was first used for medicinal purposes more than 4,000 years ago 'to restore the five internal organs, tranquillize the spirit, calm agitation of the mind, allay excitement, and ward off harmful influences. The continual use of ginseng makes for long life with light weight of the body.' It is probably the most well known and highly respected natural medicine in the world.

Useless in Perfect Harmony

Traditionally ginseng has been prescribed only in states of imbalance. It is used to treat toxicity in the body, sluggishness, anaemia, weakness and fatigue. But like most of the nutritional and natural tools for health, in a perfectly healthy and balanced person it is supposed to have no effect whatever. Because, as your body ages, its ability to withstand stress and to maintain homeostasis declines, ginseng has become a prime anti-ageing remedy. For generations in the west the value of ginseng has largely been dismissed as an old wives' tale. In part this is because the very notion of a medicine for health finds no place in the thinking behind western orthodox medicine. But in part too it is probably because some of the few studies which have been carried out to test claims made for it have been done on inferior crops or on ginseng which had been heat-treated, and heat-treating destroys many of the beneficial effects of most of the adaptogens.

A number of well-conducted studies, both on animals and humans, carried out by Brekhman and others in the Soviet Union and by European researchers in Switzerland, Sweden, Germany and Britain show quite conclusively that ginseng has extraordinary adaptogenic properties. It improves the body's ability to use oxygen – important in staving off ageing – as well as increasing mental and physical stamina and in enhancing athletic performance, all of which it has been shown to do. It helps lower blood pressure that is too high, but doesn't affect normal readings. It offers protection against radiation-caused damage, also important in slowing down the rate at which your body ages. It increases your resistance to illness and against harmful effects of chemicals in the environment. It heightens mental faculties and is a natural stimulant to the central nervous system, improving reflexes, long-term and short-term memory, and making learning easier. But unlike coffee and most other stimulants, it does not produce a sudden rise in body activity followed by an unpleasant dip in energy, or depression. Nor is there any danger of becoming dependent on it. Like all of the adaptogens, ginseng has a gradual build-up effect on the body when you take regular doses of it over about three weeks.

Staving off Exhaustion

If, like me, you like to work long hours but still be reasonably fresh and responsive afterwards, you can use ginseng as a means of staving off exhaustion, while improving mental and physical functioning and maintaining a sense of mental and physical balance. At the Maudsley Hospital in London, Stephen Fuller gave ginseng to nurses involved in stressful and exhausting shifts and an identical placebo to others. He found that although performance in psychological as well as physical tests, and overall mood, vitality and competence were undermined by the stressful conditions in which they worked, ginseng improved many of these parameters in those who took it. In the then Soviet Union ginseng was given to fifty soldiers on a 3km race while to another fifty a placebo was given. Those who had taken the ginseng finished an average of 53 seconds sooner than the rest. At the University of Minnesota researchers tested the exam-taking abilities of students by giving some ginseng and some a placebo. The exam results from the ginseng group were significantly higher than the placebo-takers. In repeated animal trials Brekhman and others have found that ginseng acts as a stimulant without causing insomnia and that not only does it help stave off fatigue and strengthen the organism's ability to cope with stressors of all sorts, the beneficial effects of taking ginseng appear to multiply and build up over the period in which it is taken. Also, ginseng's benefits last long after you stop taking it. As Brekhman says:

> After a series of experiments on men it was established that daily doses of ginseng preparations during 15–45 days increase physical endurance and mental capacity for work. The increase was noted not only during the treatment itself, but also for a period of time (a month to a month and a half) after the treatment had been over. The increase in work capacity was attended by a number of favourable somatic effects and a general improvement of health and spirits (appetite, sleep, absence of moodiness, etc).

Siberian Ginseng

Another adaptogen which has now been widely investigated, particularly in the Soviet Union, is eleutherococcus or Siberian ginseng. Unlike ginseng, eleutherococcus has not been used for generations for health. Indeed its therapeutic properties have only been discovered in the past fifty years. Siberian ginseng is a prickly plant known as 'devil's shrub' with leaves similar to ginseng and beautiful yellow and purple flowers. It is the plant's hot and spicy roots which are used medicinally. Like ginseng it has an ability to strengthen the body's ability to resist illness, degeneration and fatigue while never upsetting your body's natural physiological functions. It is a mild stimulant. Take it now and this stimulant action will last between six and eight hours. Its tonic effects are accumulative – they come gradually over a few weeks. They include increased stamina, better sleep patterns, better memory, clearer thinking and improved athletic performance. Eleutherococcus has particular relevance to any anti-ageing programme because it is a natural protector against the kind of free radical oxidation which leads to cross-linking of proteins and, among other things, skin sagging and wrinkling. It also appears to have potent anti-cancer properties. Brekhman and many Russian researchers believe that eleutherococcus is a better adaptogen than ginseng. It has been shown both to increase the work capacity of people in factories and also to reduce the incidence of absence from work because of illness.

And it is considered by Russian physicians to be a treatment of choice for both high and low blood pressure thanks to its ability to harmonize bodily functions. It is also used widely to treat anaemia and to treat arteriosclerosis in the CIS. Like ginseng and all of the adaptogens it is best taken regularly over a period of several weeks. It can however be taken year round without any loss in beneficial effects.

Stringent Demands for Adaptogens
Ginseng and eleutherococcus are the two adaptogens most widely available in Britain and America (not, alas, always in active forms however – you have to be careful what you buy). But there are others too: pantocrine (an extract of deer horn); *Schizandra chinensis* (the red berries of a Chinese plant which are widely used as a tonic); and many more, including the Scandinavian Arctic Root, and *Kvann* – a Norwegian variety of Angelica – still under rigorous investigation. *Schizandra chinensis* has protective properties for the liver, increases the ability to use oxygen at a cellular level and stimulates brain function. Acantha Root or *Acanthopanax senticocus* is used to build physical strength, regulate blood pressure that is too high or too low, improve adrenal action and heighten cerebral function. Each has its unique properties but they have a great deal in common both in the way they act on the body and in their safety even when used regularly over long periods of time.

The most exciting herb I have come across for a long time is suma

(*Pfaffia paniculata*). Locally known as *para todo* – 'for everything' – suma has been used by Brazilian Indians for centuries as an aphrodisiac and general tonic. Recent research shows that, like good ginseng, the wild root of the suma plant also has strong adaptogenic properties. Amongst its other constituents, suma is rich in the saponins, some of which show anti-tumour activity, and in a plant hormone called *ecdysone*. At the University of São Paulo, Dr Milton Brazzach, chairman of pharmacology, has treated thousands of patients with serious ailments, including both diabetes and cancer, and verified the plant's potent healing and preventative powers. Researchers have found that a major source of the plant's energy-enhancing and stress-protective properties lies in its ability to detoxify connective tissue of what are called *homotoxins*. These are wastes which can interfere with the active transport of nutrients to the cells and in the production of cellular energy, and lead long-term to changes in the DNA associated with premature ageing and the development of degenerative diseases. What all of this means to the active man or woman is that suma is well worth looking at as a nutritional support to raise your energy levels, enhance your ability to be very active both mentally and physically without fatigue or damage, and to detoxify your cells as a prevention against premature ageing and degeneration.

Russian scientists are very careful about the requirements that need to be fulfilled if a natural medicine is to qualify as an adaptogen. In Brekhman's own words:

1. The substance, whether herbal or animal in origin, must be absolutely safe to the body. It must also have a wide range of therapeutic and protective properties while only bringing about minimal alteration to bodily functions.

2. Its action must be non-specific. That is, it must increase resistance to a wide variety of harmful chemical and biological influences.

3. It must have a normalizing action regardless of the direction of pathological changes it may meet within the person's body. In other words, in a person with blood pressure which is too high it should help lower it while it should have just the opposite effect on an organism in which blood pressure is too low.

When you think just how remarkable these requirements are you begin to realize why the Chinese have traditionally believed many of the adaptogens to be worth their weight in gold. It is also easy to understand why the western mind has such difficulty grasping the idea of an adaptogen at all. After all, we are used to a totally different approach: mostly this is because of our strong emphasis on symptomatic medicine.

Our science has investigated a number of pharmacological preparations designed to do specific things, such as improve circulation or increase oxygen uptake by cells during surgical operations. However most of these drugs, such as the derivatives of phenothiazine and ganglio-blocking agents, bring about side effects which make them inappropriate for any healthy person to use as part of a programme for increasing vitality, promoting high-level health and encouraging ageless ageing. We take substances such as the phenylalkylamines, like amphetamines and their analogues, as a means of suppressing an overactive appetite, or we drink coffee with its caffeine or other purine derivatives to pep us up, and we can turn to the bromides and sedatives such as the herb valerian to calm us down, but we find it hard to conceive of something that could do both or either depending upon our specific mental and physical state when we take it. As a result little investigation of possible new adaptogenic substances is going on here. Good candidates would be bee products such as pollen, propolis and royal jelly and even honey itself.

Bee Power

'Use thou honey,' commanded Solomon, 'for it is good.' Just as ginseng has a long history of being used to increase vitality and protect from ageing, so folklore is filled with advice about the medicinal use of honey and other bee products such as pollen, propolis and royal jelly, which have been employed throughout history to increase stamina, heal sickness, beautify skin and retard ageing. A natural antiseptic with a proven ability to kill bacteria, honey and all its 'by-products' – pollen, propolis and royal jelly – have antibiotic properties. And although honey has been scientifically analyzed for the last fifty years, there appears to be a number of its constituents which remain unidentified. Scientists who have attempted to break it down into its parts and then to put it together again have failed. Although honey is made up of 75 per cent natural sugars and 17 per cent water it is also a good source of many of the B group of vitamins, vitamin C, carotene and organic acids, and of many important minerals including potassium, magnesium, iron, sodium, calcium, sulphur, phosphorus and lime. This sweet golden substance has a reputation for prolonging life. While researching longevity another famed Russian scientist, biologist and experimental botanist, Dr Nicolai Tsitsin, discovered that of the 200 people in Russia claiming to be over 100 whom he surveyed, a large number were beekeepers. All of them claimed their principal food was honey.

Natural unprocessed honey has been shown to increase calcium retention and to raise haemoglobin count – it is traditionally used to treat anaemia. It also appears to speed the healing process in a great many conditions from arthritis and poor circulation to liver and kidney disorders, poor skin and insomnia. Some researchers even believe that, thanks to its high aspartic-acid content – an amino acid important in the proper functioning of sex glands – it has rejuvenating properties. But just in case you're tempted to rush to your local supermarket and buy the first jar of golden stuff you come across you should know that it is not the honey itself which appears to be the most potent source of health-promoting qualities but the pollen-rich waste matter which lies at the bottom of honey containers. Tsitsin found that beekeepers tended to sell the 'good' honey and to eat the 'dirty residue' themselves. The dirty residue – which is a constituent of natural unfiltered and unprocessed honey and appears to have such exceptional properties for health – is too often filtered off from commercial honeys. Most have also been heated, which further limits the structural information they carry and therefore depletes their health-promoting value. Honey, by the way, keeps indefinitely thanks to its anti-microbial properties and its preserve-like concentration of sugars, so you need never worry about it spoiling.

Royal Bee Power

Even more interesting than honey are the other bee-based products – propolis, royal jelly and pollen. Propolis is a sticky resin made out of the substance bees gather from the leaves and bark of trees. It is secreted via their pharmageal glands. They use it as a binding material when making hives. It has strong antibiotic properties and is much used in Sweden and Denmark to combat minor infections. Royal jelly is a white jelly-like substance produced by glands in the heads of very young worker bees. It contains almost every life-supporting element known. The queen bee, who lays over 2,000 eggs a day, lives on the stuff and it appears to have remarkable benefits for beauty both when it is taken internally and when it is used in beauty products. The problem is that most royal jelly on the market is pretty worthless. The total weight of royal jelly sold considerably exceeds the amount available! To be active it needs to be fresh, not processed into pills and potions, and it must be properly extracted from the hive and kept under refrigeration at all times – including while it is being transported. Royal jelly contains virtually all the life-supporting elements plus an unidentified 3 per cent which scientists have been unable to break down. In the south of France royal jelly is a common sight for sale by the roadside. People take a 'cure' of it for a month or so twice a year. It is also said to be beneficial for anyone suffering from stress or exhaustion or for people recovering from an illness. Bulgaria is often called 'the country of royal jelly' because beekeeping and all its products have formed an important part of the economy since feudal times. The Bulgarians have also done a great deal of research to establish the health benefits from royal jelly, pollen, honey and propolis. They have found, for instance, that royal jelly has an ability to protect against radiation, that it increases fecundity in animals, that it improves the body's use of oxygen, lowers blood pressure, speeds regeneration of damaged tissue, lowers cholesterol and, like the official adaptogens, increases tolerance to stress. It even stimulates and encourages better functioning of the immune system.

Priceless Pollen

Pollen is the male germ seed of flowering plants. A fine powder that plants need to make seeds, it is gathered by bees in the process of collecting nectar for honey and harvested by pollen collectors as the bees fly back into the hive. Not only does it contain all the water-soluble vitamins including the elusive B12, it is a good source of carotene and vitamins E and K and it offers a rich supply of minerals, trace elements and enzymes as well as hormonal substances beneficial to human beings. As such it is probably the perfect 'skin food'. Pollen is a rich natural source of *rutin* as well – one of the bioflavonoids which, together with vitamin C and zinc, is particularly important in the formation of collagen (the structural protein which gives skin its contours and much of its strength). A thrice daily dose of raw pollen can do wonders for ailing skin, whether the problem is acne, excessive dryness or hypersensitivity.

It can also improve the look and feel of normal healthy skin. But pollen's health-promoting properties don't stop there. It has been a favourite of Olympic athletes since ancient times and still is. Those who use it claim it increases strength and endurance, improves performance and helps prevent minor infections.

A Cure for Allergies?

One of pollen's more curious attributes – particularly important in springtime – is its ability to render many hay fever sufferers free of symptoms, provided oral doses of the stuff are taken regularly for several weeks before the season begins: another example of one of those folk remedies which is supported by the experience of a number of physicians who still use it successfully every year. One more interesting attribute of pollen of interest to anyone concerned about preventing premature ageing is its ability to protect the body from some of the damaging effects of radiation. It has been tested on irradiated animals and given to cancer patients subjected to radiation doses, with excellent results. Finally, and most important, pollen taken in this way, like many of the natural substances which are high in structural information, seems to possess an ability to restore balance to a body. It is said to be particularly helpful in weight regulation – whether the person taking it is underweight or too fat.

Bee products – all of them – are best taken unheated in small quantities daily. In the case of pollen and propolis, which usually come in tablets, the recommended dose is usually two to three tablets a day on an empty stomach. Royal jelly is best bought raw, kept refrigerated and taken in amounts of between 250 and 500mg a day under the tongue where it is absorbed by the mucosa in the mouth and bypasses the digestive system. It can also be bought in less biologically active forms as capsules and suspended in tonic solutions.

The Proof of the Pudding

Using any adaptogen as a tool for increasing vitality, protecting health and resisting ageing is simple. It is taken every day, usually on an empty stomach, and an average long-term restorative dose is usually 1–2g a day in the case of ginseng and Siberian ginseng. Benefits tend to accrue over the time one is taking it and the best results come from taking it regularly over a period of a month to six weeks at least. Often people take it twice a year as a 'cure'. What is not so simple is making sure that the product you are taking has been properly grown, harvested and processed in order to preserve its biological activity. For instance, there are dozens of ginseng preparations on the market which are virtually empty of ginsenosides – the active ingredients in ginseng. And if eleutherococcus has been heated too much in its processing its effectiveness is either reduced or completely destroyed.

Panax ginseng comes from Korea or China and the best quality are the big red roots which are six years old. Second are the white roots and third are the red grown in Japan, so look for country of origin when buying them and also for the Korean 'Office of Monopoly' seal on the pack. The whole roots are the best, with root pieces and extracts following in that order. Ginseng tablets and powders often contain 'fillers' and are much less potent. American ginseng – *Panax quinquefolium* – is usually less effective than *Panax ginseng* unless you can get large old roots, and they are hard to come by.

The best form of *Eleutherococcus senticosus* (Siberian ginseng) comes in extract direct from the CIS. It has been carefully low-heat processed to preserve its biological activity. This form of extract is used in some of the German Siberian ginseng preparations. Most experts in adaptogens insist that *Panax ginseng* is primarily a man's preparation, although it can be useful for women past menopause, and that eleutherococcus is excellent for both men and women. People with very high blood pressure are usually given eleutherococcus instead of ginseng. It is best to steer clear of coffee while on a course of ginseng or you may have trouble sleeping, and to follow a light diet without too much meat.

Certain herbs and plants such as *astragalus* and *echinacea* now also appear to offer excellent immune support. Known as Purple Coneflower, echinacea is a member of the *Compositae* (daisy) family with potent antibiotic and anti-viral effects. The roots of two species, *E. purpurea* and *E. angustifolia*, have long been used against infection and in detoxifying the body by native people including the American Plains Indians, who also used it for poisonous snake and spider bites, abscesses, diphtheria, measles, chicken pox, septic wounds and many other infectious or immune-compromising conditions.

In recent years the herb has been heavily researched in Germany where numerous scientific studies now verify its health-promoting abilities. In Germany there are now more than 200 prescription products based on echinacea or its derivatives. The herb can inhibit the growth of viruses and bacteria that cause colds and 'flu, increase the number of valuable B-cells in the body and enhance the protective functions of macrophages – white blood cells – which are the guardians of the immune system. In short, echinacea is able to amplify the activity of the immune system not only by helping an ailing body recover swiftly, but by helping protect from infections such as colds and 'flu during the long winter months.

I find particularly interesting some recent research in the treatment of vaginal thrush where the herb was used. All the women in the study were treated with conventional anti-fungal drug agents. Some were also given echinacea – the equivalent of 100–200mg a day. As any woman who has ever suffered from it knows only too well, one of the major problems with thrush is although you can knock it out, it tends to recur, especially when you are under stress. Researchers discovered that amongst the echinacea-supplemented group there was a significantly lower recurrence of infection than amongst the rest. And the protection went far beyond thrush. They also found a heightened immune response to tetanus, diphtheria, streptococci and tuberculin. What is exciting about their findings is that they concluded that, unlike antibiotic drugs, echinacea does not attack germs directly. Instead it strengthens your body's own ability to resist them and heightens your defences. I find it a welcome friend taken daily as a preventative during 'the 'flu season' as well as a great boon to recovery.

28
Think Young

ALMOST EVERYBODY HAS heard of death curses. Psychological literature is laced with accounts of how Aboriginal witch doctors have quite literally brought about the death of the young and healthy by cursing them. No sooner do these people learn of the fate which has been cast for them than they begin inexplicably to sicken and eventually to die. It appears that through complex biological processes, their simple belief in the curse brings about destruction of their organism.

Modern-Day Death Curses

In civilized society we tend to look upon such phenomena as anthropological curiosities – products of primitive superstition which simply don't touch us in our more enlightened age. What we are not aware of however is that many of us in the civilized world are also under our own brand of 'death curses'. They may be subtler than those issued by witch doctors but they can be every bit as potent in bringing about the physical and mental decline which we have come to associate with ageing. Common (and usually unconscious) notions such as 'retirement', 'middle-age', 'It's all downhill after forty', and 'At your age you must start taking things more easily', are widely held. They can exert a powerful effect on the process of ageing by creating destructive self-fulfilling expectations about age decline. Instead of facing the future full of confidence and excitement about what lies ahead, optimism is replaced by anxiety as we are warned to 'Be careful', or 'Don't take chances on a new career at your age'.

The list of commonly proffered 'sensible' advice is a long one. Such well-meaning suggestions often lead people to make changes in their lifestyle which encourage physical decline – for instance decreasing the amount of exercise they get, altering their eating habits away from fibre-rich natural foods towards 'softer' foods, and even decreasing the amount of social and intellectual stimulation they have been used to. Even worse, this kind of advice can undermine your self-image and destroy self-confidence, which in turn interferes with the proper functioning of the immune system which plays such a central role in protecting your body from ageing. An essential ingredient in ageless ageing is a strong awareness of just how powerfully your emotions, state of mind, and your unconscious assumptions can influence both your susceptibility to illness and the rate at which you age. Once that awareness has penetrated your consciousness then you can begin to make use of some simple and pleasant mind-bending techniques in aid of ageless ageing.

Mind–Body Connections

The notion that your state of mind can influence your health and the rate at which you age was once something which had to be taken on faith. Now it is not only being scientifically proven, it is even being put into effective practical use thanks to a rapidly developing scientific discipline with a tongue-twisting name: *psychoneuroimmunology* (PNI). PNI has discovered that your body's immune system, that bulwark of defence, is undeniably affected by your unconscious assumptions, your emotional states and your behavioural patterns. They can lead either to an increased resistance to ageing or to an increased susceptibility to degeneration and illness. In simple terms the happier you are, the better you feel about yourself and the more positive are your expectations about the future, the more likely you are to age slowly and gracefully and the less likely you are to fall prey to degeneration and illness of whatever sort – from a common cold to a life-threatening disease.

No area of ageless ageing is more fun to explore than this one. I always think of its positive side as 'Zorba the Greek' consciousness. It can make possible the most amazing physical and mental feats by quite ordinary people living quite ordinary lives. Take the man who is able to work eighteen hours a day, drink whisky by the tumblerful, dance on tables until the early hours of the morning and still live to be 110 thanks to the sheer joy of his experience of life. I have seen it too amongst saints and holy men who carry out their day-to-day activities, from writing letters to peeling potatoes, in a state of bliss – *samadhi*. Take a look at their superbly unlined faces. They could as easily be thirty as seventy. Psychoneuroimmunologists are working to find out why.

So new is the PNI discipline (the name was only coined in 1981) that the average physician is unlikely even to have heard of it. But so profound and wide-reaching are the consequences of its findings that they threaten to revolutionize medical theory about the origins and development of degeneration. Research into psychoneuroimmunology is already describing the pathways through which mind and body are inextricably bound together. These pathways include neurological connections linking glands and organs with the brain, the anti-oxidant system and the blood, thanks to hormonal secretions triggered by thought patterns and emotions and – most important of all – via the immune system. PNI researchers have discovered for instance that several kinds of lymphocytes involved in your body's immune response carry receptors which recognize hormones found in the brain that alter mind and mood. They have also found that some of these neurotransmitters or peptide hormones stimulate T-cells to produce more lymphokines, such as interferon, while others have the opposite effect. In fact listening to leading PNI researchers talk about mind-body connections makes you realize there is probably no state of mind which is not faithfully reflected by a state of the immune system.

Beyond Psychosomatic Consciousness

Western medicine has long acknowledged that emotional states such as anxiety and depression can make a limited number of illnesses worse. These include asthma, diabetes, peptic ulcer, ulcerative colitis, migraine and cardiovascular problems. But until the advent of PNI it has paid little attention to examining the nature of their psychological components nor has it explored ways and means of improving these conditions by altering a patient's mental state or behavioural patterns. Meanwhile it has almost completely ignored possible psychological components in the vast majority of other illnesses – from lung disease and cancer to rheumatism and allergic reactions – treating them instead as pure physiological occurrences little affected by whether the patient experiencing them felt good or bad in himself.

This is mostly because Western medicine, bound by the Cartesian notion of a split between mind and matter, has failed to consider the people it treats as psychobiological units – total beings whose feelings, thoughts, expectations and perceptions are intimately bound to their physiology and biochemistry. Happily this is now changing, in no small part thanks to a few visionary scientists who began asking some penetrating questions. Why for instance do some people who smoke forty cigarettes a day for twenty years end up with lung cancer while others following exactly the same pattern don't? The first, most obvious answer is that the former have an hereditary disposition to the disease. True, genetics are important, but these scientists found that they were by no means the whole answer. A large and very important piece of the puzzle was still missing. So they began to look at psychological factors.

Let Go and Live Longer

In a pioneering study carried out over twenty years ago, Scottish researcher Dr David Kissen examined more than 1,000 Glaswegian industrial workers suffering from respiratory complaints. Before diagnosing them he gave each man a psychological test designed to delineate personality patterns. He came up with some quite fascinating and highly significant results. He discovered that those who were later found to have cancer showed a striking inability to express their emotions. Intrigued by Kissen's study and other similar investigations which suggested that emotional repression was an important component in the development of cancer, two doctors, R.L. Horne and R.S. Picard, at the Washington University School of Medicine in the United States, decided to carry out an in-depth study of the psychosocial risk factors in lung cancer as measured on a psychological scale developed from the findings of previous studies, including Kissen's. They confirmed that emotional repression was indeed the central component of a complex personality pattern which led to the development of the disease. In fact, so important were the relationships between psychological states and the development of lung cancer which they uncovered that the two researchers found they could predict with an amazing 73 per cent accuracy which men had cancer and which men had simple lung disease, from psychological testing alone. They discovered that cancer sufferers, because of their emotional repression, tended to find great difficulty coping with life's challenges and sorrows. After losing an important relationship such as a job or a wife the cancer victims often suffered profound depression for from six to eighteen months before the discovery of the illness. These findings have been confirmed by others.

Mind and Biochemistry

Similar studies linking other psychological factors to other diseases, including infections, arthritis, allergies and premature ageing, have also recently appeared. One of the best known is that done by Meyer Friedman and Ray Rosemann which demonstrated that what they called 'type A behaviour' – a behaviour pattern characterized by a fierce and unrelenting struggle to do ever more things in less time against harsh competition – appears to cause a number of bodily changes predisposing one to coronary heart disease. They include alterations in blood-fat and blood-sugar levels, changes in circulation and increased levels of the hormone noradrenaline. And each disease is beginning to appear to have its own collection of psychological characteristics.

Studies have now established that psychological factors are primary determinants in a host of illnesses, while in others psychological factors appear to interact with biological ones determining whether disease tendencies, initiated either by heredity or your environment or both, will in fact turn into degeneration or whether your body will be able to fight them off. But how does it all work? Through what physiological mechanisms do emotional repression in the case of cancer, a frustrated power drive in the case of high blood pressure, and all the various other psychological and behavioural traits linked with their illnesses help create their respective illness and age decline? Perhaps even more important, once one can find these physiological mechanisms, how can we make use of them first to prevent ageing and even perhaps to reverse some of its processes once they have occurred? The key to both questions appears once again to lie in the immune system.

Rat Magic

You'll remember that the immune system exists to defend your body against *antigens* – foreign invaders such as bacteria, viruses and chemical toxins. It is also a watchdog against the development of cancer cells and premature ageing, both of which can be induced by chemical damage, radiation, viruses and other bodily changes. It does this by being able to recognize 'self' – that which belongs naturally to the body – from 'non-self' that which is foreign to it. If your immune system is underactive you will find yourself highly susceptible to infection and to cancer. If it is working too hard you will be prone to allergies. If it is simply misfunctioning and unable to differentiate 'self' from 'non-self' you can end up with one of the auto-immune diseases such as arthritis. Until quite recently scientists assumed that the immune system was an independent physiological entity – something beyond the influence of psychological influences. Then Dr Robert Ader, professor of psychiatry and psychology at the University of Rochester School of Medicine in the United States (who himself coined the word *psychoneuroimmunology*) carried out some mysterious experiments with animals. He gave rats saccharin-flavoured water and at the same time injected them with a drug known to cause digestive disturbances and to suppress immune function. The rats rapidly developed an aversion to the flavoured water, as he expected them to. But what was surprising was that a number of the rats also died when later they were offered the flavoured water even without the drug. Why? Perhaps, Ader reasoned, it was a brain-triggered response. Perhaps the rats died because they had been conditioned, rather as Pavlov's dog was conditioned to salivate at the sound of a bell, so that their immune system reacted to the flavoured water as it would have done to the immuno-suppressive drug, thus dramatically reducing their susceptibility to disease.

To check out this theory Ader then conditioned another group of rats, challenging their immune system with a common antigen after first conditioning them with water flavoured with saccharin and the drug. They were divided into three groups. The first received another injection of the drug and, as researchers predicted, their antibody production was suppressed. The second group, which was neither treated further with the drug nor given the flavoured water, had normal antibody responses. But the third group who got only the flavoured water without the drug showed a marked decrease in immune reaction – their antibody response to the challenge was significantly less than normal. They had learnt to react to the flavoured water in the same way as they did to a chemical that suppressed the immune system. Ader concluded, 'The fact that learning could alter antibody response in this manner demonstrates a clear, direct link between the brain and the immune system.' His conclusion has since been firmly supported by a host of scientific studies showing how anxiety, depression and discouragement interfere with good immune functions and create susceptibility to illness and ageing.

Mysteries of Mind and Immunity

You may recall that the immune system has two major branches, each with its own particular kind of defence cells or *lymphocytes*. It also includes other less important factors such as large scavenger-type cells called *macrophages* which gobble up antigenic material. The first branch confers on your body what is known as *cell-mediated* immunity and is responsible for about half of your body's resources for defence. It is centred around T-cell leucocytes – warrior cells produced in the thymus which battle the thousands of potentially lethal organisms, cancer-inducing ultraviolet radiation from the sun and toxic chemicals from our highly industrialized environment. T-cells also produce a group of hormone-like substances such as interferon. They are called *lymphokines* and are considered the immune system's natural drugs. Some are poisonous to foreign tissue, others trigger white blood cells to keep an immune reaction going. The second branch of the immune system offers *humoral-mediated* immunity. It relies on what are known as B-cell lymphocytes, which produce antibodies specific to whatever invaders the body is being challenged by. B-cells are carried in the blood. They can combine with antigens in the body and neutralize them or they can coat them, making it simple for white blood cells to destroy them.

The actions of both T- and B-cells are mediated through the thymus gland – often called the master gland of immunity. As we have seen, the rate at which you age appears to be very much influenced by the function of the thymus gland and the state of the immune system which it governs. It has also been well established that immune functions can be disrupted or depressed by such things as malnutrition, free radicals, infection and certain drugs. Recent research shows too that lymphocytes from people suffering from all kinds of stress and from grief, say after the death of a close relative, have a markedly decreased ability to rise to the occasion when challenged by antigens threatening the health of the body. What psychoneuroimmunologists are now trying to explore in experiments with animals and in studies of people are the pathways between brain and body through which this occurs – to delineate the means by which mind affects immunity both as a result of direct input from the brain and the indirect influence of hormones associated with specific emotional states and personality patterns.

Stress and Immunity

One of the questions currently being most seriously investigated by PNI researchers is how biological changes associated with stress diminish immune response and increase susceptibility to illness. Stress of any kind triggers the 'fight or flight' response – a matrix of hormonal reactions designed to prepare the body for action. Adrenaline is released, for instance, along with corticosteroid hormones from the adrenal glands. They in turn trigger other hormonal reactions. PNI researchers have now found that within fifteen minutes of its hitting the bloodstream even a small dose of adrenaline challenges the immune system and triggers the release of lymphocytes. It also inhibits the function of mature white blood cells needed to ward off invasion. Other studies have shown that the corticosteroids can also seriously depress immune functions and increase your susceptibility to disease. They inhibit the functions of both lymphocytes and macrophages and they undermine the ability of lymphocytes to reproduce themselves in the body. In fact if stress is prolonged enough and the levels of corticosteroids become high enough in the body they even cause a withering away of lymphoid tissue altogether.

Stress has been shown to increase susceptibility to cancer in mice and to exacerbate the condition once it is present. And cancers appear to grow fastest and to result in earliest deaths in animals with no way of coping with stress. The same appears to be true of people. At St Luke's Medical Center in Chicago, Dr Richard Shekelle headed a research project which examined death certificates of more than 2,000 men who had been tested psychologically for depression and other emotional states seventeen years before. He found that the death rate of men who had been very depressed at the time of testing was twice that of the rest.

One of the most widely held theories about cancer states that each of us develops small malignancies all the time in our body but that these are rapidly destroyed in a healthy person thanks to the actions of his immune system. If however you have strong feelings of helplessness or depression this can result in elevated corticosteroid levels and other changes which impede your immune system from doing its proper job and rejecting the cancer cells before they can take hold.

PNI Alters Paradigms
The mind-body links which PNI research is uncovering are beginning to have far-reaching consequences, consequences which ultimately will go far beyond helping people avoid life-threatening diseases and slow the ageing process. There is a strong resonance to

be found between PNI and much of the new physics which is busily exploring the view that the observer is essential to the creation of the universe just as the universe is creator of the observer. As Nobel laureate Roger Sperry has said, 'Current concepts of the mind-brain relation involve a direct break with the long-established materialist and behaviourist doctrine that has dominated neuro-science for many decades. Instead of renouncing or ignoring consciousness the new interpretation gives full recognition to the primacy of inner conscious awareness as a causal reality.'

It is a causal reality that you can begin using to your advantage right now. For just as prolonged unmitigated stress, depression and anxiety can suppress immune functions, a positive frame of mind and a sense that you can cope with whatever comes your way offers potent protection against illness and age-degeneration.

Another researcher, Dr Stephen Locke, has used psychological tests to evaluate students' abilities to cope with the shocks and challenges of their lives. He has found that the 'poor copers' – those who tend to succumb to anxiety, depression and a sense of helplessness when life difficulties arise show suppressed immune functions, while the 'good copers' – people who feel they can deal effectively with whatever comes their way – had normal immune functions even when faced with major life changes. Meanwhile in a well-controlled study of women suffering from breast cancer who underwent mastectomy, British researcher Dr Steven Greer discovered that women who react to their diagnosis with a denial that they are ill or with a determination to conquer the illness are far more likely five years later to be free of the disease than those who stoically accepted the diagnosis or who felt hopeless or helpless.

Making Immunity Work for You

What can you do, starting right now, in the way of using your mind as a tool for ageless ageing? You can begin by exploring the benefits of mind/body techniques which can help alter your mental attitudes and emotional states from negative to positive and therefore encourage good immune functions and hence slow down the rate at which you age. There are many. Dr Herbert Benson of Harvard Medical School developed the simple meditative technique, called the relaxation response, which consists of sitting with your eyes closed for fifteen or twenty minutes morning and night and repeating a single word – say 'one' or 'peace' – over and over again silently. Practised regularly it will not only counter the immune-suppressing tendencies of stress but even bring about major psychological shifts in belief systems that can gradually change a self-defeating 'poor coper' into an optimistic 'good coper'.

You can also explore just how many negative expectations you have connected with ageing. Then you can quite simply and methodically go about changing them. For instance, how many of the following notions would you agree with? They have been adapted from a quiz designed by well-known gerontologist Erdman Palmore from Duke University Medical Center in the United States and they appeared in the scientific journal *The Gerontologist* not long ago. Do the quiz and then check your answers at the end. It is a good way of helping you become aware of how many false ideas you have about ageing. (In each case tick 'T' for 'true' or 'F' for 'false'.)

Quiz: How Much Do You Know About Ageing?

T F   1. The majority of old people (past age sixty-five) are senile (i.e. defective memory, disoriented or demented).

T F   2. All five senses tend to decline with age.

T F   3. Most old people have no interest in sex.

T F   4. Lung capacity tends to decline in old age.

T F   5. The majority of old people feel miserable most of the time.

T F   6. The majority of old people are seldom irritated or angry.

T F   7. At least one-tenth of the aged are living in long-stay institutions (i.e. nursing homes, mental hospitals, homes for the aged, etc).

T F   8. Aged drivers have fewer accidents per person than drivers under age sixty-five.

T F   9. Most older workers cannot work as effectively as younger workers.

T F 10. About 80 per cent of the aged are healthy enough to carry out their normal activities.

T F 11. Most old people are set in their ways and are unable to change.

T F 12. The majority of old people are working or would like to have some kind of work to do (including housework and volunteer work).

T F 13. It is almost impossible for most old people to learn new things.

T F 14. The reaction time of most old people tends to be slower than reaction time of younger people.

T F 15. In general, most old people are pretty much alike.

T F 16. The majority of old people are seldom bored.

T F 17. The majority of old people are socially isolated and lonely.

T F 18. Older workers have fewer accidents than younger workers.

T F 19. Older people tend to become more religious as they age.

T F 20. Most medical practitioners tend to give low priority to the aged.

The answers to this quiz are that the even-numbered questions are true and the odd numbered ones are false.

Contrary to popular opinion only 2 or 3 per cent of old people are institutionalized because of psychiatric disorders. Neither do the vast majority of old people have memory defects. Most people over sixty-five continue to be interested in sex, and sexual relations continue well into the eighties between healthy men and women. Studies made of morale and happiness amongst the elderly show no difference between their enjoyment of life and that of younger people.

People over sixty-five have fewer accidents per person driving than do younger drivers. They also have fewer accidents at work. The majority of old people are not set in their ways although it does take them longer to learn something new than the young. Studies show that few old people suffer from boredom. Neither are they socially isolated or lonely. More than 10 per cent of old people work and two-thirds of those who don't would like to. Finally old people are seldom irritated or angry. This has been determined by three separate studies.

Visualize Age Anew

Becoming aware of false assumptions about ageing is a good first step. The next is to create a new vision of what it means to have time passing. Make use of creative visualization techniques where in a state of relaxation you allow your mind to play on positive images of yourself five, ten, thirty years from now. There are some excellent books available on the subject which you can use as a guide. But really the technique is very easy. It is only a matter of letting yourself indulge in positive daydreaming. Or practise a meditation or deep-relaxation technique a couple of times a day and finish off by repeating silently to yourself Coue's formula for personal growth and healing, 'Every day in every way I am getting better and better.' It is exquisitely simple yet enormously powerful when practised daily in a deeply relaxed state so that it is your imagination rather than your will which is brought into play.

Affirm Youth and Well-Being

Another simple technique which has real power for altering unconscious expectations and creating new realities is that of writing out 'affirmations' – seven times seventy – for a week or two. This can be something as simple as 'I am well and will continue to be so as the years pass' or 'I let go of past confusion and day by day make my life anew.' The mere act of writing out such words over and over for several days helps break through old thought patterns and negativity that may be hampering you from realizing your full psychobiological potentials. You might be surprised at how quickly they penetrate your consciousness and bring about positive shifts in expectations and in your reality. For they can generate positive mental states and emotions and make them your common everyday experience of reality. And, just as PNI researchers have been discovering, it is the simple positive experiences and emotions like love, hope, faith, laughter, playfulness and creativity which can not only make life worth living, they can actually keep us alive, youthful and well. As effective as massive doses of anti-oxidant nutrients, fresh-cell therapy and all the other biological methods of age-retardation available to you? Very probably. Besides, they'll cost you absolutely nothing but a smile.

29
The Ageless Brain

OF MAJOR CONCERN to age-researchers is the brain. Many believe that alterations in the brain are central to age-related changes elsewhere in the body. Others focus on the way in which the behaviour can alter when people get older so that they show signs of confusion or memory loss or some curtailments in mental facility. Such impairments can be responsible for the irritability, depression, restlessness and even withdrawal which some older people experience, as well as for alterations in sleep patterns – the wake-often-and-sleep-little syndrome associated with ageing. Just what does happen in your brain as you get older? What relationship do these happenings have to the state of your body as a whole? And most important – can some or all of the age-related brain changes and mood alterations which accompany them be halted or reversed?

Loss of Brain Cells
At about age twenty your brain weighs about 1,400g if you are a man and about 1,300g if you are a woman. Although this can vary considerably from person to person, brain weight tends to decline in your sixties. Mostly this is because of a loss of protein and fats and to a lesser degree because it also loses water. Accompanying this loss in weight, which amounts to about 3g between the ages of thirty-five and seventy-five, a loss in volume takes place. Both may be due to the fact that most people lose about 100,000 cells – cells which are never replaced – from their brain each and every day from their mid-thirties onwards.

This may sound like a great deal, and the loss of certain cells can be important to brain and body function, but since within this 3lb or so of grey material are woven tens of billions of nerve cells and since so much of our brain's resources remain untapped throughout our

IDEAS OF THE BRAIN: OLD AND NEW

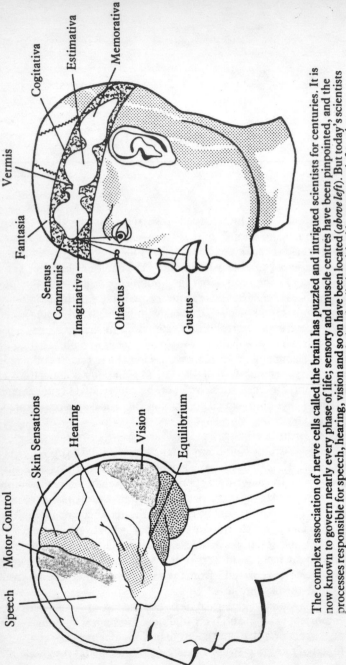

The complex association of nerve cells called the brain has puzzled and intrigued scientists for centuries. It is now known to govern nearly every phase of life; sensory and muscle centres have been pinpointed, and the processes responsible for speech, hearing, vision and so on have been located (*above left*). But today's scientists are not as bold as sixteenth-century savant Georg Reisch, who distinguished between such functions as 'imagination' and 'fantasy' (*above right*). However, while we know that his ideas were wrong, our own understanding of the brain is still far from complete.

whole life anyway, it is likely to be far less important to brain function than it might seem. As the brain gets older its ridges and convoluted patterns grow deeper and more well defined. There are other brain changes which appear to be of more concern. For instance, in the brains of most older people a substance called *lipofuscin* or 'age pigment' builds up as they get older. This pigment, which many gerontologists believe is a kind of build-up of waste products in the cells, also accumulates in other tissues of the body too, such as the heart and the skeleton, causing a kind of cellular constipation which is important because it interferes with normal cell functions and leads to further age-related changes in the body.

Finally, since the hypothalamus, which is buried within the brain tissue, and the pituitary are involved in the control of so many bodily functions, a few researchers have postulated that changes in these two glands which occur in time may trigger the release of some kind of 'age hormone' which acts as a biological clock, causing age-related damage throughout the body. But so far this is only speculation.

What is interesting about the brain in relation to ageing is the fact that much of what used to be considered inevitable mental and emotional changes connected with ageing such as senility, depression, and an inability to learn rapidly now appear to be much less time-dependent than they have always seemed. Only some 10 per cent of the population have the slightest tendency towards senility and many of the moods and mental restrictions which naively used to be considered an inevitable consequence of ageing are nothing of the sort. Instead they usually stem from two causes, both of which can be relatively easily dealt with: either they are part of the expectations people have about getting older and therefore become self-fulfilling prophecies, or they are a direct result of a decline in certain brain hormones called neurotransmitters, a state which with relative ease can be altered by nutritional means.

Oxygen-Induced Brain Damage

Senility is also unquestionably a result of excessive oxy-stress and free radical damage to tissues, and the anti-oxidant nutrients which form an important part of any effective programme for ageless ageing will help protect the brain from damage. As Bruce Ames, chairman of the biochemistry department of the University of California and an expert on ageing and cancer, says, 'The brain uses 20 per cent of the oxygen consumed by man and contains an appreciable amount of unsaturated fat. Lipid peroxidation (with consequent age pigment) is known to occur readily in the brain, and possible consequences could be senile dementia or other brain abnormalities.' Abram Hoffer, the Canadian expert in ortho-molecular treatment of mental disorders, believes as Ames does that anti-oxidant nutrients are important in protecting against age-related brain degeneration. But then so are certain specific nutrients which are not generally classified as anti-oxidants such as niacin (vitamin B3), and vitamin B1.

Deficiencies Cause 'Age' Symptoms

Although your brain accounts for less than 2 per cent of your total body weight an amazing 25 per cent of the body's total metabolic activity takes place there. That may be why it is so sensitive to even the slightest nutritional deficiency. And as people get older, unless they follow a lifestyle for ageless ageing or have an extraordinary genetic inheritance which is looking after them, nutritional deficiencies become common. One of the very first places they show up is in the brain.

James Goodwin of the University of New Mexico School of Medicine is a leading geriatrician with a particular interest in brain chemistry and its relation to ageing. He points out a long string of so-called psychiatric symptoms associated with ageing which are in reality signs of subclinical deficiencies of essential nutrients which have not been well enough supplied or well enough absorbed in the diets of older people. For instance, even mild vitamin B12 deficiencies can result in a wide range of psychiatric symptoms from indifference and irritability to hallucinations and obvious psychotic behaviour. A vitamin B1 deficiency can result in the person simply being unable to learn anything new. Lack of folic acid can result in symptoms of senility or dementia and so forth. These symptoms are certainly not a sign of normal ageing as most of us have been led to believe. Neither need they be permanent. But, as a number of recent studies in Britain and America show, such nutritional deficiencies are widespread and they tend to get worse the older people get.

In an interesting study carried out by British researcher J.C. Brocklehurst, eighty residents of an old people's home were selected and half of them were put on to a multiple-vitamin formula with the other half taking a placebo. Neither patients nor staff knew which was which. Reasoning that the vitamin group would perhaps improve in subtle ways in their behaviour, six months later researchers asked the staff to guess which old people had been getting the vitamin supplement and which the placebo – thus making them rely on their overall impression of behaviour and not on any specific test. The attending doctor guessed all of those who had been receiving vitamins because the improvement in their behaviour and mental acuity had been so dramatic.

New Life for Ageing Brains
Many symptoms of neuropsychiatric disorders result from imbalances in the functioning of the brain's neurotransmitters and/or from a deficiency in the specific nutrients needed to manufacture them for the brain. A nerve cell or *neuron* has a very special structure in order to enable it to carry information quickly from one part of the body to another. It has long projections called *axons* which reach out from the cell body to make contact with another nerve cell, creating a kind of relay system of circuitry in the brain. But they never directly contact each other because there is a tiny gap called a *synapse* between each neuron and its neighbour. The way that messages get passed on from one to the next is that the neuron's axon releases a chemical messenger – a *neurotransmitter* – which diffuses across the gap and stimulates a receptor site, causing a minute electrical current on the next neuron which in turn passes the message on to the next and so on in a process so rapid and so efficient that it occurs in virtually no time at all.

It is thanks to the actions of these neurotransmitters that motor messages get carried, that thoughts link up and that emotions can be felt. Some are excitatory in character – they rapidly trigger another electrical discharge. Others are inhibitory, in which case they suppress the spontaneous electrical firing of the nerve cells they come in contact with. Science has now identified some forty neurotransmitters but there could be hundreds as yet undiscovered. They are made in the body out of nutrients from the foods you eat and there is very good evidence that many of the most important neurotransmitters are diet-dependent – the levels of them in your brain are directly related to how many of the specific nutrients such as amino acids, vitamins and minerals needed for their manufacture are supplied through your diet.

There is much evidence that there is absolutely no reason for brainpower to decline with age. Neither should you expect that feelings of depression or apathy or even long-standing fatigue are a

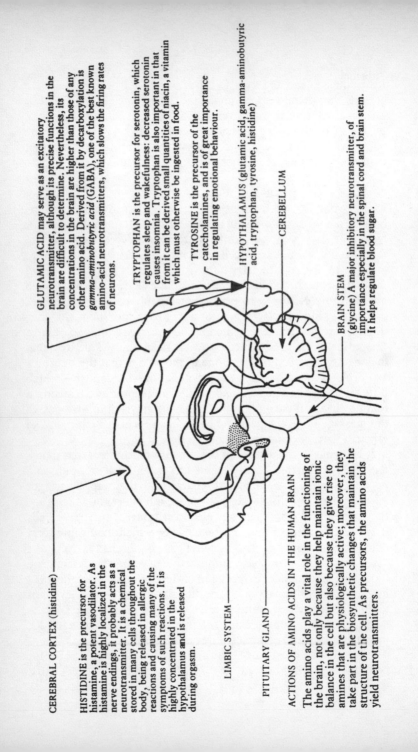

CEREBRAL CORTEX (histidine)

HISTIDINE is the precursor for histamine, a potent vasodilator. As histamine is highly localized in the nerve endings, it probably acts as a neurotransmitter. It is a chemical stored in many cells throughout the body, being released in allergic reactions and causing many of the symptoms of such reactions. It is highly concentrated in the hypothalamus and is released during orgasm.

LIMBIC SYSTEM

PITUITARY GLAND

ACTIONS OF AMINO ACIDS IN THE HUMAN BRAIN

The amino acids play a vital role in the functioning of the brain, not only because they help maintain ionic balance in the cell but also because they give rise to amines that are physiologically active; moreover, they take part in the biosynthetic changes that maintain the structure of the cell. As precursors, the amino acids yield neurotransmitters.

GLUTAMIC ACID may serve as an excitatory neurotransmitter, although its precise functions in the brain are difficult to determine. Nevertheless, its concentrations in the brain are higher than those of any other amino acid. Derived from it by decarboxylation is *gamma-aminobutyric acid* (GABA), one of the best known amino-acid neurotransmitters, which slows the firing rates of neurons.

TRYPTOPHAN is the precursor for serotonin, which regulates sleep and wakefulness: decreased serotonin causes insomnia. Tryptophan is also important in that from it can be derived small quantities of niacin, a vitamin which must otherwise be ingested in food.

TYROSINE is the precursor of the catecholamines, and is of great importance in regulating emotional behaviour.

HYPOTHALAMUS (glutamic acid, gamma-aminobutyric acid, tryptophan, tyrosine, histidine)

CEREBELLUM

BRAIN STEM (glycine) A major inhibitory neurotransmitter, of importance especially in the spinal cord and brain stem. It helps regulate blood sugar.

'normal' sign that you are getting older. They are nothing of the kind. They are rather a sign that something needs to be done to improve things and there are so many possibilities.

Brainfood – Phosphatidyl Choline plus Lecithin

One of the most important of the precursor nutrients with power to alter mental tendencies usually associated with getting older is phosphatidyl choline. Studies show that taken as a dietary supplement, granular lecithin enriched with extra phosphatidyl choline can enhance learning, improve memory, stimulate lagging brain functions in older people and even help regulate the dramatic mood-swings of manic depressives. Healthy brain function, on which clear thinking and feeling rely, is dependent on the action of many neurotransmitters. And perhaps the most important of all of these is *acetylcholine*. When there is too little of it available the ability to reason, remember and control muscles all over the body goes awry. Insufficient acetylcholine is also associated with a number of illnesses as well as with the development of senility. It can result in a number of symptoms in otherwise healthy people as well, from foggy thinking to nervousness, anxiety, hyperactivity in children, slowed reflexes and sluggishness.

Your body manufactures acetylcholine from the vitamin choline, one of the few nutrients which can be transferred directly from blood to brain. The amount of acetylcholine produced is entirely dependent upon how much phosphatidyl choline is available for its production. Researchers at Massachusetts Institute of Technology showed that if students were given 3g of choline a day their learning abilities and memories improved. But taking choline on its own as a nutritional supplement has its disadvantages, one of the main ones being it tends to give your breath and skin a fishy smell. Not so when it is taken in the form of lecithin, of which it is a major constituent. In fact granular lecithin itself, which is an emulsifier, appears to enhance the actions of the phosphatidyl choline it contains. It has recently been used successfully as a part of treatment for manic depression and vascular diseases. There are now available some excellent formulas of phosphatidyl choline – the best come in the form of enriched lecithin granules which you can sprinkle on to cereals, soups or salads or mix in fruit juice. They provide as much choline as twelve high-potency lecithin capsules and are quite pleasant-tasting. The other use for such a product is in helping to lower cholesterol levels in people whose blood fats tend to be high.

Precocious Precursors

Some of the free amino acids (see Chapter 18) are themselves either neurotransmitters or precursors to neurotransmitters. When taken as nutritional supplements they can be very useful as mind-stimulants, mood-enhancers, natural relaxers and even pain-killers. Probably the most important of all the natural mood-elevators is DL-phenylalanine. It is a highly effective natural anti-depressant and is also useful in the control of chronic aches and pains such as those of stiff joints or of arthritis. It is also very safe, non-toxic both in short-term and long-term therapy; unlike coffee and pep-up pills it does not bring about excessive arousal; toxic overdose of DL-phenylalanine is virtually impossible; and finally, it does not appear to have adverse side-effects for normal, healthy people.

Statistics show that depression tends to increase with age and also to be higher in women than in men (although the suicide rate is higher in men). Its symptoms can be as diverse as changes in sleeping or eating patterns, early morning waking or prevailing sleepiness or insomnia. The body seems low in energy and the person often feels a lack of direction or meaning in life. Doctors have had remarkable results using DL-phenylalanine as an antidote to depression, particularly what is known as endogenous depression (depression which is long-standing and very difficult to treat) and involutional depression – the sort that is associated particularly with ageing. In fact this amino acid has been found to be 89–100 per cent effective in the treatment of such depression and without the dangerous side effects associated with anti-depression drugs such as the MAO inhibitors. To my knowledge there is no other substance, natural or otherwise, which can claim similar results. How does it work ?

The Perfect Anti-Depressant?

DL-phenylalanine appears to have three quite separate anti-depressant effects on the brain. First it increases the levels of *endorphins* in the brain by inhibiting enzymes which break down endorphin hormones. These are the body's natural opiates which give runners their euphoric high, eliminate pain from the experience of natural childbirth, and appear to be an important biochemical reason for the bliss that comes in certain states of meditation. Second, DL-phenylalanine increases the production of phenylethylamine or PEA – a neurotransmitter-type natural brain-stimulant. Finally, DL-phenylalanine can also be converted in the brain into the neurotransmitter noradrenaline which is a natural stimulant and mood-elevator. (Athletes tend to produce a lot of it and depressed people to have very low levels. DL-phenylalanine can change all that.) Many anti-depressant drugs aim to increase the levels of noradrenaline in the central nervous system as well. But this they do in very different ways than DL-phenylalanine – ways which produce in many people serious side-effects, from nausea and drowsiness to anorexia – and these drugs also prevent reabsorption of the neurotransmitters into nerve terminals. What this eventually does is deplete the cells' stores of neurotransmitter material and therefore interfere with good brain function. Not only does DL-phenylalanine not have these negative effects, it can even help restore brain levels to normal. But this is by no means its only use either. Many women find it helpful in relieving the symptoms of premenstrual tension. One study using it reports that over 80 per cent of women using it for this purpose gained 'good to complete relief'. It also appears to be an effective natural painkiller – particularly useful for chronic pain such as that from arthritis.

The Nuts and Bolts of Use

DL-phenylalanine is available in white crystal-powder form or made into tablets – usually of 375mg each. Most physicians and nutritionists using it suggest that to start with you take three tablets of this size each day – each one just after a meal. The dosage needs to be divided up, they claim, in order to get the full anti-depressant effect. Once this occurs then they often reduce the dose to one tablet per day. Some people don't even need to continue taking it at all to maintain benefits of mood improvement because, like a lot of the natural substances used in orthomolecular health (and unlike drugs) they help restore normal functioning to tissues so they are no longer needed. DL-phenylalanine is most effective taken with the vitamins which encourage its conversion to brain chemicals. They are vitamins B1, B2, B6 and C. How long does it take to get results? Many people notice them within a few days but if the depression is longstanding it is usually four to six weeks before it lifts. There are three important cautions: DL-phenylalanine should not be taken by pregnant or lactating women nor by people who suffer with *phenylketonuria* (an inborn error which can result in a mentally retarded condition that occurs when the body cannot convert phenylalanine into tyrosine naturally). It should be used with caution in the case of anyone with high blood pressure as well. Something that I find DL-phenylalanine particularly good for is in helping people who feel discouraged about themselves and their life to experience the new hope and enthusiasm and energy necessary to make lifestyle changes, such as improving their diet or getting more exercise, which will eventually lead them towards a permanently heightened experience of wellness and vitality.

The Tryptophan Connection

Another free amino which has been used to treat depression is tryptophan. Tryptophan, which is also an excellent natural tranquilliser and sleep-inducer, and which for many psychologically 'normal' people appears to enhance their sense of mental and emotional well-being, is a precursor of *serotonin*. Serotonin is a neurotransmitter which is involved in many metabolic processes. Studies show that when serotonin levels are low in animals they tend to be aggressive, to overreact to stimuli and even show signs of abnormal sexual behaviour. Many authorities believe that because tryptophan is the least abundant amino acid in most foods, many people don't get enough of this substance to experience the natural stress-relief, sleep improvement and relief from anxiety and depression which it can offer.

W.M. Ringsdorf and E. Cheraskin, authors of *Psychodietetics*, believe that the standard recommended daily requirement of 500mg of tryptophan for adults every day is not enough for many people. In an experiment where sixty-six normal people increased their daily intake of tryptophan to 1,001–1,331mg a day they report 'a remarkable decrease in the number of psychological complaints'. A number of studies have demonstrated how effective tryptophan supplementation can be in dealing with insomnia when you take 1g of the amino acid twenty minutes before going to bed. The problem with tryptophan however is that it is no longer available. It was withdrawn from the market by the United States' Food & Drug Administration when an impure batch of the amino acid caused serious damage to some who used it. It has never returned.

Natural Tranquillizers

All of the brain's natural opiates – substances such as *enkephalin* and the endorphins, which uplift mood while they calm a restless mind and leave you feeling exceptionally well, are made from amino acids. And one of the most useful things you can do with the free amino acids is to apply them as natural tranquillizers. There are four which can be particularly helpful because either directly or as precursors they form the inhibitory neurotransmitter. These brain hormones will calm an overactive mind and create a mental state akin to that which comes from deep relaxation or meditation. They are L-tryptophan, L-glycine, L-taurine and L-histidine. A mixture of these four aminos has been used clinically to alleviate anxiety and depression, calm anger, banish phobias, halt obsessive-compulsive behaviour, and treat high blood pressure. It can also be simply an excellent way to switch off when you are under stress, without the help of alcohol or drugs.

A Look at L-Glutamine

L-glutamine is the amide form of glutamic acid, a 'non-essential' amino acid which has generally been considered nutritionally unimportant but which acts as a high-energy brain fuel and can have some remarkable effects on the body, such as detoxifying it of ammonia which is poisonous to living cells. It has also been shown to improve intelligence, speed the healing of ulcers, help control alcoholism, schizophrenia and the craving for sweets. And it is one of the best banishers of fatigue you will find anywhere.

Because glutamic acid itself does not pass easily through the blood-brain barrier but the amide L-glutamine does, and once there it is transformed into glutamic acid for use as fuel, it is in this L-glutamine form that it is usually taken. American biochemist Roger Williams first discovered that L-glutamine helps protect the body against the poisonous effects of alcohol and that for many people it even banishes the craving for it altogether. He and others have used it in doses of 14g daily for this purpose. L-glutamine's ability to help many people who have a craving for sweets probably works through the same mechanism as it does in helping to eliminate addiction to alcohol – via the hypothalamus. Abram Hoffer has used L-glutamine against senility, schizophrenia and mental retardation with good success, and H.L. Newbold, author of *MegaNutrients for Your Nerves* uses it regularly to treat fatigue. As a brain fuel to increase intelligence or for eliminating cravings it is usually taken in 500mg capsules twice a day for the first week, and then 500mg three times a day, working up to 2,000mg a day in split doses the third week until you find the level which seems to work best for you.

Make Brain Aminos Work Hard

Experts in amino acid supplements such as Robert Erdmann (author of *The Amino Revolution*) say that it is a good idea to take ascorbic acid – from 1 to 10g a day – and vitamin B6 when taking any amino acid product, because these two vitamins work synergistically with the aminos. It is also wise to ensure you drink plenty of water when using amino acids regularly. You also need to make sure, they say, that you have a good supply of all the known nutrients – vitamins, minerals, essential fatty acids and so forth – to work with them. There is no such thing as a single pill which will do everything or solve a particular problem. The body is a complex organism whose functioning depends on a good balance of essential nutrients and the right kind of structural information not only to function in optimum health but also to make the best use of these quite remarkable natural products in any programme for ageless ageing. Free-form amino acids should not be taken by diabetics except under the guidance of a nutritionally trained physician since some of them can influence insulin levels. And because each of us is a biochemical individual there are no set quantities of each which are right for everyone. They take a little experimenting.

30
Ageless Ageing for Life

IN THIS WORLD of sophisticated biochemistry, psychoneuro-immunology, complex treatments for face and skin and body, and mind-bending nutrients, how do you gather together what you need in order to begin creating a lifestyle for yourself which will help you live long and well and look your best year after year? Probably the best way to start is to consider what you need most help with and begin there. For instance, you may already be eating well and sparsely, and it may be only a matter of cutting out the negative things in your diet such as coffee or sugar and increasing the number of fresh foods on your table to bring you in line with the low caloric-high-potency nutrition which appears ideal for ageless ageing. But, perhaps you have sadly neglected the state of your muscles and the conditioning of your body through exercise. And perhaps you have a tendency to become easily stressed by overwork or worry. Then you might start by promising yourself a brisk walk for at least half an hour four days a week as well as learning some simple weight-training exercises and promising yourself to use them a couple of times a week too. And you might consider exploring what some of the natural anti-anxiety antidotes can offer you. Someone else, a marathon runner, for example, might be superbly fit and have lots of energy, yet be suffering (as so many athletes do) from haggard-looking skin and a diet which is not supplying all of the essential nutrients in optimum quantities. (And strenuous physical exercise can dramatically increase body demand for many of them.) In this case a substantial programme of nutritional supplements stressing the anti-oxidant nutrients could be a good idea. So might making use of some of the anti-oxidant treatment products for skin.

Each of us is an individual with particular needs, interests and weaknesses. And the best way for anyone to make ageless ageing a part of their life is to start with one or two techniques which are specifically applicable to their needs and then build from there – slowly. Leaping into some elaborate programme in which you try to do everything all at once is doomed to failure. For valuable and lasting change almost always has to come slowly and gradually. Then the things you take up for your benefit are not just curious fads to be tried and dropped. They become integrated parts of your life – solid, stable ways of living which can both bring you closer to the ordered harmony of *natural law* age-retardation as well as reaping the benefits from *high-tech* science.

Slow and Not So Steady Change

For many of us, change also comes in fits and starts. More than fifteen years ago I first came upon a physician using a high-raw diet and was fascinated by how such a simple tool could be so transformative. But I am a compulsive experimenter and a great doubter and I have to test something out twenty times before I will believe it. I began to experiment with more fresh foods in my own diet and found that they did indeed improve the way I looked and felt. But then, because of social convention or basic cynicism, I would return to the usual stodge I had been eating before. It took several years of doubt and experiment (as well as a dawning awareness that at some level I then had a real commitment to *worseness* rather than *wellness*) for me to gradually come to a point where a high-raw way of eating has become my normal lifestyle.

Probably I am slower than most to learn. Several years ago I read in a scientific journal about experiments designed to test animal intelligence. In the 'discussion' part of the paper researchers stated that basic intelligence is directly proportionate to the number of times an animal has to experience a stimulus – say an electric shock every time it touches a switch, or a reward of grain whenever it goes through a trap door – before it learns whether the stimulus is of positive or negative value. Only then does the beneficial response become integrated into an animal's behaviour. I remember thinking at the time that I definitely belonged with the lowest level of rats since I tend to have to beat my head against a brick wall a hundred times before I finally twig to the fact it hurts. Yet, like a lot of creatures that are slow to learn, once I do, I actually *know* not just in my head the way I would know a fact but on a deeper and more permanent level – the way once you learn to ride a bicycle it becomes almost an unconscious response and you *know* it for ever.

It is that kind of knowing which is valuable in creating an ageless-ageing lifestyle for yourself. And, unless you are one of the very fortunate few who are able to grasp new ideas and techniques quickly and to integrate them into your way of life easily and sensibly, it is going to take time. It also takes experiment to separate out what works best for you from what doesn't work at all. And it may take the help of a doctor or health practitioner who is well versed in nutrition.

The Orthomolecular Approach to Ageless Ageing

The orthomolecular approach to health is based on an extremely simple nuts-and-bolts hypothesis: we are made of vitamins, minerals, amino acids, fatty acids and so forth, working together according to a living molecular logic. Because we are alive, that life provides the consciousness to utilize these nuts and bolts. It is these nuts and bolts which – when insufficient – create pathology and degeneration. This simple concept is fundamental to nutritional supplementation for ageless ageing. It is also, I believe, a concept which will eventually change the course of medicine and science.

If you want to use the anti-oxidant nutrients as part of an orthomolecular approach to ageless ageing it is a good idea to consult a nutritionally oriented doctor or health practitioner who can help you work out a supplemental programme personally tailored to your individual needs. Each of us is biochemically highly individual so that where one person may need only moderate quantities of a specific nutrient such as vitamin B6 or zinc yet high levels of vitamin C, another may need quite exceptional amounts of zinc and B6 yet have only a moderate need for ascorbic acid. There are a number of useful diagnostic tools which in conjunction with an examination of the foods you eat and your lifestyle as a whole can be useful to your nutritionally trained doctor or health practitioner in helping you establish this.

Hair and sweat analysis of minerals can also be useful, as can urine analysis of blood levels of both vitamins and minerals. All of these tools work best when used together since one offers a check against the others. Hair analysis on its own can never give a complete picture. So far there are few physicians in this country using these techniques but an awareness of what they offer in helping a person create a nutritional programme for high-level wellness and longevity is rapidly growing within the medical profession.

It can also be helpful to look at what a typical selection of supplemental nutrients designed for ageless ageing looks like. For although age-researchers can disagree about specifics, the general principles of age-retardation through supplementation are becoming well established. One thing which is absolutely vital to remember is the rule of synergy. It is no good taking large doses of a few vitamins with anti-oxidant properties unless you also provide your body with adequate supplies of *all* the other nutrients you need in smaller quantities, to create an orthomolecular environment which enables it to use them.

Because each human being is absolutely unique, if you decide to follow the mega approach to ageless ageing using supplementation you need the help of a doctor or health practitioner with access to the best medical unit for testing levels of nutrients in the blood (see Resources, page 334).

Ageless Ageing Supplements	*Conservative Approach*	*Mega Approach*
Vitamin A	5,000 IU	25,000 IU
Beta-carotene or mixed Carotenoids	15 mg	30–45 mg
Vitamin B1	25 mg	50–100 mg
Vitamin B2	25 mg	50–100 mg
Vitamin B3	25 mg	30–100 mg
Pantothenic Acid	25 mg	50–200 mg
Vitamin B6	10 mg	50–100 mg
Vitamin B12	40 mcg	100 mcg
Folic Acid	200 mcg	800–4,000 mcg
Biotin	100 mcg	300–5,000 mcg
Choline	50 mg	75–500 mg
Inositol	50 mg	75–500 mg
PABA	50 mg	100 mg
Vitamin C	500 mg	2,000–12,000 mg
Bioflavonoids	50 mg	100–500 mg
Vitamin D	300 IU	400 IU
Vitamin E	100 IU	200–2,000 IU

Ageless Ageing Supplements	Conservative Approach	Mega Approach
Calcium	100 mg	400–1,600 mg
Magnesium	50 mg	250–1,000 mg
Potassium	10 mg	50–200 mg
Iron	10 mg	25 mg
Copper	0.5 mg	3 mg
Zinc	10 mg	15–40 mg
Manganese	2 mg	5 mg
Molybdenum	50 mcg	75 mcg
Chromium	25 mcg	75 mcg
Selenium	100 mcg	200–400 mcg
Iodine	50 mcg	75–200 mcg
Boron	1 mcg	2 mcg

Amino Acids and Other Necessary Nutrients

L-Methionine	500–1,500 mg
L-Cysteine	500–1,500 mg
Ginseng	100–3,000 mg
Eleutherococcus	1,000–3,000 mg
Royal jelly	250–500 mg
Evening Primrose oil	1,500–3,000 mg
Omega 3 Fish oils EPA/DHA	1,000–4,000 mg

Guidelines for Ageless Ageing

Although nutritional supplementation is a highly individual affair, not every aspect of an ageless-ageing lifestyle is so personal. There are a few simple 'don'ts' which anybody can benefit from adhering to. And while science has not yet provided us with the knowledge which will enable us to live to 200 they should go a long way towards helping us reach 120:

- *Don't* smoke.

- *Don't* drink more than a couple of glasses of wine a day.

- *Don't* let yourself become a victim of negative expectations about ageing.

- *Don't* take drugs unnecessarily.

- *Don't* overeat.

- *Don't* eat sugar and other refined carbohydrates or highly processed foods.

- *Don't* push yourself beyond your limits.

- *Don't* put off a change of lifestyle – such as giving up smoking or getting more exercise – which you know will improve your health. Do it now.

There are also some equally important 'do's' for longevity and ageless ageing:

- *Do* increase the number of fresh (as many as possible eaten raw) vegetables and wholegrain foods – particularly organically grown – in your diet.

- *Do* exercise to between 40 and 60 per cent of your maximum capacity for at least thirty minutes three to five times a week.

- *Do* investigate what nutritional supplements (including the anti-oxidant nutrients) can do for you under the guidance of a nutritionally oriented doctor or health practitioner.

- *Do* learn to listen to the messages of your own body so that you sleep when you are tired, eat only when you are hungry and follow what your conscience tells you is right. What works for someone else may not be right for you.

- *Do* make a friend of stress by taking enough relaxation when you need it, by talking problems out with other people when they arise instead of swallowing them, and by seeking out what your own intrinsic goals are and then following them.

• *Do* go easy in incorporating any of the new approaches to ageless ageing from this book into your own life and don't try to take on more than you can handle at any one time. It's important to be circumspect and to move towards newer methods of life extension with caution, wisdom and sensitivity to your own responses.

• *Do* begin to view ageing as a positive process which can lead you to even better health, greater stamina and more creativity and happiness. These expectations help create your future.

• *Do* allow yourself to experience joy in your work and when you are at play. It is the natural birthright of every human being and can do more to improve your health and longevity than any other single thing.

• *Do* seek out new challenges which keep your mind alert and stimulate your interest in life and in other people.

• *Do*, as Hans Selye counsels, 'Reach for the highest aim yet never put up resistance in vain.'

Postscript

Thanks to our growing understanding of the natural laws of health and advanced research into high-tech biochemistry, what was once little more than a pipe dream – the notion that the length of human life can be extended – is becoming a reality. Gerontologists have now challenged the maximum lifespans of many species of animals. Man is next. Already physicians are using anti-oxidant nutrients, electromagnetic techniques and other anti-ageing tools to prevent physical degeneration and to restore health and balance to ailing bodies. Meanwhile psychiatrists and psychologists trained in biochemistry and in the orthomolecular treatment of the brain are not only beginning to cure mental and emotional problems associated with age, they are even using the tools of their trade to expand consciousness. It becomes important to ask the question, 'With what consequences?'

Boon or Burden?
The first worry about life extension for most people is usually, 'What will we do with these old people we are creating?' 'Won't they be yet a further burden to society?' Naturally they want to know about the effect that longevity will have on housing, medical costs and the rest. Such questions are valid. But it is also important to penetrate the point of view from which they come – the assumptions and paradigms which underlie them.

Our society has imprinted its members with negative concepts about being old. In the book for which he won a Pulitzer Prize, *Why Survive? Being Old in America*, Dr Robert Buffer outlined the enormous practical problems of dealing with the aged: housing, pensions, personal security, need for meaningful occupations and the rest, and the horrific conditions in which many old people in modern western society live. He also pointed out that we hold many unconscious assumptions about the aged which continue to create these conditions. They are always with us, and they greatly distort our view of ageing, old people and their place in society. These assumptions include a belief that the aged are inflexible, senile, unproductive people waiting for the inevitable arrival of the Grim Reaper. Basically not interesting, of little value, they are people worthy of being assigned to a foreclosed existence. Alex Comfort refers to these common views of age and the elderly as *ageism* which he defines as 'the notion that people cease to be people, to be the same people or become people of a distinct and inferior kind, by virtue of having lived a specified number of years'. The assumptions of ageism lie behind many of the most often asked questions about the social and political consequences of ageless ageing. They make such questions impossible to answer adequately from our current perspective and with our current views of reality. They also force us to ignore a number of important realities.

We forget, for instance, that chronological age at its very best is only a limited indication of biological and functional age. Even our present old people are capable of far more than society allows them to express or contribute – indeed more than they themselves allow. We also forget that every major disease is age-dependent and all of the major causes of death and disability are secondary to the progressive degeneration of ageing. Little wonder, for until now, after the age of 30 we have been witnessing a steady and inexorable increase in the probability of morbidity and mortality from one disease or another. But people living by the principles of ageless ageing will be different. Highly resistant to the ravages of degeneration which manifest themselves in our major destructive chronic diseases such as cancer, coronary heart disease, arthritis and the rest, they will be *less* rather than *more* of a burden to the state in terms of medical, social and psychiatric care. Application of these life-lengthening and life-enhancing principles to health on a wide scale should lead to an increase in the ratio of productive to non-productive men and women with prolonged life spans. This has been the conclusion of Yale's Professor Larry Kotlikoff, one of the few academics to look seriously at the issue. Kotlikoff initiated an inquiry into the economic effects of increased lifespan. He also concluded that this increase in the ratio of productive to non-productive people would result in an increased *per capita* output, whether or not the working period increased year for year with life expectancy.

With the increased longevity and the improved resistance to degeneration which are the natural outcome of applying the findings of age-researchers to our everyday lives, the population of our old people will also change. So will our attitudes to them. No longer a burden, like the Vilcabamba Indians or the Abkhazians of the Caucasus, they will become not 'old people' but 'long-lived people'. Such a simple shift in attitude could revolutionize us as human beings not only in terms of politics and economics but by shifting us towards a more value-oriented society. At that point the question of 'What will we do with all these old people?' begins to take on quite a different meaning. For the challenge now becomes not how we house, feed, and care for a growing sector of the non-productive population but rather how we can best use the energy and wisdom of the older members of our society.

A Time for Reaping

At the moment we have about a quarter of a century allotted to us in which to grow to adulthood. The next forty years are generally directed towards accomplishment in the outside world, realizing the goals of adulthood, procreation and raising a family. Then we tend to slide headlong downhill until we die. The character Vitek in Karel Capek's celebrated play *The Makropoulos Secret* describes the plight of modern man:

> ' . . . he hasn't had time for gladness, and he hasn't had time to think, and he hasn't had time for anything except a desire for bread. He hasn't done anything. No, not even himself. . . What else is immortality of the soul but a protest against the shortness of life? A human being is something more than a turtle or a raven; a man needs more time to life. Sixty years – it is not right. It's weakness, it's innocence, and it's animal-like.'

Within the confines of our three score and ten years and under the pressures of contemporary social values, modern man and modern woman have become quite extraordinarily obsessed with accomplishment. Since for most of us the time for worldly accomplishment is limited to this middle period, we push ourselves forward, often at health-breaking and heart-breaking speed. To many of us the concern with fulfilling ourselves in our career, paying the rent, buying the baby a new pair of shoes, during what are supposed to be the best years of our lives, forces us to postpone the pleasures of a time to dream, a time to think and a time to play – in the very highest sense of the word. If we are to find a means of coping with the problems of our society – problems of poor statesmanship, overpopulation, Third World famine, pollution and economic inequities – we desperately need this time to dream. We need this time to recreate our own world and to take our destiny responsibly into our own hands, aside from the demands of adult life.

Connectedness – A Priority

Nobel laureate novelist Hermann Hesse wrote about such a time-expanded world in his *The Glass Bead Game*. There, time's limits become the rules of the game of life and each human being is freed to order his existential choices. Such a time-expanded world could help us draw together our learning and re-synthesize our knowledge. It might enable the coming together of disciplines such as mathematics, physics, philosophy, biology, medicine, psychology, anthropology, art, literature, politics, theology and law – in fact the whole gamut of human concerns and disciplines – into a kind of connectedness which is urgently needed in the excessively fragmented post-industrial society which has become our home. Healthy longevity – ageless ageing – would make available to us the steadily maturing wisdom of our old people – people whose experience and awareness have not become distorted by ill-functioning minds and rapidly waning energies. Such wisdom is, I believe, exactly what we need to help guide our species into its further evolution. Moreover, such time expansion takes hold of our personal sense of the present and in a very real way draws it into the future. For when we are able to project ourselves into the future, that future becomes not an abstract consideration but of active concern to all of us. The future of the earth is our future. We become responsible for it and we will live to see it as caretakers instead of as irresponsible tenants of a rented property. Ageless ageing will help us become its owners and like all owners we are far more likely to look after our property.

In George Bernard Shaw's preface to *Back to Methuselah* – the play in which his character Dr Conrad Barnabas promotes an extended lifespan of 300 years – he writes: 'Men do not live long enough; they are, for the purposes of high civilization, mere children when they die.' He then goes on to consider some of the creative possibilities of our being able to lengthen life:

This possibility came to me when history and experience had convinced me that the social problems raised by millionfold national populations are far beyond the political capacity attainable in three score and ten years of life by slow growing mankind. On all hands as I write the cry is that our statesmen are too old, and that Leagues of Youth must be formed everywhere to save civilization from them. But despairing ancient pioneers tell me that the statesmen are not old enough for their jobs . . . We have no sages old enough and wise enough to make a synthesis of these reactions, and to develop the magnetic awe-inspiring force which must replace the policeman's baton as the instrument of authority.

Creators of Destiny

For me this magnetic awe-inspiring force of which he speaks is nothing less than man's potential to become the creator of his destiny on earth. The situation in which we live with all the global dangers to which we are exposed, from the possibility of mass nuclear extinction to world economic collapse, are not accidents of nature. They have been created by us. And no act of God can suddenly remove their potential destructiveness from our future. Only we ourselves have the possibility of doing that. If we are to succeed, we will need to call forth every resource which we have – intelligence, wisdom, strength, courage, patience, wit, compassion – and work with them. Ageless ageing can help us do that.

Life extension, the freedom from mental and physical degeneration, is no curious artifact of twentieth-century science. Who cares if, at the age of 85, we are all capable of running a marathon or if we look 30 years younger? Such things matter little on their own. But the high-level health, mental clarity and wellbeing which are rewards of ageless ageing are of urgent concern to our future as residents of the earth. They form the foundation on which we as human beings can build if we are to make use of our full potential for creativity. In the full use of such creativity lies the future of ourselves, our children and our planet. Again in the words of Capek's Vitek:

Let's give everyone a three-hundred-year life. It will be the biggest event since the creation of man; it will be the liberating and creating anew of man! God, what man will be able to do in three hundred years! To be a child and pupil for fifty years; fifty years to understand the world and its ways and to see everything there is; and a hundred years to work in; and then a hundred years, when we have understood everything, to live in wisdom, to teach, and to give example. How valuable human life would be if it lasted for three hundred years! There would be no fear, no selfishness. Everything would be wise and dignified. Give people life! Give them full human life!

An idealistic plea in the midst of the profound disillusionment with man that is so much a part of late twentieth-century life? A dream? Perhaps. Yet our dreams become the myths by which we live. And right now we urgently need new myths to give our life direction – dreams which, having been tempered by the wisdom of age and experience, are large enough and rich enough to take us forward. Such dreams have power. They also have a remarkable way of becoming reality:

> All men dream; but not equally. Those who dream by night in the dusty recesses of their minds wake in the day to find it was vanity: but the dreamers of the day are dangerous men, for they may act their dream with open eyes, to make it possible.
>   T.E. Lawrence

Resources

Bee Products: The Garvin Honey Company have a good selection of set and clear honeys from all over the world. These can be ordered from The Garvin Honey Company Ltd, Garvin House, 158 Twickenham Road, Isleworth, Middlesex, TW7 7LD. Tel: 081 560 7171. The New Zealand Natural Food Company have a good range of honey and propolis products, in particular Manuka honey, known for its anti-bacterial effects. The New Zealand Natural Food Company Ltd, Hold Close, Highgate Wood, London, N10 3HW. Tel: 081 444 5660.

Cell Therapy: For further information contact Dr. Claus Martin, Die Vier Jahreszeiten Klinik Dr. C Martin, Farberweg 3, D-8183 Rottach-Egern, Postfach 244, Germany.

Herbs: Many good quality herbs, including suma, are available from Solgar (see under nutritional supplements). A good tincture of echinacea is Echinaforce. It is available from Bioforce. For stockists contact Bioforce UK Ltd, Olympic Business Park, Dundonald, Ayrshire, KA2 9BE. Tel: 0563 851177. For stockists of Siberian ginseng contact RH& M Victuals Ltd, Gardiner House, Broomhill Road, Wandsworth, London, SW18 4JQ. A good ginseng comes in the form of Jinlin Ginseng Tea, Jinlin *Panax ginseng* Dried Slices, and Jinlin whole root, available from health-food stores. If you have difficulty finding it, contact Alice Chiu, 4 Tring Close, Barkingside, Essex, IG2 7LQ. Tel: 081 550 9900.

Herb Teas: Some of my favourite blends include Cinnamon Rose, Orange Zinger, and Emperor's Choice by Celestial Seasonings; Warm & Spicy by Symmingtons; and Creamy Carob French

Vanilla. Yogi Tea, by Golden Temple Products, is a strong spicy blend perfect as a coffee replacement.

Impedance Units: For further information on measuring lean body mass to fat ratio contact: Bodystat Ltd, PO Box 50, Douglas, Isle of Man, IM99 1DG. Tel: 0642 629 571.

Marigold Low Salt Swiss Vegetable Bouillon Powder: This instant broth powder based on vegetables and sea salt is available from health-food stores or direct from Marigold Foods, Unit 10, St. Pancras Commercial Centre, 63 Pratt Street, London, NW1 0BY. Tel: 071 267 7368.

Nutritional Analysis: Biolab Medical Unit in central London is a referral centre for Nutritional Medicine. Patients can be referred by their GP or hospital consultant. Doctors can also contact the unit for advice on laboratory investigations and the correction of nutrient deficiencies or imbalances. Biolab Medical Unit, The Stone House, 9 Weymouth Street, London W1N 3FF. A list of practitioners whose reputation I know to be good is available by writing to Leslie Kenton, c/o Ebury Press, Random House, 20 Vauxhall Bridge Road, London SW1V 2SA.

Nutritional Supplements: Solgar do a good selection of high potency nutritional supplements. For stockists contact Solgar Vitamins Ltd, Solgar House, Chiltern Commerce Centre, Asheridge Road, Chesham, Bucks, HP5 2PY. Tel: 0494 791 691. For lower potency supplements with high bio-availability, Nature's Own do a good range of vitamins and minerals. For stockists contact Nature's Own, 203–205 West Malvern Road, West Malvern, Worcs, WR14 4BB. Tel: 0684 892 555.

Personal Trainers: For help with personal exercise you can contact the National Register of Personal Fitness Trainers, Cecil House, 52 St Andrew's Street, Hertford, Hertfordshire SA14 1JA. Tel: 0992 504336. They will supply you with a list of personal trainers in Britain. However, not all the best people belong to an organisation. A personal trainer I highly recommend was my own. He is Welsh champion weightlifter Rhodri Thomas, 90 Cherry Grove, Derwen Fawr, Swansea SA2 8AX. He is often willing to spend either a weekend or a week or two working out your own personal programme in your own home which he will then monitor and readjust regularly.

Royal Jelly: Good, fresh European royal jelly is sold at Harrods. It is also available mail-order – refrigerated and sent in insulated boxes – from: Ortis, PO Box 223A, Thames Ditton, Surrey, KT7 0LY. Tel: 081 398 9888.

Skin care anti-wrinkle tablets: Imedeen by Ferrosan based on fish cartilage is available from leading chemists and health-food stores.

Water: Friends of the Earth have an excellent briefing sheet, 'Drinking water: is it up to standard?'. Contact Friends of the Earth, 26–28 Underwood Street, London N1 7JQ.

If you wish to keep informed of Leslie Kenton's forthcoming books, videos, workshops and other activities, please write to her, c/o Ebury Press, Random House, 20 Vauxhall Bridge Road, London SW1V 2SA, enclosing a stamped, self-addressed A4 envelope.

References

Chapter One

Bjorksten, J. 'Approaches and prospects for the control of age-dependent deterioration', *Annals of the New York Academy of Sciences*, 7 June 1971, 184:95–102.

Compendium of Health Statistics, 4th ed, Office of Health Economics, London, 1981.

Coronary Heart Disease: The Scope for Prevention, Office of Health Economics, London, 1982.

Gruenberg, E. M. 'The Failures of Success', *Millbank Memorial Fund Quarterly*, winter 1977, 55(1):3–24.

Harris, A. *Handicapped and Impaired in Great Britain*, HMSO, London, 1971.

Leaf, A. 'Every Day Is a Gift when You Are Over 100', *National Geographic*, 1973, 143(1):93–119.

Leaf, A. *Youth in Old Age*, McGraw-Hill, New York, 1975.

Medvedev, Z. A. 'Caucasus & Altay Longevity: A Biological or Social Problem?', *The Gerontologist*, 1974, 14:381.

Mortality Statistics, 1979, DHI, No 8, Table 22 series, Office of Population Censuses and Surveys, London, 1979.

Special Report on Ageing, 1979, NIH, Pub No 79–1907, Washington DC, 1979.

The Surgeon General, *Healthy People: The Surgeon General's Report of Health Promotion and Disease Prevention*, DHEW, Pub Nos 79-55071 and 79–55071A, Washington DC, 1979.

Thoms, W. J. *The Longevity of Man: Its Facts and Fictions*, John Murray, London, 1873.

Walford, Roy. *Maximum Life Span*, W. W. Norton & Co, New York, 1983.

Chapter Two

Brown-Séquard, Charles E. *Société Biologique*, Vol II, Paris, 1851.
Codellas, P. S. 'Rejuvenation and Satricons of Yesterday', *Ann. of Med. Hist.*, Vol IV, 1934.
Comfort, A. *The Biology of Senescence*, Routledge & Kegan Paul, London, 1956.
Comfort, A. et al. *The Process of Ageing*. Signet/NAL, New York, 1964.
Hayflick, L. *Scientific American*, March 1968: 218.
Hayflick, L. 'Cell Biology of Ageing', *Federal Proceedings*, 1979, 38(5):1851–1856.
Hayflick, L. and P. S. Moorhead, *Expl. Cell. Res.*, 1961, 25:585.
Lambert, Gilbert. *Conquest of Age*, Souvenir Press, London, 1960.
Niehans, Paul. *Introduction to Cell Therapy*, Pageant Books Inc, New York, 1960.
Niehans, Paul. *Die Endokreinen Drusen des Gehirns, Epiphyse und Hypophyse*, Hans Halen, Berne, n.d.
Rosenfeld, A. *Pro-Longevity*, New York: Avon, 1977.
Trimmer, Eric J. *Rejuvenation*, Robert Hale, London, 1967.

Chapter Three

Bender, A. D. et al. *Expl. Gerontol.*, 1970, 5:97.
Bjorksten, J. 'Cross Linking: Key to Ageing?', *Chemical and Engineering News*, 9 May 1955, 33:1957.
Bjorksten, J. *Longevity: A Quest*, Bjorksten Research Foundation, Madison, Wisconsin, 1981.
Bjorksten, J. 'Biochemistry of Ageing', in *Clinical Biochemistry: Contemporary Theories and Techniques*, Vol 2, ed H. Spiegel, Academic Press, New York, 1982.
Bjorksten, J. *Dialogue on Death*, Bjorksten Research Foundation, Houston, Texas, n.d.
Cranton, E. M. and J. P. Frackelton. 'Free Radical Pathology in Age-Associated Diseases: Treatment with EDTA Chelation, Nutrition and Anti-oxidants', *Journal of Holistic Medicine*, spring/summer 1984, 6(1).
Frank, B. S. and P. Miele. *Dr Frank's No-Ageing Diet*, Dell, New York, 1976.
Haugaard, Niels. 'Cellular Mechanisms of Oxygen Toxicity', *Physiological Reviews*, April 1968, 47(2).
Kent, Saul. *The Life Extension Revolution*, Quill, New York, 1983.

Kugler, Hans. *Slowing Down the Ageing Process*, Pyramid, New York, 1974.

Levine, Stephen and Jeffrey Reinhardt. 'Biochemical-Pathology Initiated by Free Radicals, Oxidant Chemicals and Therapeutic Drugs in the Etiology of Chemical Hypersensitivity Disease', *Journal of Orthomolecular Psychiatry*, third quarter 1983, 12(3).

Levine, Stephen. *Anti-oxidant Biochemical Adaptation: Doorways to New Science and Medicine*, Publication preview copy from author, 1984.

Mann, John A. *Secrets of Life Extension*, Harbor Publishing, San Francisco, 1980.

Passwater, Richard, *Supernutrition*, Pocket Books, New York, 1976.

Pelletier, Kenneth. *Longevity: Fulfilling Our Biological Potential*, Delacorte Press/Lawrence, New York, 1981.

Rosenfeld, Albert. *Pro-Longevity*, Avon, New York, 1977.

Tappel, A. L. 'Will Anti-oxidant nutrients slow aging processes?' *Geriatrics*, October 1968.

Williams, R. J. 'Medical Research Leading to the Acceptance of the Orthomolecular Approach', *Journal of Orthomolecular Psychiatry*, 4(2):99.

Chapter Four

Bjorksten, J. 'Cross Linking: Key to Ageing?' *Chemical and Engineering News*, 9 May 1955, 33:1957.

Bjorksten, J. *Longevity: A Quest*, Bjorksten Research Foundation, Madison, Wisconsin, 1981.

Bjorksten, J. *Dialogue on Death*, Bjorksten Research Foundation, Houston, Texas, n.d.

Demopolos, H. B. 'The Basis of Free Radical Pathology', *Federation Proceedings*, 32:1859–1861, symposium issue.

Goodhart, Robert S. and Maurice Shils. *Modern Nutrition in Health and Disease*, Lea & Febiger, Philadelphia, 1978.

Guyton, Arthur C. *Textbook of Medical Physiology*, W. B. Saunders, Philadelphia, 1976.

Levine, Stephen, 'Oxidants, Anti-Oxidants and Chemical Hypersensitivities', Parts I and II, *International Journal of Biosocial Research*, 4:51–54 and 4:102–105.

Levine, Stephen and Parris M. Kidd. *Anti-Oxidant Biochemical Adaptation: Doorway to the New Science and Medicine*, Biocurrents Research, San Francisco, 1984.

Rosenfeld, Albert. *Pro-Longevity*, Avon, New York, 1977.

Chapter Five

Amkraut, A. and G. F. Solomon. 'From the symbolic stimulus to the pathophysiologic response: Immune mechanisms', *International Journal of Psychiatry in Medicine*, 1975, 5(4):541–63.

Anderson, R. et al. *American Journal of Clinical Nutrition*, 1980, 33:71.

Barton, G. M. G. and O. S. Roath. *International Journal of Vitamins and Nutritional Research*, 1976, 46:271.

Bjorksten, J. In *Theoretical Aspects of Ageing*, ed. M. Rockstein et al, 43–59, Academic Press, New York, 1974.

Brook, M. et al. *American Journal of Clinical Nutrition*, 1968, 21:1254.

Chandra, R. K. *Nutrition Immunity and Infection*, Plenum Press, New York, 1977.

Colgan, Michael. 'Strong Immunity', *Colgan Institute Lecture Series No 15*, Colgan Institute, 531 Encinitas Blvd, No 19, Encinitas, Calif. 92024, USA, September 1992.

Hayflick, Leonard. 'On the Facts of Life', *Executive Health*, June 1978, XIV, 9.

Herbert, V. and K. C. Das. In *Vitamins and Hormones*, Vol 34, eds P. L. Minson et al, Academic Press, New York, 1976.

Holland, J. J. *Scientific American*, Feb 1974:32.

Hume, R. and E. Weyers. *Scott. Medical Journal*, 1973, 18:3.

Lewin, S. *Vitamin C: Its Molecular Biology and Medical Potential*, Academic Press, London, 1976.

Milne, J. S. et al. *British Medical Journal*, 1971, 4:383.

Pisciotta, A. V. et al. *Nature*, 1967, 215:193.

Scrimshaw, Nevin S. 'Synergistic and Antagonistic Interactions of Nutrition and Infection', *Federation Proceedings*, Nov–Dec 1966, 25:1679–1681.

Siegel, B. V. and J. I. Morton. *Experientia*, 1977, 33:393.

Stein, M. et al. 'Influence of brain and behavior on the immune system', *Science*, 6 Feb 1976, 191:435–440.

Walford, Roy. *The Immunologic Theory of Ageing*, Williams and Wilkins, Baltimore, 1969.

Walford, Roy. *American Journal of Clinical Pathology*, 1980, 74:247.

Walford, Roy. *Maximum Life Span*, W. W. Norton, New York, 1983.

Wilson, C. W. M. and H. S. Loh, *Lancet*, 1973, 1:1058.

Yonomoto, R. H. *International Journal of Vitamins and Nutritional Research*, 1979, Suppl 19.

Chapter Six

'It's Not the Amount of Stress You Have, It's How You Respond to It', *Executive Health*, February 1983, XIX(5).

Khorol, I. S. 'Einstein and Selye', *Rejuvenation*, July 1978, VI(3):54ff.

Selye, Hans. *The Story of the Adaptation Syndrome*, Acta Inc Medical Publishers, Montreal, 1952.

Selye, Hans. *In Vivo: The Case for Supramolecular Biology*, Liveright, New York, 1967.

Selye, Hans. *Stress Without Distress*, Hodder & Stoughton, London, 1974.

Selye, Hans. *The Stress of Life*, McGraw-Hill, New York, 1975.

Selye, Hans. *Stress in Health and Disease*, Butterworths Inc, Reading, Mass., 1976.

Chapter Seven

Bertalanffy, L. von. 'General Systems Theory: A Critical Review', *General Systems Yearbook*, Society of General Systems Research, 1962, 7:1.

Bertalanffy, L. von. 'The Mind-Body Problem: A New View', *Psychosomatic Medicine*, 1964, XXVI(1).

Bertalanffy, L. von. *Robots, Men and Minds*, George Braziller, New York, 1967.

Bertalanffy, L. von. *Problems of Life: An Evaluation of Modern Biological Thought*, Harper Torchbook, New York, 1980.

Bray, H. G. and K. White. *Kinetics and Thermodynamics in Biochemistry*, J. & A. Churchill, London, 1957.

Brekhman, I. I. *Man and Biologically Active Substances*, Pergamon Press, Oxford, 1980.

de la Peña, A. M. *The Psychobiology of Cancer*, Praeger Publishers, CBS Educational and Professional Publishing, New York, 1983.

Komarov, L. V. 'Life as a Notion and Gerontology', *Rejuvenation*, June 1984, XII(1–2).

Pardee, A. B. and L. L. Ingraham. 'Free Energy and Entropy in Metabolism', *Metabolic Pathways*, Vol I, ed D. M. Greenberg.

Polanyi, M. 'Life Transcending Chemistry and Physics', *Chemistry and Engineering*, 21 Aug 1967.

Schrödinger, Erwin. *What Is Life?* and *Mind and Matter*, University Press, Cambridge, 1980.

Szent-Györgyi, A. *Bioenergetics*, Academic Press, New York, 1957.
Szent-Györgyi, A. *Introduction to a Submolecular Biology*, Academic Press, New York, 1960.
Szent-Györgyi, A. *Bioelectronics*, Academic Press, New York, 1968.
Szent-Györgyi, A. *The Living State*, Academic Press, New York, 1972.

Chapter Eight

Becker, R. O. *Electromagnetism and Life*, State University of New York Press, Albany, NY, n.d.

Becker, R. O. 'Electromagnetic Forces and Life Processes', *Technological Review*, Dec 1972.

Becker, R. O. 'The Basic Biological Data Transmission and Control System Influenced by Electrical Forces', *Annals of the New York Academy of Sciences*, 11 Oct 1974, 238:236–241.

Becker, R. O. 'An Application of Direct Current Neural Systems to Psychic Phenomena', *Psychoenergetic Systems*, 1977, 2:35.

Becker, R. O. 'Electromagnetic Fields and Life', *Psychoenergetic Systems*, 1979, 3:119–128.

Becker, R. O. 'Electrical Control Systems and Regenerative Growth', *Journal of Bioelectricity*, 1982, 1(2):239–264.

Becker, R. O. 'Electromagnetic Controls over Biological Growth Processes', *Journal of Bioelectricity*, 1984, 3(1 and 2):105–118.

Becker, R. O. *The Body Electric: Electromagnetism and the Foundation of Life*, William Morrow & Co, New York, 1985.

Becker, R. O. 'Modern Bioelectromagnetics and Functions of the Central Nervous System', *Subtle Energies*, 1992, Vol 3, No 1:53ff.

Burr, Harold Saxton. *Blueprint for Immortality*, Neville Spearman, London, 1952.

Chimoskey, J. E. et al. 'Time Varying Magnetic Fields: Effects on DNA Synthesis', *Science*, 24 Feb 1984, 223:818ff.

Crile, George. *The Bipolar Theory of Living Processes*, Macmillan, New York, 1926.

Crile, George. *The Phenomenon of Life*, W. W. Norton, New York, 1936.

Galvani, Luigi, *Commentary on the Effects of Electricity on Muscular Motion: A Translation of Luigi Galvani's De Viribus Electricitatis in Motu Musculari Commentarius*, E. Licht, Cambridge, Mass., 1953.

Goodman, Reba, et al. 'Pulsing Electromagnetic Fields Induce Cellular Transcription', *Science*, 17 June 1983, 220:1283ff.

Kenton, L. and S. *The New Raw Energy*, Vermilion, London, 1995.

Komarov, L. V. 'On the possible use of permanent magnetic fields for the artificial prolongation of the specific lifespan', *Rejuvenation*, 1975, 3(4).

Lakhovsky, G. *L'Origine de la Vie*, University Press, Texas, 1947.

Lawden, D. F. 'Separability of Psycho-physical Systems', *Psychoenergetics*, 1981, 4(1):1–10.

Lawden, D. F. 'A Berkeleian Model for Psychic Phenomena', *Psychoenergetics*, 1983, 5(3):185–198.

Szent-Györgyi, A. *Introduction to a Submolecular Biology*, Academic Press, New York, 1960.

Chapter Nine

Bjorksten, J. 'The Theoretical Base of the First Law of Le Compte', *Rejuvenation*, May 1975, III(4).

Bjorksten, J. 'Pathways to Longevity', *Rejuvenation*, June 1978, VI(2).

Bjorksten, J. *Longevity: A Quest*, Bjorksten Research Foundation, Madison, Wisconsin, 1981.

Bjorksten, J. 'Biochemistry of Ageing', *Clinical Biochemistry*, Academic Press, New York, 1982.

Colgan, Michael. *Your Personal Vitamin Profile*, Quill, New York, 1982; Blond & Briggs, London, 1983.

Le Compte, Herman. 'Le Compte's Law', *Zeitschrift für Altersforschung*, 1965, Band 18, Heft 2.

Le Compte, Herman (with Northcote Parkinson). *The Law of Longer Life*, Troy State University Press, Troy, Alabama, 1980.

Le Compte, Herman. Personal communication with the author.

Nutrition Search. *Nutrition Almanac*, McGraw-Hill, New York, 1979.

Pfeiffer, C. *Mental and Elemental Nutrients*, Keats Publishing, New Canaan, Conn., 1975.

Pfeiffer, C. and J. Banks. *Total Nutrition*, Simon and Schuster, New York, 1980.

Szent-Györgyi, A. 'On a Substance that Can Make Us Sick if We Do Not Eat It', *Executive Health*, June 1977, XIII(9).

Williams, Roger J. and D. Kalita. *A Physician's Handbook on Orthomolecular Medicine*, Keats Publishing, New Canaan, Conn., 1977.

Chapter Ten

Gatsko, G. G. et al. 'Combined Effect of Periodic Feeding and Using the Vitamin B Complex upon Biological Age, and Some Metabolic Indices of the White Rat', *Rejuvenation*, January 1982, X(1).

McCay, Clive. 'Clinical Aspects of Ageing and the Effect of Diet upon Ageing', *Cowdry's Problems of Ageing*, 3rd ed, Williams & Williams Co, New York, 1952.

Ross, M. H. et al. 'Length of Life and Caloric Intake', *American Journal of Clinical Nutrition*, Aug 1972, 25:834–838.

Ross, M. H. et al. 'Food Preference and Length of Life', *Science*, 10 Oct 1975, 190:165–167.

Ross, M. H. et al. 'Dietary practices and growth responses as predictors of longevity', *Nature*, 12 August 1976, 262(5569):553–584.

Ross, M. H. et al. 'Dietary Behavior and Longevity', *Nutrition Reviews*, Oct 1977, 35(10).

Ross, M. H. et al. 'Dietary Practices of Early Life and Spontaneous Tumours of the Rat', *Nutrition and Cancer*, 1982.

Schlenker, E. D. *American Journal of Clinical Nutrition*, Oct 1973.

Walford, Roy. *Maximum Life Span*, W. W. Norton, New York, 1983.

Walford, Roy. 'On Retarding Ageing by Nutrition', *Executive Health*, Sept 1983, XIX(12).

Young, Vernon. 'Diet as a Modulator of Ageing and Longevity', *Federation Proceedings*, 6 May 1979, 38(6).

Chapter Eleven

Ames, Bruce. 'Dietary Carcinogens and Anticarcinogens', *Science*, Sept 1983, 221:1256ff.

Bircher, Franklin. 'The Relationship Between Clinical Symptoms and Disturbances in Microcirculation', 9th European Conference on Microcirculation, Antwerp, 1976, *Bibl. anat.* 16:249–252, Karger, Basel, 1977.

Bircher, Ralph. 'A Turning Point in Nutritional Science', Lee Foundation for Nutritional Research, Milwaukee, Wisconsin, reprint, n.d.

Bircher-Benner, Max. 'The Healing Community', unpublished translation by Hilda Marlin.

Bircher-Benner, Max. 'The Prevention of Incurable Disease', unpublished translation by Hilda Marlin.

Bircher-Benner, Max. 'The Meaning of Therapeutic Order', unpublished translation by Hilda Marlin.

Brekhman, I. I. *Man and Biologically Active Substances: The Effect of Drugs, Diet and Pollution on Health*, Pergamon Press, Oxford, 1980.

Brekhman, I. I. and M. G. Kublanov. 'The Concept of Structural Information in Pharmacology and Nutrition', Vladivostok, 1983.

Eppinger, H. et al. 'Transmineralisation und vegetarische Kost', *Ergebnisse der Inneren Medizin und Kinderheilkunde*, 1936, 51.

Eppinger, H. et al. 'Über Rohkostbehandlung', *Wiener Klinische Wochenshrift*, 1 July 1936.

Eppinger, H. et al. *Die Permeabilitätspathologie als Lehre vom Krankheitsbeginn*, Vienna, 1949.

Goodhart, Robert S. and Maurice Shils. *Modern Nutrition in Health and Disease*, 6th ed, Lea & Febiger, Philadelphia, 1980.

Hall, R. H. 'Is Nutrition a Stagnating Science?', *New Scientist*, 2 January 1975:7ff.

Heddle, J. A. (ed). *Mutagenicity: New Horizons in Genetic Toxicology*, Academic Press, New York, 1982.

Kenton, L. and S. *The New Raw Energy*, Vermilion, London, 1995.

Kenyon, Julian. 'Food Sensitivity – A Search for Underlying Causes: A Case Study of Twelve Patients', photocopy from the author.

Liechti von Brasch, Dagmar. 'Seventy Years of Experience in the Bircher-Benner Therapy of Order', unpublished translation by Hilda Marlin.

Stich, H. F. et al. *Mutat. Res.*, 1981, 90, 201 and 1983, 116, 333.

Sugimura, T. and S. Sato. *Cancer Research supplement*, 1983, 43, 2415s.

Szent-Györgyi, A. *Introduction to a Submolecular Biology*, Academic Press, New York, 1960.

Chapter Twelve

Balfour, E. B. *The Living Soil*, Universe Books, New York, 1943.

Blackburn, G. L., G. T. Wilson, B. S. Kanders, et al. 'Weight Cycling: The Experience of Human Dieters', *American Journal of Clinical Nutrition*, 1989.

Boyd, Eaton S. and Melvin Konner. 'Palaeolithic Nutrition: A Consideration of its Nature and Current Implications', *New England Journal of Medicine*, 1985.

Burkitt, Denis. *Refined Carbohydrate Foods and Disease*, Academic Press, New York, 1975.

Carson, Rachel. *Silent Spring*, Penguin, London, 1962.

Colgan, Michael, *Prevent Cancer Now*, CI Publications, San Diego, 1992.

Cousins, N. *The Healing Heart*, Avalon Books, New York, 1983.

Howard, Sir Albert. *The Soil and Health*, Schocken Books, New York, 1975.

Hur, Robin. *Food Reform: Our Desperate Need*, Heidelberg Publishers, Austin, Texas, 1975.

Jenkins, D. J. A., A. L. Jenkins, T. M. Wolever, et al. 'Simple and Complex Carbohydrates', *Nutrition Review*, 1984.

Kenton, L. 'What Price Convenience?', *Harpers & Queen*, Feb 1978.

Kenton, L. 'Sprayscape', *Harpers & Queen*, July 1985.

Lappé, Frances Moore, *Diet For a Small Planet*, Ballantine, New York, 1971.

McCarrison, Sir Robert. *Nutrition and Health*, The McCarrison Society, London, 1953.

Ornish, Dean. *Reversing Heart Disease*, Random Century, London, 1991.

Price, Weston. *Nutrition and Physical Degeneration*, Price-Pottinger Nutrition Foundation, San Diego, 1939, reprinted 1971.

Pritiken, N. *The Pritiken Program for Diet and Exercise*, Grosset & Dunlap, New York, 1979.

Siegel, B. *Love, Medicine and Miracles*, Harper & Row, New York, 1986; Rider, London, 1986.

Trowell, H. C. and D. P. Burkitt, *Western Diseases: Their Emergence and Prevention*, Harvard University Press, Cambridge, Mass., 1981.

Chapter Thirteen

Bircher, Ralph. 'The Question of Protein', typed paper from author.

Challem, Jack Joseph and Renate Lewin. 'Keeping the Mind Young', *Feldmore Newsletter*, No 44.

Colgan, Michael. *Your Personal Vitamin Profile*. Quill, New York, 1982; Blond & Briggs, London, 1983.

Eastwood, M. A. and W. D. Mitchell. 'The Place of Fibre in the Diet', *British Journal of Hospital Medicine*, Jan 1974:123.

Ershoff, B. H. 'Antitoxic Effects of Plant Fiber', *American Journal of Clinical Nutrition*, 27:1395–1398.

Horrobin, David. *Clinical Uses of Essential Fatty Acids*, Eden Press, London, 1982.

Issel, Josef. 'Nutritional Protection against Cancer', *Tjidskrift fur Halsa*, Stockholm, 1975, 1–3.

Karstrom, Henning. *Ratt Kost*, Skandinavska Bokforlaget, Gavle, Sweden, 1982.

Katenkamp and Stiller. *Histochemistry of Amyloid*, VEB Gustav Fischer Verlag, Jena, Germany, 1975.

Katenkamp and Stiller. 'Das Amyloid', *Hippokrates*, 41(1):5–23.

Kelsay, J. 'A Review of Research on Effects of Fibre Intake on Man', *American Journal of Clinical Nutrition*, Jan 1978, 31:142-159.

Kruiswijk, H., H. A. Oomen and E. H. Hipsley. *Voeding*, 1969, 30/5:225–230.

McCully, Kilmer S. *American Journal of Pathology*, 1970, 59:181–193 and 61:1–8.

McCully, Kilmer S. *American Journal of Clinical Nutrition*, May 1975, 28.

Spiller, Gene. 'Interaction of Dietary Fiber with Other Dietary Components: A Possible Factor in Certain Cancer Etiologies', *American Journal of Clinical Nutrition*, Oct 1978:231–232.

Winick, M. 'Slow the problems of Aging and Quash its Problems – With Diet', *Modern Medicine*, 15 February 1978:68–74.

Chapter Fourteen

Kenton, L. & S. *The New Raw Energy*, Vermilion, London, 1995.

Kenton, L. & S. *Raw Energy Recipes*, Ebury Press, London, 1994.

Kunz-Bircher, Ruth. *Eat Your Way To Health: The Bircher-Benner Approach to Nutrition*, Allen & Unwin, London, 1984.

Polunin, Miriam. *The New Cookbook*, Macdonald, London, 1985.

Chapter Fifteen

Ash, J. E. 'The Blood in Inanition', *Arch. Inter. Med.*, July 1914, 14:8–32.

Buchinger, Otto. *About Fasting*, Thorsons, Wellingborough, 1961.

Buchinger, Otto. *Über Moderne Heilfasten Kuren*, Turm-Verlag, Beitigheim, Germany, 1970.

Carlson, A. J. 'Hunger, appetite and gastric juice secretion in man during prolonged fasting', *American Journal of Physiology*, 1918, 45:120–46.

Child, C. M. *Senescence and Rejuvenescence*, University Press, Chicago, 1915.

Cott, Alan. *Fasting As a Way of Life*, Bantam Books, New York, 1977.

Cott, Alan. *Fasting: The Ultimate Diet*, Bantam Books, New York, 1981.

De Vries, Arnold. *Therapeutic Fasting*, Chandler Book Co, Los Angeles, 1963.

Hazzard, L. B. *Fasting for the Cure of Disease*, Physical Culture Pub Co, 1910.

Hills, Christopher. *Rejuvenating the Body*, University of the Trees Press, Boulder Creek, Calif., 1979.

Kent, Susannah, 'Fasting', *The Vegetarian*, Nov 1974.

Maleskey, Gale. 'The Truth about Fasting', *Prevention Magazine*, Oct 1984.

Morgulis, S. *Fasting and Undernutrition*, E. P. Dutton & Co, New York.

Morgulis, S. 'Contributions to the physiology of regeneration', *J. Exp. Zool.*, 1909, 7:595–642.

Shelton, H. *The Science and Fine Art of Fasting*, Natural Hygiene Press, Chicago, 1978.

Sinclair, U. P. *The Fasting Cure*, M. Kennerly, 1913.

Szekely, Edmond Bordeaux. *The Essene Science of Fasting and the Art of Sobriety*, International Biogenic Society, Cartago, Costa Rica, 1978.

Chapter Sixteen

Airola, P. O. *Health Secrets from Europe*, Arco, New York, 1972.

Airola, P. O. *How to Get Well*, Health Plus Publishers, Phoenix, Ariz., 1974.

Dalas, Nergis. *Yoga for Rejuvenation*, Thorsons, Wellingborough, 1984.

Dhillon, Sukhraj. *Health, Happiness and Longevity*, Japan Publications, Tokyo, 1983.

Guyton, A. C. 'Interstitial fluid pressure-volume relationships and their regulation' in G. E. W. Wolstenholms and J. Knight (eds), *Ciba Foundation Symposium on Circulatory and Respiratory Mass Transport*, J. & A. Churchill, London, 1969.

Guyton, A. C. *Basic Human Physiology: Normal Function Mechanisms of Disease*, W. B. Saunders Co, Philadelphia, 1971.

Kluger, M. J. 'On Fever: Does it really harm or help?', *Executive Health*, March 1984, XX(6).

Knowles, William. *Knowles Breathing Course*, privately published, 1960.

Lederman, E. K. *Good Health through Natural Therapy*, Pan, London, 1978.

Lindlahr, Henry. *Natural Therapeutics*, Vol 2, C. W. Daniel, Saffron Walden, 1981.

Powell, Eric. *The Natural Home Physician*, Health Science Press, Saffron Walden, 1962.

Turner, R. N. *Naturopathic Medicine*, Thorsons, Wellingborough, 1984.

Wareland, Are. *In the Cauldron of Disease*, A. G. Berry, London, 1934.

West, Samuel C. *Trapped Protein: The Major Cause of Pain, Loss of Energy and Degenerative Disease*, The New Way of Life Health Foundation, Mesa, Ariz.

West, Samuel C. *Excess Protein*, The New Way of Life Health Foundation, Mesa, Ariz., Jan 1978.

Yoffrey, J. M. and F. C. Courtice. *Lymphatics, Lymph, and Lymphoid Tissue*, Williams & Wilkins, Baltimore, 1967.

Chapter Seventeen

Bjorksten, J. 'A Theoretical Base for Multivitamin Therapy', *Rejuvenation*, Oct 1976, 4(4).

Cameron, Ewan and Linus Pauling. *Cancer and Vitamin C*, Warner Books, New York, 1981.

Cathcart, R. 'The method for determining proper doses of Vitamin C for the treatment of disease by titrating to bowel tolerance', *Journal of Orthomolecular Psychiatry*, 10(2):125ff.

Committee on Animal Nutrition, *Nutrient Requirements for Laboratory Animals*, Publication No 990: National Academy of Science.

Cranton, E. M. and J. P. Frackelton. 'Free Radical Pathology in Age-Associated Diseases: Treatment with EDTA Chelation, Nutrition and Anti-oxidants', *Journal of Holistic Medicine*, spring/summer 1984, 6(1).

Crary, E. et al. 'Potential Clinical Applications for High-Dose Nutritional Anti-Oxidants', *Medical Hypothesis*, 1984, 13:77.

Davis, A. *Let's Eat Right to Stay Fit*, Signet Books, New York, 1970.

Demopolus, H. B. et al. 'Theoretical Basis for Free Radical Damage and Review of Experimental Data', *Neural Trauma*, Raven Press, New York, 1979.

Gilbert, D. L. *Oxygen and Living Process*, Springer-Verlag, 1981.

Halliwell, B. and J. Gutteridge. *Lancet*, 23 June 1984, p 1396.

Pauling, L. 'For the Best of Health: How Much Vitamin C Do You Need?', *Executive Health*, Dec 1975, 12(3).

Pauling, L. *Vitamin C and the Common Cold*, Berkley Books, New York, 1982.

Roos, D. et al. 'Oxygen Free Radicals and Tissue Damage', Ciba Symposium, 65, Amsterdam: Excerpta Medica – New Series.

Stone, Irwin. *The Healing Factor: Vitamin C Against Disease*, Grosset & Dunlap, New York, 1972.

Chapter Eighteen

Bjorksten, J. *Longevity: A Quest*, Bjorksten Research Foundation, Madison, Wisconsin, 1981.

Colgan, Michael. 'Anti-Oxidants, Health and Ageing, *Colgan Institute Lecture Series No 4*, Colgan Institute, 531 Encinitas Blvd, No 19, Encinitas, Calif. 92024, USA, March 1992.

Goodhart, Robert S. and Maurice E. Shils. *Modern Nutrition in Health and Disease*, Lea & Febiger, Philadelphia, 1980.

Hoffer, Abram and Morton Walker. *Orthomolecular Nutrition*, Keats Publishing, New Canaan, Conn., 1978.

Kent, Saul. *The Life Extension Revolution*, Quill, New York, 1983.

Kirschmann, John D. (ed) *Nutrition Almanac*, McGraw-Hill, New York, 1985.

Kraus, V. K. and L. K. Mahan. *Food, Nutrition and Diet Therapy*, W. B. Saunders Co, London, 1979.

Kugler, Hans. *Slowing Down the Aging Process*, Pyramid, New York, 1974.

Levine, Stephen A. and Parris M. Kidd. *Anti-Oxidant Adaptation: Its Role in Free Radical Pathology*, Biocurrents Division, Allergy Research Group, San Leandro, Calif., 1985.

Newbold, H. L. *Mega-Nutrients*, Peter H. Wyden, New York, 1975.

Rosenfeld, Albert. *Pro-Longevity*, Acorn, New York, 1977.

Stryer, Lubert. *Biochemistry*, W. H. Freeman and Company, San Francisco, 1975.

Tappel, A. 'Will Anti-oxidant nutrients slow ageing processes?', *Geriatrics*, Oct 1968.

Williams, Roger. *Physicians' Handbook of Nutritional Science*, Charles C. Thomas, Springfield, Illinois, 1975.

Williams, Roger. *Biochemical Individuality*, University of Texas Press, London, 1979.

Chapter Nineteen

Brown, P. E. *Nature*, 1967, 213:363.

Cutting, W. C. *Handbook of Pharmacology*, 5th ed, Appleton-Century-Crofts, New York, 1972.

Erdmann, Robert. Private communications with the author.

Freidman, H. et al. *Nature*, 1965, 205:1050ff.

Goodhart, R. S. and M. E. Shils. *Modern Nutrition in Health and Disease*, Sixth edition, Lea & Febiger, Philadelphia, 1980.

'Growth Hormone Releasers', *Newsletter 53*, Feldmore Health Publications, Tunbridge Wells. Has excellent list of references on free amino acids used for GHR.

Guyton, A. C. *Textbook of Medical Physiology*, W. B. Saunders, Philadelphia, 1976.

Hoffer, A. and H. Osmond. *How to Live with Schizophrenia*, University Books, New Hyde Park, NY, 1966.

Journal of Clinical Nutrition, 1953, 1:232.

Meiss, D. et al. 'Amino Acid Analysis: An Important Nutritional and Clinical Evaluation Tool', *Nutritional Perspectives*, 1983, 6(2):19–24.

Orthomolecular Psychiatry, Vol 4, 1975, 4:297ff.

Pearson, D. and S. Shaw. *Life Extension and The Life Extension Revolution*, Warner Books, New York, 1984.

Pfeiffer, C. *Mental and Elemental Nutrients*, Keats Publishing, New Canaan, Conn., 1975.

Philpott, William H. and Dwight K. Kalita. *Victory over Diabetes*, Keats Publishing, New Canaan, Conn., n.d.

Pryor, W. A. *Scientific American*, Aug 1970, 70ff.

Schauss, A. *Diet, Crime and Delinquency*, Parker House, Berkeley, Calif., 1981.

Science, 1973, 179:588–591.

Sprince, H. et al. *Federal Proceedings*, 1974, 33:233.

Svacha, A. J. et al. *Federal Proceedings*, 1974, 33:690.

Williams, R. et al. (ed) *A Physician's Handbook on Orthomolecular Medicine*, Keats Publishing, New Canaan, Conn., 1979.

Williams, R. *Nutrition Against Disease*, Bantam Books, New York, 1981.

Chapter Twenty

Barry, A. et al. 'The Effects of Physical Conditioning on Older Individuals', *Journal of Gerontology*, 1966.

Bortz, Walter M. 'Effect of Exercise on Ageing – Effect of Ageing on Exercise', *Journal of the American Geriatric Society*, Feb 1980, XXVIII(2):49ff.

Bortz, W. 'On Disease, Ageing, and Disuse', *Executive Health*, Dec 1983, XX(3).

British Journal of Dermatology, Aug 1978.

Colgan, M. *Your Personal Vitamin Profile*, Quill, New York, 1982; Blond & Briggs, London, 1983.

Colgan, Michael and Ben Weider. *Bodybuilding for a Healthy Heart*, International Federation of Bodybuilders.

deVries, Herbert A. *Physiology of Exercise*, William C. Brown Co, Dubuque, Iowa, USA, 1966.

de Vries, H. 'On Exercise for Relieving Anxiety and Tension', *Executive Health*, Sept 1982, XVIII(12).

'Exercise and Longevity: A little goes a long way', *New York Times*, 1989.

Finch, C. E. and L. Hayflick. *Handbook of the Biology of Ageing*, Van Nostrand, New York, 1977.

Franklin, B. A., E. R. Buskirk and P. C. Mackeen. 'Eighteen Month Follow-up of Participants in a Physical Conditioning Program for Middle-aged Women', *Med. Sci. Sports*, 1978.

Franklin, B. A. and M. Rubenfire. 'Losing Weight Through Exercise', *Journal of the American Medical Association*, 1980.

Gutin, Dr Bernard. *The High Energy Factor*, Random House, New York, 1983.

Journal of the American Medical Association, 16 Nov 1979 and 27 July 1984 (252(4):491).

McCartney, N. A. et al. 'Usefulness of Weightlifting Training in Improving Strength and Maximal Power Output in Coronary Heart Disease', *American Journal of Cardiology*, 1991.

Moorehouse, L. *The Physiology of Exercise*, 7th ed, Mosby, St. Louis, 1976.

Nieman, David C. *The Sports Medicine Fitness Course*, Bull Publishing, Calif. 1986.

Oscai, L. B. 'The Role of Exercise in Weight Control', *Exercise and Sport Sciences Reviews*, J. H. Wilmore (ed), Academic Press, New York, 1973.

Polednak, A. P. *The Longevity of Athletes*, C. C. Thomas, Springfield, Illinois, 1979.

Psychosomatic Medicine, Oct 1983.

Quas, Dr Vince. *The Lean Body Promise*, Synesis Press, Oregon, 1989.

'On Walking: Nature's True – and Painless – Elixir', *Executive Health*, June 1984, XX(9).

Sidney, K. H. et al. *American Journal of Clinical Nutrition*, 1977, 30.

Wood, P. D. and W. L. Haskell, *Lipids*, 1979, 14.

Chapter Twenty-One

'On Walking: Nature's True – and Painless – Elixir', *Executive Health*, June 1984, XX(9).

Belozerova, L. M. 'Ageing and Motor Activity', *Rejuvenation*, Apr 1982.

Bortz, Walter. 'On Disease, Ageing and Disuse', *Executive Health*, Dec 1983.

de Vries, Herbert. 'On Exercise for Relieving Anxiety and Tension', *Executive Health*, Sept 1982, XVIII(12).

Kenton, L. 'Secret Sources', *Harpers & Queen*, Feb 1985.

Leonard, George. *The Ultimate Athlete*, Avon Books, New York, 1974.

Sperryn, Peter. *Sport and Medicine*, Butterworths, London, 1983.

Spino, Mike. *Beyond Jogging*, Celestial Arts, Milbrae, Calif., 1976.

Sprague, Ken. *The Athlete's Body*, Tarcher, Los Angeles, 1981.

Syer, John and Christopher Connolly. *Sporting Body, Sporting Mind*, Cambridge University Press, London, 1984.

Chapter Twenty-Two

Angele, K. H. *Your Daily Health Care with Kneipp*, Kneipp-Verlag, Bad Worishofen, 1980.

Bruggemann, W. *Kneipp Vademecum Pro Medico*, Sebastian Kneipp Publications, Würzburg, 1982.

Broughman, J. 'The Pure Truth', *Health*, 1991.

Brooks, S. M. *The Sea Inside Us: Water in the Life Processes*, Meredith Press, New York, 1968.

Campion, Kitty. 'Water, not a drop to drink', *What Doctors Don't Tell You*, U.K., Vol 3, No 12.

Carpenter, B., S. J. Hedges, C. Crabb, M. Reilly and M. C. Bounds. 'Is Your Water Safe?', *US News & World Report*, 1991.

Consumer Reports. 'The Pollutants that matter Most: Lead, Radon, Nitrate', 1990.

Consumer Reports. 'Bottled Water: Any Better than Tap Water?', 1991.

Craig, Winston, J. *Nutrition for the Nineties*, Golden Harvest Books, Michigan, 1992.

Fagliano, J. M. Berry, et al. 'Drinking Water Contamination and the Incidence of Leukemia: An Ecological Study', *American Journal of Public Health*, 80, 1990.

Gershoff, S. N. 'Water, Water Everywhere, But is it Fit to Drink?', *Tufts University Diet & Nutrition Letter, No 9*, 1991.

'How Safe is Your Water?', *Newsweek*, 1982.

Hunt, J. *The Conquest of Everest*, E. P. Dutton, New York, 1954.

Kneipp, Sebastian. *My Water Cure*, Thorsons, Wellingborough, 1979.

la Peña, A. de *The Psychobiology of Cancer*, Praeger Publishers, CBS Educational and Professional Publishing, New York, 1983.

Lederman, E. K. *Good Health Through Natural Therapy*, Pan, London, 1976.

Leibold, Gerhard. *Practical Hydrotherapy*, Thorsons, Wellingborough, 1980.

Lindlahr, Henry. *Natural Therapeutics*, Vol 2, C. W. Daniel, Saffron Walden, 1983.

Oglesby, P. 'Stimulants and Coronaries', *Postgraduate Medicine*, 1968.

Ostertag, W., E. Duisberg and M. Sturman. 'The Mutagenic Actuary of Caffeine in Man', *Mutation Research*, 1965.

Pitts, G. C. et al. 'Factors Affecting Work Output in Hot Environments', *American Journal of Physiology*, 1944.

Sargent, F. and K. Weiman in *Physiological Measurements of Metabolic Functions in Man*, (eds) C. F. Consolazio, et al. McGraw-Hill, New York, 1963.

Slater, D. 'Bottled Waters. The Beverage of the Future', *Dairy and Food Sanitation*, 1991.

Taylor, Mary. *Water Pollution: Finding the Facts*, Friends of the Earth, London, 1993.

Tufts University. 'Bottled Waters' Muddied Image', *Diet and Nutrition Letter*, 1991.

University of California. 'In the Heat, Drink Up', *Wellness Letter*, Vol I, Berkeley, Calif., 1985.

US Food and Nutrition Board. 'Water Deprivation and Performance of Athletes', *American Journal of Clinical Nutrition*, 1974.

Vogel, A. *Swiss Nature Doctor*, Edition A, Vogel, Teufen, Switzerland, 1980.

Chapter Twenty-Three

Acta Dermato-Venereologica, 1980, 60 and 1975, 55, suppl 74; *British Journal of Cancer*, 1983, 48; *British Journal of Dermatology*, 1981, 104; *Lancet*, 6/4/74.

Bjorksten, J. *Longevity: A Quest*, Bjorksten Research Foundation, Madison, Wisconsin, 1981.

Frank, B. S. and P. Miele. *Dr Frank's No-Ageing Diet*, Dell, New York, 1976.

Goodhart, Robert S. and Maurice Shils. *Modern Nutrition in Health and Disease*, Lea & Febiger, Philadelphia, 1978.

Guyton, Arthur C. *Textbook of Medical Physiology*, W. B. Saunders, Philadelphia, 1976.

Kent, Saul. *The Life Extension Revolution*, Quill, New York, 1983.

Kugler, Hans. *Slowing Down the Ageing Process*, Pyramid, New York, 1974.

Maleskey, Gale. 'Vitamins for External Use Also', *Prevention*, July 1984.

Mann, John A. *Secrets of Life Extension*, Harbor, San Francisco, 1980.

Passwater, Richard. *Supernutrition*, Pocket Books, New York, 1976.

Pelletier, Kenneth. *Longevity: Fulfilling Our Biological Potential*, Delacorte Press/Lawrence, New York, 1981.

Rosenfeld, Albert. *Pro-Longevity*, Avon, New York, 1977.

Stryer, Lubert. *Biochemistry*, W. H. Freeman, San Francisco, 1975.

Chapter Twenty-Four

Blum, H. F. *Carcinogenesis by Ultraviolet Light*, Princeton University Press, Princeton, NJ, 1959.

Johnson, B. E. et al. 'Response of Human Skin to Ultraviolet Light', *Photophysiology*, Vol IV, A. C. Giese (ed), Academic Press, London, 1968.

Magnus, I. A. *Dermatological Photobiology*, Blackwell, Oxford, 1976.

Urbach, F. (ed) *The Biological Effects of Ultraviolet Radiation With Emphasis on the Skin*, Pergamon Press, Oxford, 1969.

Chapter Twenty-Five

Bircher, F. 'Thérapie cellulaire des troubles circulatoires terminaux', report of the Third French Congress of Cellular Therapy, Paris: Edition du Centre Méd. d'Etudes, ed de Rech., 1959, 65–67.

Bircher, F. Private communications and conversations.

Kment, A. Third International Cell Therapy Congress, Paris, 1961.

Kment, A. 'The objective demonstration of the revitalization effect after cell implantations', *Cell Research and Cellular Therapy*, (eds) F. Schmid, et al., Ott, Thun, Switzerland, 1967.

Kuhnau, W. *My Three Decades with Live Cell Therapy*, Kuhnau, Tijuana, Mexico, 1983.

Lumière, Cornel. *The Fountain of Youth: Not a Legend*, Editions Mont-Blanc, Geneva, 1971.

Niehans, Paul. *Einführung in die Zellular Therapie*, Huber, 1957.

Osband, M. et al. 'Demonstration of abnormal immunity, T-cell histamine H-2 receptor deficiency, and successful treatment with thymic extract', *New England Journal of Medicine*, Jan 1981, CCIV: 146.

Schmid, F. 'Down's Syndrome: Treatment and Management', *Cytobiol. Rev.* 1978, 2:25–32.

Chapter Twenty-Six

American Journal of Anatomy, 1913, 15:431; *Berl. Klin. Wochenschr.*, 1887, 5(371); *British Medical Journal*, 1920, 2:807; *Comp. Ther.*, 1978, 2:49; *Endocrinology*, May–June 1934; *Journal of the American Medical Association*, March 1922, and 1924 (83:1380); *Journal of Chiropractic Economics*, 1983, 26(2); *Med. Record*, 3 March 1917; *Medico-Chir. Trans.*, 1878, 81:57; *Rev. Med.*, 1886, 6(297); *South. Med. J.*, 1979, 72(5):593; *World J. Surg.*, 1977, 1:605ff.

'Antigen Absorption in the Gut', MTP, Lancaster, 1978.

Birch, T. W. et al. *Nature*, 1936, 138:27.

Bland, Jeffrey. *Glandular-Based Food Supplements: Helping to Separate Fact From Fiction*, Bellevue-Redmont Medical Laboratories, 1980.

Callahan, E. J. et al. *Med. Rec.*, 1936, 149, 167.

Frank, B. S. *A New Approach to Degenerative Disease and Aging*, Patria Press, New York, 1964.

Frank, B. S. *Nucleic Acid Therapy in Aging and Degenerative Disease*, 3rd ed, Fiquima, Lisbon, 1975.

Frank, B. S. and P. Miele. *Dr Frank's No-Ageing Diet*, Dell, New York, 1976.

Gardner, T. S. J. *Gerontol.*, 1946, 1:445.

Goodhart, Robert S. and Maurice Shils. *Modern Nutrition in Health and Disease*, Lea & Febiger, Philadelphia, 1978.

Guyton, Arthur C. *Textbook of Medical Physiology*, W. B. Saunders, Philadelphia, 1976.

Hemmings, W. A. (ed). *Antigen Absorption by the Gut*, University Park Press, Baltimore, 1978.

Hemmings, W. A. (ed). *Protein Transmission Through Living Membranes*, Elsevier/North Holland Biomedical Press, Oxford, 1979.

Kugler, H. J. *Slowing Down the Ageing Process*, Pyramid, New York, 1973.

Kugler, H. J. *American Laboratory*, Nov 1976, 8:24.

Ralli, E. P. *Recent Advances in Nutritional Research*, National Vitamin Foundation, New York, 1952.

Robertson, T. B. *Australian Journal of Expl. Biol. Med. Sci.*, 1928, 5:47.

Stryer, Lubert. *Biochemistry*, W. II. Freeman, San Francisco, 1975.

Vorhaus, M. G. *Acta. Rheumatol.*, 1938, 10, 8.

Chapter Twenty-Seven

Brekhman, I. I. *Man and Biologically Active Substances*, Pergamon Press, Oxford, 1980.

Brekhman, I. I. 'New Substances of Plant Origin which Increase Nonspecific Resistance', *Annual Review of Pharmacology*, 1969, 9.

Brekhman, I. I. 'Pharmacological Investigations of Glycosides from Ginseng and Eleutherococcus', *Lloydia*, March 1969, 32(1).

Brekhman, I. I. 'Ginseng, Eleutherococcus and Another Adaptogen', speech given at Chelsea College, 1979.

Curtze, A. 'Eleutherococcus senticosus Maxim: Officinal plant of adaptogenic effect', *Der Deutsche Apotheker*, 1977, 29, 8.

'Experimental rationale and trial of the therapeutic use of bee-raising products in cardiovascular disease', *Kardiologiia*, May 1983, 23(5).

Forgo, I. et al. 'The effect of different ginsenoside concentrations on physical work capacity', *Notabene Medici*, 1982, 12(9):721–727.

Fuller, Stephen. *An End to Ageing*, Thorsons, Wellingborough, 1983.

Hacker, B. and P. Medon. 'Cytotoxic Effects of Eleutherococcus senticosus', *Journal of Pharmaceutical Sciences*, Feb 1984, 73(2).

Medon, P. J. and P. W. Ferguson et al. 'Effects of Eleutherococcus senticosus Extracts on Hexobarbital Metabolism in Vivo and in Vitro', *Journal of Ethnopharmacology*, 1984, 10:235–241.

Peichev, P. et al. 'Results of the Complex Use of Certain Apiary Products – Honey, Royal Jelly and Pollen from Bees – In Elderly Persons', *Folia Medica* (Bulgaria) 1966, 8(6).

Petkov, V. 'Effect of Ginseng on the Brain Biogenic Monoamines and 3', 5'-AMP System', *Arzneimittel-Forschung/Drug Research*, 1978, 28(3):388–393.

Sandberg, Finn. 'The Ginseng Root: A New Examination of an Old Drug', *Oesterreichische Apotheker-Zeitung*, 1971, 25(12):205–209.

Sandberg, Finn. 'Vitality and Senility: The effect of the ginsenosides on performance', *Svensk Farmaceutisk Tidskrift*, 1980, 84(13):499–502.

Selye, Hans. *Stress Without Distress*, Hodder & Stoughton, London, 1974.

Selye, Hans. *The Stress of Life*, McGraw-Hill, New York, 1976.

Wilson, R. B. 'Royal Jelly: The Medical Aspects', *American Bee Journal*, 97(9 and 10):356–359 and 396–399.

Chapter Twenty-Eight

Benson, Herbert. *Beyond the Relaxation Response*, Times Books, New York, 1984.

Brain Mind Bulletin, 10 Dec 1984, 10(2).

Cousins, Norman, 'How Doctors Cause Disease', *Medical Self Care*, 1983.

Frank, J. D. 'Psychotherapy of bodily disease', *Psychotherapy and Psychosomatics*, 1975, 26:192–202.

Frank, J. D. 'The Faith That Heals', *Johns Hopkins Medical Journal*, 1975, 137:127–131.

Frank, J. D. 'The medical power of faith', *Human Nature*, Aug 1978: 40–49.

Hammer, Signe. 'The Mind as Healer', *Science Digest*, Apr 1984.

'Hope, That Sustainer of Man', *Executive Health*, Dec 1983, II, XX(3).

Maddox, John. 'Psychoimmunology Before Its Time', *Nature*, 31 May 1984.

Mason, L. John. *Guide to Stress Reduction*, Peace Press, Culver, Calif., 1980.

Morton, Marion. 'Attitudes and Responsibilities to the Elderly and of the Elderly', *Rejuvenation*, June 1984, XII(1–2).

Pelletier, Kenneth. *Mind as Healer – Mind as Slayer*, Delta, New York, 1977.

Pelletier, Kenneth. 'A Long and Happy Life', *Medical Self Care*, winter 1983.

Simonton, Carl O. *Getting Well Again*, Tarcher, Los Angeles, 1978.

Chapter Twenty-Nine

Ames, Bruce. 'Dietary Carcinogens and Anticarcinogens', *Science*, 23 Sept 1983.

Aprison, M. et al. 'Glycine, Its Metabolic and Possible Transmitter Role in Nervous Tissues', *Handbook of Neurochemistry*, Vol 3: 391, Plenum Press, New York, 1969.

Bartus, R. T. et al. 'Age-Related Changes in Passive-Avoidance Retention: Modulations with Dietary Choline', *Science*, 1980, 209:301.

Bland, J. (ed). *Medical Applications of Clinical Nutrition*, Keats Publishing, New Canaan, Conn., 1983.

Cheraskin, E. and W. M. Ringsdorf. *Psychodietetics*, Bantam, New York, 1976.

Clark, Michael. 'Obsessive-Compulsive Behavior Linked to Low Serotonin Levels', *Medical Tribune*, 21 June 1978: 19.

'Clinical Symptoms Developed During Histidine Deprivation', *Nutritional Review*, 1975, V(33):201.

Goodwin, J. S. et al. 'Association between nutritional status and cognitive function in a healthy elderly population', *Journal of the American Medical Association*, 3 June 1983.

Goodwin, J. S. 'On Nutrition and Memory', *Executive Health*, Oct 1984, XXI(I).

Growdon, J. H. and R. J. Wurtman. 'Dietary Influences on the Synthesis of Neurotransmitters in the Brain', *Nutrition Reviews*, 1979, 37:129.

Jackson, I. V. et al. 'Treatment of Tardive Dyskinesia with Lecithin', *American Journal of Psychiatry*, 11/79, 136:11.

Kalita, D. and W. H. Philpott. *Brain Allergies*, Keats Publishing, New Canaan, Conn., 1980.

Mesulam, M. and S. Weintraus. 'Cholinergic Therapy for Dementia', presented at the International Study Group on Memory Disorders, Zürich, 1979.

Nutrition Search Ltd., *Nutrition Almanac*, Revised edition, McGraw-Hill, New York, 1979.

Pfeiffer, Carl. *Mental and Elemental Nutrients*. Keats Publishing, New Canaan, Conn., 1975.

Williams, R. *Physician's Handbook of Nutritional Science*, Charles C. Thomas, Springfield, Illinois, 1978.

Chapter Thirty & Postscript

Butler, R. N. *Why Survive? Being Old in America*, Harper & Row, New York, 1975.
Baines, J. *Ageing and World Order*, The Whole Earth Papers, No 13, Global Education Associates, East Orange, NJ, 1979.
Capek, Karel. *The Makropoulos Secret*, International Pocket Library, Boston, 1925.
Comfort, Alex. *A Good Age*, Simon and Schuster, New York, 1976.
Erikson, E. H. 'Identity and the Life Cycle', *Psychological Issues*, 1:18, 1959.
Fontana, A. *The Last Frontier: The Social Meaning of Growing Old*, Sage Publications, Beverley Hills, Calif., 1977.
Hesse, Hermann. *The Glass Bead Game*, Penguin, London, 1972.
Kotlikoff, L. J. 'Some Economic Implications of Life Span Extension', *Ageing, Biology and Behaviours*, J. March, et al. (ed), Academic Press, New York, 1982.
Lawrence, T. E. *Seven Pillars of Wisdom*, Brodie, 1963.
Rendricks, J. and C. D. Hendricks. *Ageing in Mass Society: Myth and Realities*, 2nd ed, Winthrop Publishing, New York, 1981.
Shaw, George Bernard. *Back to Methuselah* in *Complete Plays with Prefaces*, Vol II, Dodd, Mead, New York, 1963.

Index